Advanced Practice in Mental Health Nursing

Advanced Practice in Mental Health Nursing

Edited by

Michael Clinton
RN, RPN, BA (Hons), PhD, PGCertEd, FRCNA, FANZCMHN, AFAIM
Professor of Nursing, Curtin University of Technology,
Professorial Fellow, Sir Charles Gairdner Hospital, Western Australia,
Emeritus Professor, Queensland University of Technology

Sioban Nelson
BA (Hons), PhD, RN
Research Fellow, School of Postgraduate Nursing,
University of Melbourne, Australia

Blackwell
Science

© 1999 by
Blackwell Science Ltd
Editorial Offices:
Osney Mead, Oxford OX2 0EL
25 John Street, London WC1N 2BL
23 Ainslie Place, Edinburgh EH3 6AJ
350 Main Street, Malden
   MA 02148 5018, USA
54 University Street, Carlton
   Victoria 3053, Australia
10, rue Casimir Delavigne
   75006 Paris, France

Other Editorial Offices:

Blackwell Wissenschafts-Verlag GmbH
Kurfürstendamm 57
10707 Berlin, Germany

Blackwell Science KK
MG Kodenmacho Building
7–10 Kodenmacho Nihombashi
Chuo-ku, Tokyo 104, Japan

First published 1999

Set in 10/12 Palatino
by DP Photosetting, Aylesbury, Bucks
Printed and bound in Great Britain by
MPG Books Limited, Bodmin, Cornwall

DISTRIBUTORS

Marston Book Services Ltd
PO Box 269
Abingdon
Oxon OX14 4YN
(*Orders:* Tel: 01235 465500
       Fax: 01235 465555)

USA
   Blackwell Science, Inc.
   Commerce Place
   350 Main Street
   Malden, MA 02148 5018
   (*Orders:* Tel: 800 759 6102
          781 388 8250
       Fax: 781 388 8255)

Canada
   Login Brothers Book Company
   324 Saulteaux Crescent
   Winnipeg, Manitoba R3J 3T2
   (*Orders:* Tel: 204 837-2987
          204 837-3116)

Australia
   Blackwell Science Pty Ltd
   54 University Street
   Carlton, Victoria 3053
   (*Orders:* Tel: 03 9347 0300
       Fax: 03 9347 5001)

A catalogue record for this title
is available from the British Library

ISBN 0-632-04892-1

Library of Congress
Cataloging-in-Publication Data
is available

For further information on
Blackwell Science, visit our website:
www.blackwell-science.com

Contents

Foreword

Advanced Practice in Mental Health Nursing is the first book of its kind which succeeds in the ambitious work of identifying common international concerns, both clinical and professional, while emphasising the vital role of the psychiatric and mental health nurse in diverse health care delivery systems. Michael Clinton and Sioban Nelson, the editors, emphasise that all nurses must keep abreast of the unprecedented changes within the mental health care delivery systems. Nurses also need actively to develop or to adapt interventions and knowledge from other fields. The editors focus attention on three main areas of interest: the social context of practice; specific approaches to practice situations; and clinical and diagnostic issues.

This organising strategy allows for discussion of important themes throughout the book: the development of a new framework for advanced practice through the recognition of a contemporary social context of practice; the adoption of a strengths-focused, person-centred perspective; the identification of the value of therapeutic communication within this contemporary practice context; and the creation of a climate for dialogue with consumers as participants in their own mental health care.

Individual authors capture the essence of advanced practice with an historic focus on the discipline as a holistic and biopsychosocial practice. They also raise conceptual, professional and clinical issues, from an international perspective, linking similar trends in the USA, Canada, Europe and Australia. This international focus on the contemporary context of advanced psychiatric and mental health nursing practice begins with the move from the traditional role of 'patient' to the up-to-date role of 'consumer' of mental health services, and includes discussions of the consumer's contribution in services delivery, quality assurance, and staff training.

Consumers of mental health and rehabilitation services have expressed interest in self-care and wellness, and in alternative approaches to the treatment of acute and chronic medical and psychiatric illnesses. The reader will find that portions of the book address important issues in consumer self-care, involvement and empowerment. Questions such as: Is it possible to recover from serious mental illness? Can consumers play a key role in designing and implementing their own individualised plans for recovery? are considered.

Recognising that there is no one plan for recovery that suits everyone, the authors illustrate the many ways in which advanced practice in psychiatric and mental health nursing assumes greater responsibility for engaging consumers in the recovery process, collaborating in the management of therapeutic interventions, and providing care for people with mental illness within the community.

Throughout the book, the authors place the social context of life with a mental disorder squarely within the latest debates emphasising the current research findings about neurobiological illnesses. Discussions balance the value of greater understanding about a neurobiological basis for mental disorders with the recently re-emerging controversy about the potential for lasting and damaging effects. The value of holding and maintaining hope, and the use of hope-inspiring strategies to build relationships is also discussed. These strategies facilitate potential successes and provide connections with other successful consumer oriented approaches in the community.

The theme of innovative approaches for advanced practice continues with the authors examining the complexities and current challenges in collaborating with specific, at-risk client groups. These client groups include those who are depressed, elderly or neurologically impaired, children and adolescents, and clients with personality disorders. Each chapter identifies strategies to engage members of these at-risk groups by creating therapeutic environments which nurture recovery. In this context, the authors emphasise staff attitudes that can be helpful or harmful in creating a climate for recovery. Psychiatric and mental health nurses are encouraged to understand that each person's journey toward improved mental health is unique, and to recognise the gifts each person can bring and share with each other along the way, such as the pooling of knowledge, skills, supports, and learning from each other's life experiences.

The editors and contributing authors of *Advanced Practice in Mental Health Nursing* are all recognised experts with substantial experience. They present a series of well-researched, well-written chapters which weave the themes of the healing strengths of the therapeutic relationship, emphasising the value of the individual, and identifying holistic and humanistic principles associated with advanced practice in psychiatric and mental health nursing. Psychiatric and mental health nurses of all experience levels will find many ideas to stimulate their thinking and enhance their clinical practice.

Victoria K. Palmer-Erbs, *PhD, RN, CS*
Boston, Massachusetts, USA
August 1998

List of Contributors

Phil Barker   PhD, RN, FRCN
Professor of Psychiatric Nursing Practice, University of Newcastle-upon-Tyne, United Kingdom

Pierre Baume   RN, RMN, DipAppSoc, MHP, DipCh, FRCNA, FANZCMHN
Director, Australian Institute for Suicide Research and Prevention, Griffith University, Brisbane, Australia

Charlotte Clarke   BA, MSc, PGCE, PhD, RGN
Research Fellow (Practice Development), Faculty of Health, Social Work and Education, University of Northumbria at Newcastle-upon-Tyne, United Kingdom

Michael Clinton   RN, RPN, BA (Hons), PhD, PGCertEd, FRCNA, FANZCMHN, AFAIM
Professor of Nursing, Curtin University of Technology, Professiorial Fellow, Sir Charles Gairdner Hospital, Western Australia, Emeritus Professor, Queensland University of Technology

Merinda Epstein   DipTeach, BEd (Melb)
Consumer Activist, sits on the Australian National Community Advisory Group on Mental Health, and has worked for Victorian Mental Illness Awareness Council (Australia).

Mary E. Evans
College of Nursing, University of South Florida, USA

Ruth Gallop   BScN, MScN, PhD, RN
Associate Professor, Faculty of Nursing and Clarke Institute of Psychiatry, University of Toronto, Canada

Kevin Gournay   MPhil, PhD, CPsychol, AFBPsS, RN
Professor of Psychiatric Nursing, Institute of Psychiatry, University of London, United Kingdom

Helen Kirkpatrick   RN, MScN, MEd
Program Director, Schizophrenia Psychosocial Rehabilitation Program, Hamilton Psychiatric Hospital, Ontario, Canada

Jan Landeen   BScN, MEd, PhD
Assistant Professor, School of Nursing, MacMaster University, Ontario, Canada

Tom Mason   PhD, BSc (Hons), RMN, RNMH, RGN
Senior Lecturer, Department of Nursing, University of Liverpool, United Kingdom

Dave Mercer   BA (Hons), PGCE, RMN, MA
Lecturer, Department of Nursing, University of Liverpool, United Kingdom

Sioban Nelson   BA (Hons), PhD, RN
Research Fellow, School of Postgraduate Nursing, University of Melbourne, Australia

Astrid Norberg   RN, PhD
Professor, Head of Department of Advanced Nursing, Umeå University, Sweden

Anne M. Olsen   BA(Hons), Dip Ed
Consumer Activist; has worked for Victorian Mental Illness Awareness Council (Australia)

Jennifer Pyke   RN, MHSc
Director, Community Support Services, Community Resources Consultants of Toronto, Toronto, Canada

Jan Reed
Lecturer, Faculty of Health, Social Work and Education, University of Northumbria at Newcastle-upon-Tyne, United Kingdom

Sandry Speedy   BA (Hons), DipEd, EdD, RN, PAPS, FANZCMHN, FRCNA
Dean, Faculty of Health, University of the Southern Cross, Lismore, Australia

Catherine H. Stein   PhD
Associate Professor, Department of Psychology, Bowling Green State University, Ohio, USA

Acknowledgements

The field of mental health is well served by authors from many disciplines, including mental health nursing, who have become expert in fields of practice and scholarship. We are grateful that we have been able to draw on the vast experience of contributors from such diverse backgrounds, and for their cooperation in preparing this book for publication. We should also like to thank Helen Nicholl and Bron Lloyd at the Centre for Education and Research at Ashford Community Hospital for their assistance in following up queries. Finally, we would like to thank Griselda Campbell and Sue Moore at Blackwell Science in Oxford for their encouragement and expertise.

Introduction

Michael Clinton and *Sioban Nelson*

There are few areas of practice as diverse and multiple as that of advanced mental health nursing practice. Increasingly, for the nurse starting out in the speciality, there are choices that need to be made. These choices embrace philosophical, therapeutic, social and political issues. The therapeutic milieu of an acute in-patient facility is markedly different to that of private practice. Similarly, working in the community, or alongside co-workers who are themselves consumers, demands of the nurse a philosophical, if not a political commitment to notions of empowerment and equity.

Within these frameworks and positionings we still confront the clinical reality of illness, but the status we accord to this reality depends on our perspective and the context of practice. As practitioners we find that particular diagnostic categories confuse and frustrate us, that certain client populations challenge our internal resources. Often it is our own helplessness that thwarts our capacity to care for clients. Still more challenging are the issues inherent in the management of such a political 'problem' as mental illness. Workforce issues, the forensic movement and the relationship between nurses and non-nurses working in mental health are major issues that the profession needs to confront. However, to examine these issues we need to take a longer, more global approach to problems that we might otherwise be too close to. Our careers and professional lives are, after all, bound within a particular way of relating to, managing or dealing with mental illness and those who have been created into patients or consumers by the mental health systems of our respective countries. How clearly, then, can we see the picture?

This book represents a collection of perspectives and viewpoints on these important matters. It is necessarily a heterogeneous piece of work, as, indeed, is mental health nursing practice. Psychiatry is vilified by some authors and left unchallenged by others; the nurse–patient relationship is considered the centrepiece of practice by several contributors, whereas others focus on programmatic issues or on consumer autonomy and empowerment. 'Difficult' diagnostic categories, such as personality disorder and dementia, are tackled. The young and the elderly are given their due as clients requiring skilled and qualified care by nursing clinicians with advanced practice skills.

This concept of advanced practice is often taken to refer to technical skills that are difficult to acquire, and moreover, to require knowledge that would normally be gained in studying for a higher degree. However, the term 'advanced practice' is used here to refer to the 'second order' reflection that brings into question the assumptions on which such technical interventions are based. If day-to-day practice is a 'first order' activity, in which the everyday understandings of the practitioner link theory and practice in the immediate sense of the judgements and beliefs embedded in practice, 'second order' reflection is the process of scrutinising and challenging these conceptualisations. Therefore, the contributors have taken advanced practice to mean the reflective skills involved in examining ways of thinking about mental health nursing interventions. By reflecting on the nature of nursing practice, the contributors have demonstrated that they are exponents of the forms of advanced practice they are seeking to promote. To the extent that they present different perspectives on advanced practice, without exhausting the possibilities, they leave open possibilities for further reflection. We hope that the 'third order' reflections of readers will lead to the practical application of the insights gleaned.

The book begins, as it must, with a consumer perspective. Chapter 1 offers us a correct starting point from which to approach mental health nursing practice. But this chapter delivers more than that. It brings us up to date with approaches, perspectives and resources that have been utilised by consumers to turn what has been, too often and for too long, the monster of the mental health system, into something that does what it should do – aid, nurture and assist those in need.

We stay with our eye fixed firmly on the outcome of mental health nursing for the next two chapters. Helen Kirkpatrick and Jan Lanean's Chapter 2 provides an inspirational account of rehabilitation, reminding us that the greatest damage our systems of care have done is to destroy hope. Catherine Stein's chapter (3), too, shows us that much more can be done to break down the division between the consumer of mental health services and the rest of the community. Her collaborative education program in Ohio, and its replication in Brisbane, Australia, brings home the message that *everyone* can do with a little help from their friends when it comes to social skills and support networks.

Sandra Speedy (Chapter 4) brings us back to the therapeutic nature of the nurse–patient relationship. Her discussion highlights the values that underpin the therapeutic alliance and sets the scene for the detailed discussion of practice that follows. The values that are clarified also raise the question of how discussions of mental health nursing practice are to be understood. It is far too simplistic to believe that such discussions can be accepted uncritically, for as Tom Mason and David Mercer show in Chapter 13, everything is not always what it seems, and there are dilemmas that nurses face in acting on the values they believe in, especially in practice settings over which they have little control.

In Jennifer Pyke's Chapter 5 we begin to concentrate on the resources necessary for recovery and the sets of skills that the nurse requires to work within the community. Case management, in its various forms, is reviewed and its importance to nurses in the field is affirmed. In Chapter 6 Kevin

Gournay provides us with an even more delineated appraisal of the skills required for nurses to work in community mental health. Gournay introduces the complex issue of the mental health workforce and brings skill mix and training into our discussion. He also brings to the surface the uneasy relationship between mental health nurses and non-nurses in the field.

Mary Evans continues our focus on intervention. In Chapter 7 on adolescence and mental health nursing, she provides us with a thorough and practical guide to approaches to nursing care. She gives wide scope to programmatic, social and research issues and makes the reader aware that it is possible to provide exemplary nursing care in this most challenging area of mental health.

Phil Barker retains our focus on nursing care and therapeutic skill in Chapter 8 on depression. Barker situates his therapeutic encounter in the tradition of humanistic psychology and carries the reader through from a philosophical position to nurse–patient interaction. Astrid Norberg, in Chapter 9 on dementia, commences from a different philosophical space. Through existential phenomenology, she allows us to explore the non-verbal world of carer interaction with a person with dementia. Jan Reed and Charlotte Clarke are also concerned with older people in Chapter 10, but for these authors the care of older people is derived from a more overtly political standpoint.

Ruth Gallop brings us back into the clinical setting in Chapter 11 on personality disorder and nursing care. She confronts us with the very great challenge that the nurse so often fails to meet with this group of clients, and shows us how skilled, intelligent, and theoretically sound nursing care can make a difference. In Chapter 12 Pierre Baume and Michael Clinton grapple with one of the major challenges of contemporary mental health nursing and of society in general – suicide. Australian data on suicide in young males provides us with an exemplar study of disturbing western social trends. Issues of prevention and crisis intervention are canvassed and a model of prevention is proposed. Tom Mason and David Mercer problematise the status of the mentally ill offender and provide a provocative account of the place of forensic psychiatry and forensic nursing in a contemporary society.

With Chapter 14 we end where we began, with the idea of recovery, but this time we do not have the consumer in focus, but the way disease, illness and recovery have been historically understood and mental health nurses' special relationship to these understandings. The final two chapters emphasise a post-structuralist reading of advanced mental health nursing practice. However, this is not intended to privilege post-modernism or to give authors with this perspective the last word, but to leave open the possibility of other interpretations.

In summary, we bring together the experiences and expertise of consumers, leading practitioners and academics in the United States, Canada, Great Britain, Australia and Scandinavia to provide a text aimed at advanced practitioners, and masters and doctoral program students. We hope that its international scope emphasises the consistent concerns that frame practice, approaches to practice and clinical challenges.

1 An Introduction to Consumer Politics

Merinda Epstein and *Anne M. Olsen*

Introduction

In recent years the consumer movement has become a force in mental health care. The emphases and activities of consumer groups vary locally as well as from country to country but converge on common themes. Of particular importance to this chapter is the international trend towards consumer involvement in the planning, design, and implementation of government and private sector mental health services. In this context the changing role of the consumer is examined with special reference to the role of consumer consultants and the introduction of a consumer perspective into service delivery, quality assurance, staff training, and research. Underpinning these discussions are different notions of consumer advocacy and the recurrent themes of political power, legitimacy, accountability, and contextuality.

The authors as consumers and writers

In writing this chapter we are very much aware of our own unique experiences as consumers as well as of our authorial role as one particular public voice for the consumer movement. Therefore, it is necessary to emphasise that we do not claim to speak for all consumers everywhere about everything. Consumers of government, private sector and alternative mental health services are diverse groups of people. Differences among consumers include those of socio-economic status, ethnicity, gender, diagnosis, treatment experience, and so on. There is no such thing as a single consumer voice. It follows that the issue of 'representativeness' – of *who is being represented* – is raised whenever consumers speak out. Sometimes, the issue of who is being represented is raised by providers, and others, in order to denigrate the arguments of articulate or impassioned consumers (Hutchinson & Ausland, 1992/3, p. 17). David Crepaz-Keay (UK-based consumer activist and writer), having pointed out that one consumer (or even one consumer group) 'cannot hope to represent the "user/survivor movement" ', goes on to stress that, despite this fact, '[w]e cut across the boundaries of class and gender and culture that still grip the "mental health" professionals, particularly at the higher levels' (Crepaz-Keay, 1996, p. 185).

Interestingly, the question 'Who do they represent?' is rarely one 'that is equally applied to professional members of groups who seem no less likely to express personal opinions or outrageous views' (Hutchinson & Ausland, 1992/3, p. 17).

The most fruitful way of addressing concerns about representativeness is to ensure that a range of consumer views is heard. Groups that are active in the area of reform can be encouraged to undertake surveys and interviews with other consumers. User input from hospital wards, from organised self-help groups, and from advocacy groups can and should be sought and included in any process of advocacy or consultation. In particular the voices of consumers from marginalised and minority groups need to be heard (Hutchinson & Ausland, 1992/3, p. 17).

As consumers and authors who acknowledge the limitations of our own position we have endeavoured to take account of a range of consumer views from many different sources in writing this chapter. Despite this we need to acknowledge our own contexts of engagement with consumer politics.

Merinda's involvement with the consumer movement has been extensive. Projects with which she has been closely associated include The Understanding and Involvement (U & I) Project and The Lemon Tree Learning Project. She also sits on the Australian National Community Advisory Group on Mental Health (NCAG) and the National Mental Health Strategy Evaluation Steering Committee. Merinda's cartoons have appeared in the *Perceptions* bulletins, *Victorian Consumer Participation Guidelines*, and the U & I books.

The U & I Project grew out of a consumer evaluation project, *Understanding, Anytime*, which was carried out from late 1990 through to the end of 1991 (McGuiness & Wadsworth, 1992). U & I was a three year project funded by the Victorian Health Promotion Foundation. The project was directed towards '[e]stablish[ing] and refin[ing] processes by which staff and consumers in psychiatric hospital wards can routinely collaborate to research and evaluate the experiences of consumers and make the consequent relevant and appropriate changes to hospital practices' (Epstein & Wadsworth, 1994, p. 7). The Lemon Tree Learning Project developed and trialled strategies for training both service providers and consumers in the area of effective consumer participation. As well as writing up the project, the team created a board game called 'Lemon Looning' which constitutes an innovative training tool for learning more about the 'consumer perspective' and/or consumer participation (Epstein & Shaw, 1997).

Anne has been employed as a consumer researcher and editor by The Lemon Tree Learning Project (under the auspices of The Victorian Mental Illness Awareness Council (VMIAC)).

The consumer movement

Despite the differences between individual consumers and between various consumer groups it is possible to talk about the *consumer movement* as a world wide liberation movement with certain common concerns and aims. Consumers are attempting to claim their right to be recognised as human beings rather than as walking diagnoses or collections of symptoms (Read & Reynolds, 1996). People are becoming aware of their rights to accurate information regarding treatment, and to having a say in that treatment (Epstein & Wadsworth, 1994). Consumers are seeking to bring about changes in community attitudes towards mental illness, and they are increasingly working towards setting up and running support and advocacy groups. Janet Meagher's book *Partnership or Pretence* (1995) and its extensive bibliography provide further references on this topic. Consumers around the world are in regular and productive contact with one another through conferences, workshops, research, and (recently) through the Internet.

Common themes and differences

Differences: strength in diversity

Where the various consumer groups tend to differ most – whether between countries or within them – is in how they seek to bring about change. Some groups are dedicated to support and self-help; arguing that only those who have experienced mental illness/distress are able to give non-judgemental, non-patronising help and advice to others. Many of these groups provide temporary and emergency accommodation, crisis centres, drop-in and chat sessions, and legal advice. There has been a recent proliferation of consumer/survivor support groups to which people can subscribe on the Internet, as well as web sites dedicated to giving information about social issues, research, and current debates in the mental health field (*Websites of interest* at the end of the chapter). Among the most active consumer groups are Survivors Speak Out (UK), The National Empowerment Center (USA), and Support Coalition (USA).

These are examples of consumers *as* service providers and as such constitute alternative and/or complementary avenues for consumer participation. Other groups work in partnership with mental health professionals. Advocacy Projects such as VMIAC and consumer consultants employed in hospitals and clinics work in this way. In some countries there are co-ordinating or umbrella consumer bodies whose function it is to make sure that a variety of consumer voices are heard and taken notice of. The United Kingdom Advocacy Network (UKAN) is an example of such an umbrella group. Whatever form these groups assume each is an important source of consumer expertise and, as such, deserves to be heard in any decision-making process about mental health services.

We see these differences between consumer groups as a healthy and fruitful aspect of the consumer movement. As previously mentioned, there is no single consumer voice; neither is there a single way for consumers to participate in a liberation movement. All too often life choices are denied to people suffering from mental distress and the variety of consumer groups allows individuals to participate in whichever way they decide is best for them. In addition, encouragement of a wide range of viewpoints nourishes the exchange of ideas and promotes the strength of the movement.

Stereotyping and stigma: a fundamental problem

One of the most damaging experiences for consumers is that of stigma (Epstein & Olsen 1997). Stigma is a shameful mark of difference and one that works as a particularly effective social sanction. Stigma for those suffering from mental/emotional distress results from the way that we are 'branded' with various (and often contradictory) pejorative and/or disempowering labels. The principal effect of using labels (based on stereotypical conceptions) to categorise people is dehumanisation, and the use of such markers to stigmatise individuals and groups is enabled by social constructions of 'normality'. In order to appreciate just how artificial notions of 'normality' can be it is worth reflecting on the following definition:

> [t]o be 'normal' in Australia it is important (1) to belong to certain dominant status groups – male, Australian-born, Anglo-Saxon, middle-class, about 25 to 55 years of age, Protestant, heterosexual, *and* (2) to live in a nuclear family household in one's own house *and* (3) to be employed and believe in the work ethic for all. Precise figures are not available but it could be estimated that as many as 10% of people (100 per 1000 general population) must be included in this problem group known as 'normals' (Sargent, 1987, p. 213).

The humorous tone of this passage reminds us of the kinds of limitations and loss of perspective attached to labels. At the same time, the passage points out a (possibly unpalatable) truth regarding the unequal distribution of power in our society: that is, the very small number of people who – by virtue of their 'normality' – are able to impose their belief and value systems on the majority. For many of us it is true to say that 'normality is a figment of someone else's imagination' (anon).

Dehumanisation through stereotyping and labelling is inflicted on those groups and individuals perceived as threatening to the physical and emotional stability of society. To mark/label/identify the unknown *other* is to control our fear of *otherness*. The adverse effects of social stigma, as perpetuated and practised by our dominant culture, are felt not only by those with mental illness but also by other marginalised groups:

- Black Australians
- People who don't speak English
- Those living in poverty
- Those without work
- People who are illiterate
- Those with other disabilities
- Those who have been in gaol
- Gay men and lesbian women ... etc.

In many instances the effects of 'othering' serve the interests of the powerful and create divisions within communities by encouraging the

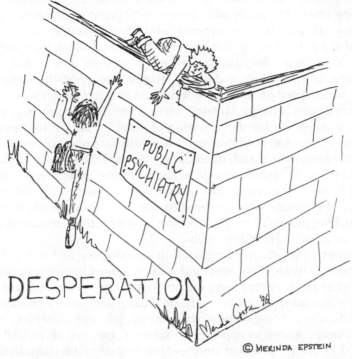

PUBLIC PSYCHIATRY

DESPERATION

© MERINDA EPSTEIN

Fig. 1.1 'Desperation'.

development of antagonistic interest groups vying for recognition and respect. This is one reason why it is so difficult to change erroneous perceptions and encourage tolerance. Negative stereotyping – as peculiar, dangerous, incompetent, and so on – of those suffering from mental health problems has resulted in an exacerbation of the difficulties we face in our lives. In addition to symptomatic distress and the often quite unpleasant side-effects of medication, we have to contend with the judgemental attitudes of those around us.

Consumers talk about various kinds of behaviours which they experience as stigmatising. For example, the way that people fail to make eye contact with them, or find it really difficult to engage in any sort of conversation about mental illness or psychiatric treatment. The use of collective nouns such as 'schizos' or 'depressives' is another example of stigmatising behaviour. Other consumers talk about how those who have not been through an experience of mental illness/serious emotional distress often offer simplistic (and potentially demoralising) advice such as, 'she just needs a good kick up the bottom', or 'he needs to pull his socks up', or 'if only she didn't think about herself all the time'. Some talk about stigma in terms of being treated like a child: being told what to do all the time or being unnecessarily monitored. Paternalistic attitudes towards consumers denies them the range of good and bad experiences, feelings and decisions taken for granted by the majority of adults in our society.

The impact of stigma can be profound. It can actually promote 'illness' by adding stress; it certainly adds unnecessary pressure to the lives of those who may already be experiencing almost unbearable strain. Stigma imposed from the 'outside' has the capacity to reproduce itself within the individual 'victim'. Because social beings absorb others' judgements, others' shame, others' fear, and others' disgust, these negative attitudes can become internalised as self fear, self disgust and self judgement.

Diagnostic and behavioural labels serve a number of purposes – some of which are *convenient* for the provision of services. But all too often these labels merely serve to reinforce social and cultural prejudices against those who suffer from mental and/or emotional distress. Those who work within the mental health system are not immune to the influence of their own cultural context. The system has its own set of assumptions and expectations about consumers. It can be difficult for mental health workers to avoid making judgements about people based on these assumptions and expectations, but it is not impossible.

We have written at some length about stereotyping and stigma because these phenomena are recognised and acknowledged by consumers all over the world as major contributing factors to disempowerment. The kinds of specific issues taken up by activists, including involuntary treatment and over-medication, homelessness, education, job opportunities, deinstitutionalisation, access to appropriate services, etc., are all related to and informed by the processes of stereotyping and stigmatisation. In the next section we will look at some of the ways in which consumers and others can battle the effects of stigma while contributing to the improvement of services.

Consumer involvement

The United Nations has developed a set of principles that emphasise the right of people with mental illness to participate fully in the life of the community, and to have assistance tailored to their individual needs. Obviously even well-defined principles are open to interpretation and subsequent modification – not only by the various government bodies but by service providers, carers, the wider community, and consumers themselves. The espousal of fine principles *at the top* does not, of itself, ensure positive changes within the system. We (as consumer activists) are often confronted with the accusation that the changes have already occurred; that the consumer movement is trying to 'reinvent the wheel'. We would argue that cosmetic and superficial alterations – as represented by high flown rhetoric and token gestures towards consumer inclusion in decision making – does not constitute genuine change. It is in service provision (in hospitals and in the community) that changes must occur; and these changes depend on a culture shift whereby deeply held attitudes and habits of thought are transformed (Epstein & Shaw, 1997).

Some practical issues

Involvement and value

With the rise and continuing growth of the consumer movements, funding bodies, whether governmental or private, have come to expect and require consumer representation in mental health projects (Epstein & Shaw 1997, pp. 65-70). However, satisfying the terms and conditions of funding is not the only reason for including consumers: 'the sharing of experiences and perspectives of providers, researchers, and consumers can enrich the project' (Ralph & Muskie, 1994, p. 2). While this sharing is an important aspect of consumer involvement, it should be remembered that the most important thing for *consumers* is to be listened to by providers and to have their views taken seriously.

There are a number of ways in which consumer contributions can be valued – and shown to be valued. Ralph and Muskie suggest the following:

- Listen without judgement;
- Be sensitive to (and be prepared to change) your own and others' stigmatising language
- Use 'person-first' language, e.g. 'persons with mental illness' rather than 'the mentally ill'
- Include consumers' ideas in decisions and written material
- Give consumers credit publicly and by name for ideas and work done
- Realise that many consumers do not have adequate income to volunteer and payment for meeting attendances, transport, child care, etc. should be managed in ways that provide choice and dignity

(Ralph & Muskie, 1994, pp. 4-5)

Financial remuneration

In our society there is a great deal of reliance on volunteers and unpaid labour. The notion that it is proper and acceptable for people to offer their labour and expertise for no payment is entrenched in our culture. It is a notion that poses a particularly insidious problem for consumers who participate – as acknowledged experts – in various sectors of the mental health system or in other advisory roles. Issues around unpaid labour create problems in many sections of the community; especially for those individuals who increasingly find themselves filling in gaps left by decreases in government funding in essential areas such as health, education, and social support. At the same time payment for consumer participants is a special case precisely because of the loss of self esteem and self confidence that so often accompany experiences of mental distress.

Financial remuneration is a medium of recognition that carries much more significance than its mere market value: there is a wealth of social value in the concept of paid work. When employing consumers it is essential that a clear job description be provided, including outlines of responsibilities and necessary credentials. The employer must be sure that she or he is 'willing to pay a salary that compensates for . . . [the consumer's] experience' (Ralph & Muskie, 1994, p. 5).

Most of the professionals and experts who sit on boards of management, reference groups, or advisory panels do so from a position of financial security in that they are also in employed positions elsewhere. This is not necessarily the case where consumers are concerned. Participation for the unpaid consumer can, in fact, place a further strain on already inadequate financial resources. In addition, the value that is attached to consumer contributions is diminished when those contributions are regarded as somehow separate from the issues surrounding what it means – materially – to be a consumer. We need to be aware of the tendency for service providers to regard expert consumer participation as *therapeutically* rewarding for the individual and, so, a favour conferred by the system upon less able members of society. This position is fundamentally disrespectful to consumers who bring to the system not only their abilities and knowledge but a unique and important perspective.

Tokenism

Tokenism is the expedient inclusion into a mainstream body of a representative from a socially marginalised group. Tokenistic appointments are frequently made to fall in with anti-discriminatory legislation or to take advantage of targeted funding opportunities. Token inclusion of consumers as researchers, as institutional staff, on advisory and evaluation boards, etc., are not genuine attempts to listen and learn from the 'other'. They are, rather, ways of avoiding such genuine attempts. Even legitimate attempts to include the consumer perspective in the planning and delivery of services run the risk of tokenism. This is due to the way in which consumers are perceived within the services that they use (see discussion of *Stereotyping and stigma* above).

Tokenism has been identified as one of the major difficulties facing consumers who work within the system. Various consumer organisations around the world have suggested ways in which the problem can be addressed. Ideally there should be at least two (preferably more) consumer representatives or employees, especially in those situations where the majority of participants are mental health professionals who might be expected to share similar opinions. A lone consumer in such situations risks becoming no more than a token presence, no matter how articulate and committed to change she or he is. Nevertheless, the danger of tokenism is 'not averted simply by having two, or three, or four users [consumers] . . . The concern is not just about numbers but about how users are treated and which decisions they can make' (Hutchinson & Ausland, 1992/3, p. 16).

Too often consumers are consulted to approve predetermined decisions with little or no opportunity to contribute to the decision making process. Clear, understandable information must be available to *all* participants and the importance of the decisions users/consumers can make must move from 'the cosmetic . . . to issues that might matter more' (Hutchinson & Ausland, 1992/3, p. 16).

Consumer involvement cannot be successfully tacked onto existing structures. This practice can be seen in many provider education and training courses that include a consumer-run presentation. This critical component is often appended to the tail end of the program: as an after-thought and a one-off. Once again such practice minimises consumer input; in fact it further *marginalises* the consumer perspective. If consumers are brought in during the planning stages of programs in which they are to participate, this problem can be avoided. Another way in which tokenism can be avoided is to 'give participation [in projects, meetings, etc.] a high profile and a clearly positive image. Don't let consultation activities slip in through the back door with only a few people knowing anything about it' (Hutchinson & Ausland, 1992/3, p. 16).

Education and training

Successful consumer participation requires adequate education and training for consumers, providers, and other involved groups. As con-sumers we need to feel that we have adequate skills to communicate with those whose social and professional status confers a kind of automatic authority. The most appropriate training for consumers probably comes from other consumers. In addition to appreciating the difficulties involved consumer-trainers can provide essential support and back-up.

One of the most important things that we need to learn as consumers is that our opinions and ideas are valuable. Consumers need to feel empowered in order to contribute to the education (in the widest sense of the word) of other consumers and of service providers. Among the many things that consumers can teach service providers, one of the most important is the value of *consumer empowerment*. The development of 'new and more empowering ways' of working with consumers will eventually be rewarding – even if initially it is difficult to 'see how to achieve neces-sary changes' (Read & Wallcraft, 1992, p. 22).

If workers are expected (by consumers or by management) to change their working practices, 'then training should be offered'; 'training gives both workers and users [consumers] the chance to step out of everyday roles and meet as equals on neutral ground' (Read & Wallcraft, 1992, p. 22). For both users and providers training can be empowering. There can be honest and open discussion of what needs to change in the system and ideas about how best to overcome obstacles to positive change can be shared on more equal terms.

It is important to appreciate that 'empowerment training' does not imply that one person can empower another – this is not possible. Such training is aimed at helping people – whether consumers, carers, or MH workers – empower themselves. Certain elements are necessary for 'good' empowerment training within various parts of the mental health system.

Read and Wallcraft have suggested the following as essential:

- Invite local consumers to become involved. Local user/consumer groups should be invited to discuss course content, provide speakers, and perhaps offered free places on the course.
- Take advantage of the fact that many groups have members who are experienced as trainers who could be asked to run a course for staff.
- If no local group exists then larger (state or national) networks should be approached to find speakers and trainers.
- Consumer-trainers, speakers, etc., should be paid at the same rate as any other trainers who would be employed.
- Training sessions should be held in pleasant, comfortable surroundings – preferably not in the workplace.
- Strict rules of confidentiality should be agreed so that all participants feel safe to be open and honest with each other.
- There must be agreed ground rules regarding considerate, non-sexist, non-racist, non-attacking behaviour.

(Read & Wallcraft, 1992, p. 22)

The changing roles of consumers

The consumer perspective

The consumer perspective is not easily defined – nor is it easily understood. There are ongoing debates regarding what such a perspective actually means in terms of consumer involvement in bringing about the improvement of services. Different consumers will give different opinions about what consumer perspective means to them, but some general observations can be made.

It has been suggested that 'consumer perspective is acquired as a result of receiving, or being unable to receive when you wish to, services in the mental health system' (Epstein & Shaw, 1997, p. 13). Perhaps, too, the perspective comes to those who see the world in ways which the dominant culture constructs as 'mad'. At another level the consumer perspective can be regarded as 'something which has developed out of a collective consciousness and political solidarity that grew from the consumer/survivor movement' (Epstein & Shaw, 1997, p. 13). This particular understanding of the consumer perspective is essentially a socio-political one, and comparable to the way in which we recognise a feminist perspective emerging from the women's movement; a particular solidarity and perspective from the gay and lesbian movement; or a sense of common identity in the various forms of the black or civil rights movement. Consumer perspective depends, therefore, on some kind of shared consciousness and identity. It is 'shaped through an awareness of "belonging" to a group of people who are marginalised and discriminated against, who have an experience of oppression' (Epstein & Shaw, 1997, p. 13).

It is important to understand that this sense of solidarity is experienced not only at the level of participation in political consumer groups or over the Internet. When consumers come together, whether in consumer-only training sessions or in hospital wards, there is often a strong feeling of shared identity. The close bonds that develop between 'patients' in the hospital setting are an example of this phenomenon that is frequently mentioned by consumers.

One of the most important – indeed fundamental – qualities of the consumer perspective is that it is respectful of the consumer experience. That is, individual consumers are acknowledged and listened to as experts in terms of their own lives and being. It is not consumer perspective to interpret someone else's behaviour using the tools (language and diagnostic categories) supplied by the medical establishment. Nor is it consumer perspective to argue that all other consumer experiences must be like your own (Epstein & Wadsworth, 1996a).

It seems useful to think of consumer perspective as being a multi-layered construction. At one level there is that respectful attention to the collective and individual experience of consumers that *some* non-consumers move closely towards and that may enable them to represent consumers' views in some contexts. At the other level is the consumer perspective that comes from the deeply felt and personalised experiences of the individual consumer that can never encompass the voices of all consumers and that can never be adequately represented by anybody else. Maintaining awareness of consumer perspective is a matter, we think, of juggling these different layers and levels of awareness – the political, collective awareness with the deeply personal (Epstein & Shaw, 1997, p. 15).

Consumer consultancy

The title consumer consultant has been applied fairly loosely to a range of positions in which consumers have been employed within the mental health system. In an attempt to remove any possible ambiguity in this name the U & I Project coined the term staff-consumer consultant (Epstein & Wadsworth, 1996a). A staff-consumer consultant is a person with both a consumer perspective *and* consumer experience who is employed by any of the mental health services in the context of quality assurance. The hyphen in this title emphasises the role of the consultant in a feedback loop that encourages communication between consumers and staff that is innately respectful to consumers. The rationale for staff-consumer consultancy is grounded in a commitment to culture change within and around the mental health system.

Training for staff-consumer consultants
One of the keys to successful and effective consumer participation in service provision is adequate and appropriate training – preferably in courses run by experienced consumer trainers. Such training needs to include discussion of specific government (national, state, and local) policy on mental health and services. Consumer perspectives, tokenism, power, and representativeness are also important topics to be covered in training

sessions. Since establishing open and equal dialogue between staff and consumers is a major aspect of the staff-consumer consultant's role, it is important that training includes sessions in which staff views and issues can be considered. Interested staff can be invited to participate in training workshops run by consumer trainers.

Other topics that need to be covered in staff-consumer training include conducting successful workshops, public speaking, building skills in policy reading and reportage, and participating in committees.

Practical considerations

There are a number of organisational matters that need to be addressed in relation to these training courses. They relate to the way time is structured, the choice of venue, the employment of 'expert' presenters, and the question of paying consumers for their participation in training courses.

One successful course was held in classrooms at a metropolitan hospital and was specifically designed to accommodate the people appointed as potential locums for consumer consultancy within the acute ward setting at that hospital. A generous room entitlement meant that participants were able to move between a classroom setting and a room which had a consumer history. This room had been thoughtfully arranged to enhance the capacity for group discussion and personal reflection. Organisers were careful to ensure extended half hour coffee breaks and an hour for lunch. This proved to be a very important feature of the program because it allowed people freedom to have some time to themselves if that was what they needed, or to spend time getting to know each other. Due to the funding arrangements of the hospital concerned it was possible to pay consumers for attending this course. We are convinced of the value in paying consumers for undertaking courses such as this. It is not simply for the obvious reason that money is a welcome and often scarce resource in this sector. The act of paying consumers for their time and effort is an important way of respecting and valuing their energies and contribution.

The final point to note here relates to the payment of expert presenters. Given that budgets may allocate one rate for consumer participation and a rate more than three times that for guest consultants – *who* should be invited to speak at various courses? The following account describes how we gained some insight into this issue. A number of the consumers undertaking a particular training course were especially interested in learning more about public speaking. Some of the consumers working in the field were experienced public speakers. They would have been prepared to lecture in this course at the consumer participation rate. On the other hand, so-called expert public speakers were quoting rates in the thousands of dollars for lecturing in the same course. We (consumer trainers) decided (for this one time) to try one of the marketed experts who agreed to cut his rate drastically for a one-off session with our project. What we learnt can be summed up as follows:

- The consumers in the course appreciated the opportunity to experience the talents of this person first hand
- They appreciated being valued enough to have such an 'expert' employed in their course.
- We all relished having someone from outside the mental health field involved in one of our courses

At the same time we also learned that this so called expert was no better a public speaker or educator than some of the people in the room, but his self-marketing strategies were a world away from our own. This was a valuable learning experience for all concerned.

Consumer advocacy

Advocacy can be defined as 'people promoting rights for themselves or others' (Meagher, 1995, p. 26). There are many different types of advocacy and much discussion about which are most appropriate and effective within the context of the consumer movement. Before looking at the types of advocacy it is important to understand why advocacy is needed. Social movements arise from the need of disempowered people to be heard; these people include members of ethnic minorities, elderly people, young people, as well as people suffering from psychiatric and other disabilities. Discriminatory laws, social mores and attitudes which lead to the social, economic, or personal disadvantage of people must first be identified and then efforts must be made to change them. Social and legislative changes are slow processes and much advocacy work is related to bringing about this sort of change. At the same time individuals who are suffering under current conditions require adequate information and support to claim their rights; or they should have access to those who can assist them in that endeavour.

Janet Meagher (consumer activist and writer) has drawn attention to the fact that traditional understandings of advocacy are inadequate to the needs of mental health consumers (1995, p. 25). Traditional advocacy in the mental health field has been left to particular interest groups such as voluntary charitable organisations, non-government 'overseers' of legislation, community visitors, patient care committees, and service providers. According to Meagher (1995, p. 25) this type of advocacy 'is not enough to protect consumers or to inform them of their place in society and their rights ... [the] way to rights, responsibility, and equity is self-advocacy'.

Self advocacy
Self advocacy is what happens when 'an individual or a group of individuals speak up for themselves or a common cause' (Meagher, 1995, p. 27). Examples of self advocacy include people challenging decisions made about them – their treatment, their needs, etc. – without their input. Perhaps they have been asked to make decisions without having been made aware of all the alternatives, or perhaps they have not been given access to all the

relevant information in a readily understandable form. Obviously it is not always easy for people to stand up for themselves. Often consumers are not taken seriously by carers – whether these are family members, friends or professionals. Consumers therefore need support and encouragement in speaking on their own behalf. Where a group of individuals speaks up regarding common concerns support comes from other group members. Group self-advocacy is carried out by unions, carers groups, parent groups, consumer groups, and voluntary organisations (Meagher, 1995, pp. 27–28).

Consumer advocacy groups

There are groups which have been formed by and for consumers and which take up social and political issues which affect their group. These groups may work with or without the collaboration of mental health workers but essentially they are consumer driven. The kinds of issues tackled by consumer advocacy groups include stigma, discrimination, accommodation, civil rights, and so on. This type of advocacy is usually concentrated on raising public awareness of these issues through various forms of campaigning.

Requirements for successful consumer advocacy

One of Meagher's most important observations is that advocacy actions and programs (of whatever kind) 'should enable consumers to be assertive about identifying their own needs and exercising their own choices from a knowledge base' (1995, p. 31). There are certain basic requirements which need to be met if this ideal is to be achieved:

- *Resources:* These include access to rehabilitation programs that emphasise and support self-determination and access to basic community services such as accommodation, transport, education, etc.
- *Information:* The availability of readily understood information and clear and open communication with professionals.
- *Choice:* The right to make choices and learn from mistakes.
- *Validity:* Consumer views, opinions, needs and experiences must be accepted as valid. This does not mean taking consumer opinions as intrinsically 'right' (a patronising and unproductive stance) but rather of acknowledging and supporting consumer views and initiatives.
- *Independent appeal, review, advocacy:* There should be avenues of appeal, review and advocacy open to consumers that are independent of service providers or legal decision makers.
- *Systemic safeguards:* These are built into organisations and processes; they include consumer evaluation and review of consumer involvement in decision making and policy development, in research and in quality assurance processes (Meagher, 1995, pp. 31–32).

Conclusion

In this chapter we have endeavoured to identify and address the central issues of consumer politics – albeit briefly. While there have been moves towards greater consumer involvement in the development and delivery of services deeper changes need to occur. In emphasising the importance of stigma and the consumer perspective we have tried to suggest how resistance to change can be a function of social and institutional processes and attitudes. In identifying education, participation, consultation and advocacy as avenues through which change can occur we have also tried to acknowledge the diversity of consumers, their experiences and their needs. We hope that the *Websites of Interest* and *References* will provide opportunities for the reader to discover more about the consumer movement. At the same time we would urge all service providers and workers in the mental health area to *listen* to what individual consumers have to say.

Websites of Interest

CSIPMH – Recovery-Self Help-Internet Sites
  http://www.rfmh.org/csipmh/recov03.html

Mental Health Consumer Concerns
  http://www.community.net/~mhcc/

Mental Health Consumers' Self-Help Clearinghouse
  http://www.libertynet.org/mha/cl_house.html

Psych Central – Dr John Grohol's Mental Health Links
  http://www.coil.com/~grohol/

Support Coalition – Human Rights and Psychiatry
  http://www.efn.org/~dendron/

FULL ACCESS
  http://members.aol.com./pbruckart/index.html

National Empowerment
  http://www.concentric.net/~power2u/

Psychiatry Information for the Public
  http://www.med.nyu.edu/psych/public.html

Clearinghouse Information – Self Help
  http://www.cmhc.com/selfhelp/clrnghse/clrnghse.html

References

Crepaz-Keay, D. (1996) Who Do *You* Represent? In: *Speaking Our Minds: An Anthology* (ed. J. Read & J. Reynolds, 184–5. Macmillan, London.

Epstein, M. & Olsen, A. (1997) One Stigma or Many. Discussion paper. Prepared by M. Epstein 27.5.95 and revised by Epstein and Olsen June/July 1997.

Epstein, M. & Shaw, J. (1997) *Developing Effective Consumer Participation in Mental Health Services: The Report of the Lemon Tree Learning Project.* VMIAC, Melbourne.

Epstein, M. & Wadsworth, Y. (1994) *Understanding and Involvement (U & I): Consumer Evaluation of Acute Psychiatric Hospital Practice – A Project's Beginnings* ... VMIAC, Melbourne.

Epstein, M. & Wadsworth, Y. (1996c) *Understanding and Involvement (U & I) ... A Project Unfolds.* VMIAC, Melbourne.

Epstein, M. & Wadsworth, Y. (1996b) *Understanding and Involvement (U & I) ... A Project Concludes.* VMIAC, Melbourne.

Epstein, M. & Wadsworth, Y. (1996a) *Orientation and Job Manual – Staff Consumer Consultants in Mental Health Services.* VMIAC, Melbourne.

Hutchinson, M. & Ausland, T. (1992/3) Learning About User Involvement. In: *User Involvement Information Pack.* MIND, London.

McGuiness, M. & Wadsworth, Y. (1992) *Understanding, Anytime.* VMIAC, Melbourne.

Meagher, J. (1995) *Partnership or Pretence.* Psychiatric Rehabilitation Association, Strawberry Hill.

Ralph, R.O. & Muskie, E.S. (1994) How to Involve Consumers in Mental Health Research and Demonstration Projects. Paper presented at the *Ohio Program Evaluation Group, Evaluation Exchange Conference.* Columbus, Ohio.

Read, J. & Reynolds, J. (1996) *Speaking Our Minds: An Anthology*, 2nd edn. Macmillan, London

Read, J. & Wallcraft, J. (1992) *Guidelines for Empowering Users of the Mental Health System.* MIND/COHSE, London.

Sargent, M. (1987) *Sociology for Australians*, 2nd ed. Longman Cheshire, Melbourne.

2 Rehabilitation for People with Enduring Psychotic Illnesses

Helen Kirkpatrick and *Jan Landeen*

'It is our job to form a community of hope which surrounds people with psychiatric disabilities. It is our job to create rehabilitation environments that are charged with hope.'

(Deegan, 1992).

Helping individuals to 'get on' with their lives despite having major psychotic illnesses has long been a focus for nurses. Psychosocial rehabilitation (PSR, also called psychiatric rehabilitation) gives nursing a framework for assisting in this recovery process. Several authors have elaborated on what PSR has to offer nursing (Boyd, 1994; Furlong-Norman, Palmer-Erbs & Jonikas, 1997; Palmer-Erbs & Anthony, 1995). The focus of this chapter is what nursing has to offer individuals with psychotic illness, exploring nursing's unique role in psychosocial rehabilitation. Nursing can move between psychosocial and biomedical paradigms, while assisting the client to negotiate those services that will most effectively meet his/her needs.

This chapter includes the following areas:

- Changes influencing psychiatric nursing
- The recovery and rehabilitation paradigm and how it fits with nursing
- Essentials of rehabilitation with a special section on hope
- Biomedical and psychosocial approaches
- Implications for nursing.

The illness addressed will be schizophrenia because it is the most common and severe of the major mental illnesses that cause ongoing psychoses. Issues related to schizophrenia are relevant to individuals with other psychotic illnesses.

This is a period of unprecedented change in the mental health system. The past 25 years have witnessed deinstitutionalisation, the consolidation or closing of inpatient units, shorter hospitalisation stays for all conditions, and the introduction of generic workers to replace nurses. Efforts to control costs co-exist with growing concerns about the quality of care and patient well-being. Consumers and families have become not just recipients of service but empowered as active partners in the development and delivery of services. Individuals who were called patients became service recipients and then citizens with rights who can be full members of their communities (Carling, 1996). Various terminology is advocated within the mental health system: patients, clients, consumers and consumer/survivors. Individuals may be each of these at different times and these terms will be used interchangeably in this chapter.

The Ontario, Canada context

Changes in health care delivery are occurring world-wide. The Ontario, Canada context is one example of evolving priorities and health care delivery systems. Canada has a single-tier system funded through the federal government but administered by each of the ten provinces. The system is based on five key criteria. It is publicly administered, comprehensive, accessible, portable across the country, and provides universal access.

In 1993, the Ministry of Health of Ontario released a ten-year plan, *Putting people first*, for the reform of mental health services in Ontario. It prioritised the needs of people who are severely mentally ill and used three dimensions to identify them: diagnosis, disability and duration. The predominant diagnoses were schizophrenia, major affective disorders, organic brain syndrome, and paranoid and other psychoses. 'Duration' referred to the chronic nature of the illness, and 'disability' to the fact that the disorder interfered with the individual's capacity to function normally. *Putting People First* identified that Ontario's mental health system was a collection of services, not a system. Ten provincial psychiatric hospitals, general and speciality hospitals, community-based programs and physician services were all Ministry of Health funded but with little coordination. The vision included a comprehensive service delivery system with a mix of institutional and community services, with all components integrated and coordinated. Consumer survivors and families would help plan and deliver overall services, and also develop alternatives to the formal services. Changes included a focus on forensic services and a shift from a hospital-based system. Funding would move from the current 80:20 institutional/community services to 40:60 (Ministry of Health of Ontario, 1993). The regional committees to develop the implementation plan for the Mental Health Plan are mandated to include 30% consumer/survivors and 20% family members (Ministry of Health of Ontario, 1995). This reflects similar initiatives throughout North America.

Changes influencing psychiatric nursing

Many changes in this decade have had, or will have, tremendous impact on psychiatric nursing. Nursing is at the junction of change in both the biomedical and the psychosocial fields. Historically, nurses have been part of multidisciplinary teams in inpatient settings, responsible for maintaining a therapeutic environment and managing patient symptoms 24 hours a day.

With new delivery models, a shift to alternative, rehabilitation-orientated, community-based settings offers new opportunities for nurses (Furlong-Norman *et al.* 1997). However, nurses must be prepared to adjust and take advantage of the changes.

Scientific knowledge is growing dramatically

Nursing leaders have described and predicted major increases in awareness about the biology of mental illness and the implications for psychiatric nursing (Hayes, 1995; Lowery, 1992; McBride, 1990). 'The decade of the brain is halfway through, and hardly a month passes without exciting news from the field of neuroscience and cognitive neuroscience' (Spitzer, 1995, p. 317.) This has been particularly dramatic in understanding schizophrenia. In fact, the question has been posed whether schizophrenia should be considered a neurological disorder rather than a mental illness (Braden, 1997). And long-term studies are challenging the traditional view that schizophrenia has a chronic deteriorating course (Harding & Zahniser, 1994).

Psychiatry is becoming more medicalised

There is a shift from the behavioural sciences to the neurosciences as the organising framework for psychiatry (Lowery, 1992; McBride, 1990). Neuropsychiatrists and neuropsychologists are replacing generalist psychiatrists in the treatment of individuals with schizophrenia. This shifting within psychiatry provides a special challenge for nurses to develop and maintain knowledge and skills that enable them to move between the biological and psychosocial paradigms.

Nursing is reconnecting to the biological model

The focus for psychiatric/mental health nurses has been and continues to be holistic, biopsychosocial practice. However, some authors believe that there has been an insufficient focus on the biological side of health and illness (Lowery, 1992; McBride, 1990; Hayes, 1995; Dunn, 1993) although others suggest too much focus on the biological aspects has caused us to lose the wholeness and integrity of the person (Palmer-Erbs, 1996). Psychiatric/mental health nurses have traditionally been trained in an interpersonal model of care with only a minor focus on biology. However there is a need to incorporate all models of knowledge, particularly at a time when increasingly sick patients require complex care (McBride, 1990). In addition to aspects of mental illness, this biological knowledge must encompass physical health (Dunn, 1993; Hayes, 1995; Krch-Cole, *et al.* 1997). Serious concern has been expressed about the poor physical health of those with chronic mental illnesses (Hutchinson, 1996). However, as patient populations change to include the more physically ill, psychiatric nurses feel inadequately prepared (Hayes, 1995).

Comprehensive systems offer both treatment and rehabilitation

Individuals with major mental illnesses who need the most comprehensive and sophisticated care have historically been given the least individualized treatments (Bachrach, 1992). The treatment of schizophrenia is most effective if medications are combined with targeted rehabilitation strategies (Munich & Lang, 1993; Palmer-Erbs, 1996). Unfortunately, there has been a lack of integrated models to incorporate all these aspects of service (Harding & Zahniser, 1994). However, this is changing (Dunn, 1993; Krch-Cole, *et al.*, 1997; Links, *et al.*, 1994; Starkey, *et al.*, 1997).

Recovery and rehabilitation

Patricia Deegan (1988), who is both a consumer and clinical psychologist, writes about recovery and rehabilitation. These processes are not specific or different for those with mental illness than those with other major disabilities. Recovery refers to the lived or real life experience of persons as they accept and overcome the challenge of the disability. It is a subjective experience of recovering a new sense of self and of purpose within and beyond the limits of the disability. Rehabilitation refers to the services and technologies made available to disabled persons so that they might learn to adapt to their world (Deegan, 1988).

Recovery

Recovery has been called the emerging vision of the mental health field (Anthony, 1993, p. 15). It 'is a way of living a satisfying, hopeful, and contributing life even with limitations caused by illness'. Deegan (1988, p. 15) refers to the paradox of recovery, 'that in accepting what we cannot do or be, we begin to discover who we can be and what we can do'. In a recovery-orientated system, each service contributes to specific outcomes (see Table 2.1). In rehabilitation, the terms impairment, dysfunction, disability and disadvantage have specific meaning with implications for both treatment approaches and for the types of services needed (see Table 2.2). The phrase, 'places to be and symptom free' captures the importance of being successful and satisfied in one's environment of choice, and also a reduction in the symptoms of severe mental illness (Anthony, 1996).

Deegan (1992) cautions that those who have passively given up should not be abandoned, which happens at some point to every person diagnosed with a mental illness. Giving up is a solution, a way of surviving in desolate environments. The task for the individual is to move from surviving to recovering. However, environments must change to nurture growth and recovery. Consumers have written about environments that nurture recovery (Deegan, 1988; Leete, 1987; Lovejoy, 1984). Such environments:

(1) Are structured to embrace, and expect, the approach/avoid, try/fail dynamic that is the recovery process
(2) Recognise that staff attitudes can be helpful or unhelpful

Table 2.1 Focus of mental health services.

Recovery: Development of new meaning and purpose as one grows beyond the catastrophic effects of mental illness.

Mental health services (and outcomes)	Impact of severe mental illness			
	Impairment (disorder in thought, feelings, and behaviour)	Dysfunction (task performance limited)	Disability (role performance limited)	Disadvantage (opportunity restrictions)
Treatment (symptom relief)	✓			
Crises intervention (safety)	✓			
Case management (access)	✓	✓	✓	✓
Rehabilitation (role functioning)		✓	✓	✓
Enrichment (self-development)		✓	✓	✓
Rights protection (equal opportunity)				✓
Basic support (survival)				✓
Self-help (empowerment)			✓	✓

Reprinted from: Anthony, W.A. (1993). Recovery from mental illness: The guiding vision of the mental health service system in the 1990s. *Psychosocial Rehabilitation Journal,* **16**(4), 10–23.

(3) Understand that each person's journey of recovery is unique
(4) Recognise the gift that disabled people have to give to each other.

Rehabilitation

Individuals with psychiatric disabilities have the same goals and dreams as anyone else. These include a decent place to live, an appropriate work environment, social activities and friends (Palmer-Erbs & Anthony, 1995). The mission of psychiatric rehabilitation is to help individuals with psychiatric disabilities to 'increase their functioning so that they are successful and satisfied in the environments of their choice with the least amount of ongoing professional intervention' (Anthony *et al.*, 1990, p.151). Within this mission, key rehabilitation values provide a focus for rehabilitation:

Table 2.2   The negative impact of severe mental illness.

Stages	Definitions	Examples	Interventions	Relationship to treatment
Impairment	Any loss or abnormality of psychological, physiological, anatomical structure or function	In physical disabilities (diabetes is an impairment in physiological function)	Treatment with medication to moderate glucose metabolism; neuroleptic medication to moderate symptoms	Treatment could moderate an impairment
Dysfunction	Any restriction or lack of ability to perform an activity or task in the manner or within the range considered normal for a human being	In psychiatric disabilities – demonstration of minimal proficiencies in the areas of self-care, social adjustment and/or work skills	Implementation of a rehabilitation program	Treatment may modify the effects of dysfunction
Disability	Any restriction or lack of ability to perform a role in the manner or within the range that is considered normal for a human being	Severity of disability is defined within the sociocultural context – unemployment, underemployment, homelessness	Implementation of a rehabilitation program	Treatment will not change a disability
Disadvantage	A lack of opportunity for an individual that limits or prevents the performance of an activity or the fulfilment of a role that is normal (depending on age, sex, social, cultural factors) for that individual	In physical disabilities – inaccessible facilities for wheelchairs. In psychiatric disabilities – stigma and assumptions about rehabilitation potential	Implementation of a societal rehabilitation/ education program on stigma and discrimination	Treatment will not change a disadvantage

Reprinted from: Palmer-Erbs, V. & Anthony, W. (1995). Incorporating psychiatric rehabilitation principles into mental health nursing. *Journal of Psychosocial Nursing*, **33**(3), pp. 36–44.

- Functioning (performance of everyday activities)
- Success (meeting requirements of other people in the client's world)
- Satisfaction (the client's feelings of happiness)
- Environmental specificity (the specific context where the person lives, learns, socialises or works)
- Choice (self-determined goals)
- Outcome orientation (evaluation based on client outcomes), support (assistance provided for as long as needed and wanted)
- Growth potential (improvement in functioning and status)

(Anthony *et al.*, 1990)

Outcomes of psychiatric rehabilitation are unique and specific compared with other mental health service interventions: improved role performance or status in consumers' living, learning, working or social environments. There may be important ancillary outcomes (e.g. symptom reduction), but consumer goals in PSR services are changes in role performance. Differentiating role performance and skill performance is important. Role performance can be affected either through skill development or environmental supports (Anthony, 1996). Psychosocial rehabilitation uses individually tailored interventions, based on active involvement of the consumer, which recognises the tremendous variation of individuals (Bachrach, 1992). This heterogeneity can be affected by gender, age, developmental tasks, education, job history, symptoms, coping skills, personality characteristics, meaning systems, and stress response besides the heterogeneity of the illness itself. And seeing the person within the context of his or her environment is essential (Harding & Zahniser, 1994). The person may be helped to meet the needs of the environment or social and physical environments may be created, modified or adapted to meet the needs of the individual (Bachrach, 1992).

Palmer-Erbs and Anthony (1995) identified basic principles of psychiatric rehabilitation that are relevant to nursing practice (see Fig. 2.1). Nursing contributes a holistic focus to psychosocial rehabilitation, with attention to the biomedical and psychosocial models. Therefore nursing can intervene in all aspects of impairment, dysfunction, disability and disadvantage (see Table 2.2). Within the basic tenets of PSR is the strong belief that hope is critical to recovery and rehabilitation. Because hope is so important, it will be considered separately.

Basic principles of psychiatric rehabilitation for nursing practice

If people with major mental illness are perceived as people with disabilities, the field of physical rehabilitation is a useful metaphor for psychosocial rehabilitation. Both may need a wide range of services for an extended period, exhibit limitations in performing roles such as worker or student, and may or may not experience a full recovery from their impairment (Palmer-Erbs & Anthony, 1995). Rehabilitation and treatment

---

- Person-centered focus to develop the competencies of persons with psychiatric disabilities.
- Interventions targeted to behavioural improvements in consumer's environment of need.
- Uses an eclectic approach.
- Relies on hope as an essential ingredient.
- Values an intentional initial increase in consumer dependency that can lead to an eventual increase in independence.
- Values an active consumer involvement as critical to the overall success of reaching a rehabilitation goal.
- Interventions focus on the development of consumer life skills and increased environmental supports.
- Long-term drug treatment often is necessary, but rarely a sufficient component of the rehabilitation process.

Fig. 2.1 Basic principles of psychiatric rehabilitation for nursing practice. (*Journal of Psychosocial Nursing.*)

Reprinted from: Palmer-Erbs, V. & Anthony, W. (1995). Incorporating psychiatric rehabilitation principles into mental health nursing. *Journal of Psychosocial Nursing,* **33**(3), 36–44.

may be delivered in different settings, with different points of emphasis, but with an occasional overlap (see Table 2.2). However, for the most severely mentally ill with the most serious impairments, it is imperative that treatment and rehabilitation are closely intertwined. It is the integration of psychosocial rehabilitation and psychiatry that can provide optimal services for those with long-term mental illnesses. Whether viewed as two separate approaches or two aspects of a single approach, they should not be considered mutually exclusive (Bachrach, 1992).

Example of a PSR program

The Schizophrenia Psychosocial Rehabilitation Program (SPRP) is one of three programs in the Schizophrenia Services at Hamilton Psychiatric Hospital (HPH). SPRP patients have a diagnosis of schizophrenia, have had prolonged or repeated hospitalisation or treatment, and a history of unsuccessful community functioning. This is a small group of the most severely mentally ill for whom short-term hospitalisation and community-based programs have been insufficient. The SPRP provides both inpatient assessment and treatment as well as intensive transitional supports until the individual is accepted into a community-based program.

The holistic framework developed in the SPRP has four major components: consumer goals, health status, functional status, and supports. The initial focus is on a new assessment (see Fig. 2.2), essential after years of illness and dysfunction, given the longitudinal nature of the illness (Harding & Zahniser, 1994). Key to all of this is partnership with the consumer. A chart review begins the process. The history of treatment may be known, but who was the person before the illness interfered? This chart review poses questions for the assessment. Goals provide the driving force

---

STANDARDS OF PATIENT CARE

Principal function: Assessing patients regarding their health status, functional status, supports, and personal goals as the basis for their rehabilitation.

Objectives:

1. To collect information required to plan, design, and evaluate effective treatment and rehabilitation interventions and strategies.
2. To establish a baseline to assess and evaluate patient progress and the effects of treatment and rehabilitation interventions and strategies.
3. To initiate the development of a working relationship with the patient.

Standard: All patients admitted to the program will be assessed by members of the multidisciplinary team in the following areas:

A. Personal goals:
   The expressed direction that the individual wants to pursue in living, working, and/or social areas.

B. Health status:
   1. *Psychiatric status:* The symptomatology that is amenable to treatment.
   2. *Medical status:* Physical illness and/or impairments, which may have an impact on the individual's rehabilitation or on the operation of the program.
   3. *Medication Response:* Responses to medication including side effects (particularly extrapyramidal and tardive dyskinesia).
   4. *Diet and nutrition:* Dietary patterns and requirements related to lifestyle or medical status.
   5. *Sleep and rest:* Sleep and rest patterns and requirements.
   6. *Health practices and beliefs:* Individual and cultural health practices and values.

C. Functional status:
   1. *Social interaction:* Skill and performance level to interact verbally and physically with individuals and groups.
   2. *Self-care:* Skill and performance level in carrying out activities of daily living independently.
   3. *Productivity:* Skill and performance level required in a meaningful role.
   4. *Leisure and exercise:* Leisure and exercise interests and activities.

D. Supports:
   Supports that are potentially useful to maximize the overall effectiveness of the rehabilitation plan. Areas to be assessed include: *family/significant others, social resources, health care services, accommodation,* and *income.*

Fig. 2.2 Schizophrenia psychosocial rehabilitation program. (*Journal of Psychosocial Nursing.*)

for the assessment and treatment, recognising one only works for what one wants. The program appreciates the importance of helping the person set goals, and of daring to dream of new possibilities after years of unsuccessful functioning. Standardised assessment measures are used so that the client's status can be documented in widely understood terms, provide a basis for systematic treatment selection and the reliable documentation of change (O'Connor & Eggert, 1994).

The role of hope

Hope is an important concept in the recovery literature. Some first person accounts of schizophrenia describe regaining hope as a turning point in recovery. However, consumers also describe treatment settings and the realities of living with the illness as situations that rob them of hope (Deegan, 1988; Leete, 1987; Lovejoy, 1984).

Judith Miller, a renowned nurse–researcher in the area of hope, defines hope as an 'anticipation of a continued good state, an improved state, or a release from a perceived entrapment (1992, p. 414). According to Miller, maintaining hope is a challenge of the chronically ill. Chronic illness, by virtue of its unpredictable nature and concomitant losses, precipitates powerlessness. When powerlessness is not contained, hopelessness can result. Suicide (the antithesis of recovery) is the leading cause of premature death for individuals with schizophrenia, with a 10% to 13% lifetime incidence. Hopelessness and depression have been identified as significant factors in such suicides (Caldwell & Gottesman, 1990; Tanney, 1992).

The role of hope for individuals with schizophrenia has recently received increased attention (Littrell, *et al.*, 1996). Work in this area by the authors includes cross-sectional studies of hope and schizophrenia in both staff (Byrne, et al., 1994; Kirkpatrick, *et al.*, 1995; Landeen, *et al.*, 1996; Woodside, *et al.*, 1994) and individuals with schizophrenia (Pawlick, *et al.*, 1997). The staff/client relationship was the most powerful hope-instilling strategy staff identified for working with clients (Byrne, *et al.*, 1995; Kirkpatrick, *et al.*, 1995). For clients, global satisfaction with quality of life and subjective measures of satisfaction in three life domains (leisure, health and social) were positively correlated with hope (Pawlick, *et al.*, 1997).

What nursing has to offer in enhancing hope

The following interventions are based on the authors' clinical work and their research on hope and schizophrenia. Staff described the importance of managing the illness and education, but the key strategies were building relationships, facilitating success and connecting to successful role models (Kirkpatrick, *et al.*, 1995).

Build and support relationships

Staff emphasised the importance of the staff/client relationship, rapport, communication and/or trust. This relationship was often described as a 'journey' by the client with the staff member as facilitator. Most staff talked about what might be called 'being present': listening to the client, understanding his/her perspective and accepting each person. This is also a basic PSR principle: hear what the person has to say; see their experience and understand what hope means through his/her eyes.

Programs can be developed or altered by listening to their clients' collective perspective. The SPRP developed a supported housing project in response to clients' goals (Kirkpatrick, *et al.*, 1995). In the example, Moving Out, (see Fig. 2.3) staff initiated the sentimental journeys in response to concerns expressed by several individuals.

The SPRP began on a 'long-stay' unit where patients had been hospitalised for an average of 14 years. The mandate was to help these institutionalised individuals successfully move into the community. Changes to the environment included consultation meetings with patients and then families, individualised reassessments and goal planning, and developing a sense of movement and change. If patients had to leave the hospital, many wanted to return to their home community. Often, the place where they wanted to live no longer existed or had changed dramatically. The team initiated monthly *sentimental journeys* for six to eight clients from a region about 100 km from the hospital. Each month one person was the 'star' and the group visited that person's hometown. If the 'star' had family in the area, the group often visited the relatives, and had coffee at a boarding home in the area. These journeys helped individuals reconnect with their past, reminisce, and explore their old community as a possible choice of living environment. As individuals prepared to leave the hospital, the team initiated *farewell teas*. The person who was leaving was the guest of honour. The tea provided everyone the opportunity to say goodbye and contributed to the sense of movement and change. The farewell teas became a 'rite of passage' and individuals often planned their own (Kirkpatrick, *et al.*, 1996). It was really no different than teas for staff retiring after long years in the hospital.

The most elaborate tea was for a young woman who had been in hosital more than ten years. She had a new dress, she invited her family and staff from other parts of the hospital, some of whom brought flowers. Her tea was videotaped and the tape given to her.

Individuals frequently took encouragement and hope from other patients. John who had been hospitalised for 45 years was asked about George who had left after 33 years hospitalisation. He said, 'He must be crazy but he likes it.' He then began to work with staff to plan his own discharge, having spent his whole adult life institutionalised. Patients cannot do it on their own without institutional supports but co-patients who successfully move out of hospital can have tremendous impact on those left behind.

Fig. 2.3 Moving out.

Facilitate success

Staff talked about assisting clients to move forward in both exceptional situations and in their day-to-day lives. Helping someone do something and being successful is empowering for the individual. In Alex's story (see Fig. 2.4) the nurse listened to his request, making something happen and facilitated a successful outcome. He was proud of *his* accomplishment.

Connect with successful role models

Help the person connect to another individual with schizophrenia who has succeeded in a relevant aspect. This can increase the person's connection with others in a similar situation and thereby decrease the feeling of aloneness. In Moving Out (see Fig. 2.3), individuals became role models for one another.

Alex was referred to the SPRP from an intensive community-based case management program. This was a unique situation in which his previous case manager retained some involvement, and he would return to that community program when he no longer required the levels of support the SPRP could offer. He was living in a supervised lodging home with supports from our program. He had been ill for many years and tended to be hopeless about his future. When he received his tax rebate, he wanted to visit his family 3000 miles away. His original case manager said he could never do it, couldn't save the money or follow through. Our community nurse told him she would help him. He did it with her help to bank the money, negotiate plans with his family, make the reservation, arrange for necessary laboratory work in Vancouver, deliver him to, and pick him up from, the airport in another city. He did it. He had a wonderful visit. He reconnected with his sister. And he is planning to do it again.

Fig. 2.4 Alex's story.

Jevne (1993) identified several other hope strategies that can be helpful for individuals with any chronic illness, including the use of hope rituals, images, and stories. She notes hope is experienced in the present but is linked to the past and the future. Strength and wisdom from the past can be used to construct a bridge to the goals of the future. This is reflected in the example, Moving Out (see Fig. 2.3). Using the sentimental journey, staff helped clients link to their past and thus begin to plan for their own future. The farewell teas were a hope ritual, a clear sign for them and others that the person was moving on to a new chapter in their life. Other rituals include celebrating birthdays or achievements. Nurses can encourage individuals to tell hope stories. John's accounting of Gordon's experience is a hope story. The video tape of the young woman's farewell tea is a hope story she can play repeatedly.

Working with individuals, nurses can help the person describe their image. Staff asked a patient why he was having a hard time working with them. He said he felt like there was a door between them. Staff asked if it were locked. He replied not just locked but with several bolts. Staff worked with this image, one bolt at a time. This approach recognised his own experience and moved at the rate he was able to cope with.

Our research indicated it is also important for staff to consider their own workplace and its impact on their hope. Hope can be contagious. Client successes were not only hope-instilling for clients but also for staff. Strategies to maintain a hopeful work atmosphere included: a supportive group that offers encouragement when needed; co-workers who make specific, helpful clinical suggestions or share the responsibility for a particularly difficult client; meetings that allow for brainstorming of alternate clinical approaches; and staff meetings that focus on clients who are improving, not only problems. Learning about new treatments and approaches, learning from other staff and programs, and sharing in a greater sense of community are important (Landeen, *et al.*, 1996).

Biopsychosocial treatments

Biological treatments

This is an exciting time in the evolution of knowledge about the severe mental illnesses, especially in schizophrenia. The invention of PET and NMR scans have allowed scientists to study the working brain, opening the doors to new areas of research and stimulating interest in biological research for mental illness (Cleghorn, *et al.*, 1991). Nursing must keep abreast of these changes to both explain the results of newsworthy studies to their clients and their families, and to take advantage of new treatments as they become available. While recovery and rehabilitation are key approaches for the seriously mentally ill, they are enhanced by the best treatment approaches possible for controlling the symptoms of the illness. Nursing, with its foundations in the biological sciences, can lead in combining these many approaches.

Medications

Nursing has a tradition of assisting their clients to maximise the benefits of medications while reducing any side effects associated with these. Research has abounded on issues of compliance and the most effective ways of teaching about medications (Corrigan, *et al.*, 1990; Awad, 1993; Eckman, *et al.*, 1990; Streicker, *et al.*, 1986). What is new in the field of psychiatry is the availability of atypical medications that hold great promise for individuals who have not responded to traditional neuroleptics (Remington, 1995). Researchers have been quick to respond to the success of Clozapine by examining the neurotransmitters activated by the drug. This has led to the discovery of multiple dopamine receptor sites that may explain some of the differential effects of the traditional and atypical neuroleptics (Seeman, 1995). In the search for new drugs, researchers have now mapped out the receptor profiles for all of the traditional and atypical drugs (Gerlach & Peacock, 1995). This allows physicians and nurses to predict more accurately and scientifically which side effects are most likely to occur with a particular drug. In nursing's search to minimise side effects, this additional knowledge is a powerful tool to assist individual clients as they search with their physicians for the medication best suited to their needs.

Neurocognitive functioning

Neurocognitive psychology is a field that is offering new insights into why some clients with similar levels of symptoms have better functional outcomes. In a review of recent neurocognitive studies that focused on functioning, Green (1996) found associations between neurocognitive deficits and specific functional outcomes. Secondary verbal memory was a strong predictor or correlate of community outcome, social problem solving and skill acquisition. Vigilance, an attentional process, was consistently associated with social skill acquisition. Individuals with schizophrenia who performed poorly on some measures did not tend to do so on all. Such knowledge holds out the hope of being able to target interventions and supports to specific deficits, tailoring the rehabilitation plan to that individual. Heinssen (1996) described the use of a 'cognitive exoskeleton' for environmental interventions. Velligan and colleagues (1996) developed a treatment approach, cognitive adaptation training, to alter the physical environment to compensate for cognitive deficits and improve adaptive functioning for individuals with schizophrenia. Fogel (1996) suggested a neuropsychiatric approach to understanding impairments in goal-directed behaviour, which is common to many psychiatric disorders. Thus, the area of neurocognitive functioning is growing in terms of understanding the particular types of deficits that an individual may experience, and also offering new approaches or modifications of approaches to best compensate for those deficits.

Genetics

The field of genetics is rapidly expanding with predictions of mapping out the entire genome within the next five to ten years. While it is now becoming increasingly clear that no one gene is the cause of schizophrenia, a picture of several genes interacting is beginning to emerge. It is also known that genetics probably play a significant role in establishing susceptibility to the illness, but not for every individual affected by schizophrenia (Buckley, *et al.*, 1996). While it is too early in this research to offer any direct benefits to clients, new information is emerging rapidly. The implications of genetic research are not solely contained to genetic counselling, but a new field of genetic therapy is emerging that holds out some hope to individuals already affected by schizophrenia.

Early intervention

There is growing evidence that early and appropriate intervention in schizophrenia may reduce relapse rates (Herz, *et al.*, 1991), and in fact, lessen the severity of the illness over the long term (Wyatt, 1991). It appears that acute, untreated psychotic episodes have a toxic effect on brain functioning, and thus on social functioning for the individual. If this is verified in repeated studies, it is imperative that nurses work actively with clients and their families to seek early intervention and to continue with appropriate medication for a period of time after an initial episode to avoid repeated relapses. While early diagnosis of schizophrenia and ongoing denial remains a problem, new programs and approaches aimed at early intervention and relationship building are being developed and researched (Wilson & Hobbs, 1995).

Psychosocial treatments

In addition to social skills training and cognitive therapy techniques, important components of PSR, other psychosocial approaches include family psychoeducation and individual psychotherapy.

Family psychoeducational approaches

There has been significant research and program development in family psychoeducational approaches (McFarlane, 1983; Mueser & Gingerich, 1994). It has been demonstrated that family participation in such programs can reduce relapse rates when combined with drug therapy (Hogarty, 1993). Many rehabilitation and treatment programs now offer such courses as one part of their services. In Hamilton, several agencies collaborated in developing and delivering such a program, the Family Education and Training Program. Staff from different agencies take turns co-leading the groups along with family graduates from the program. This strategy has been effective in having sufficient participant numbers to make the program cost effective, with the added benefit of families hearing about the different programs that are available from other families and staff. Nurses routinely run these courses with social workers and other health professionals.

Individual psychotherapy

Individual psychotherapy fell out of favour in the treatment of schizophrenia because this approach used alone did not cure schizophrenia. However, psychotherapy has again emerged as a viable treatment option for individuals with schizophrenia (McGlashan, 1994; Wasylenki, 1992). Many have had life experiences that go well beyond their illness, and require therapy to move past these difficult experiences. Other individuals require ongoing supportive psychotherapy to help them cope with the losses associated with having a chronic illness. Traditional psychotherapy approaches frequently need to be adapted to individuals who are less verbal or who have difficulty distinguishing reality. This highly skilled approach goes beyond traditional nursing training. However, a nurse may be the only one with whom the client will discuss highly personal issues, if they are the only professional with whom the client has developed a trusting relationship. In such cases, the nurse might help the client move that trust to another individual, perhaps attending sessions jointly with the client. In other instances, the nurse might receive intense supervision in providing this service.

As knowledge expands in the biological and psychosocial areas, nursing is in the position to incorporate these approaches into the rehabilitation approach, offering the best possible care to clients.

Examples of service delivery models

In providing effective rehabilitation, nurses can play an instrumental role in developing service delivery systems that integrate PSR approaches. Many models have been developed and tested that can serve as examples to consider such developments. Case management has gained in popularity across North America as a generic service delivery model with a variety of health care workers and professionals filling the role of case manager. Case management can be either individual (Mound, *et al.*, 1991) or team case management (Lachance & Santos, 1995). No matter which model of case management is used, the relationship with the client is key to effective case management. Nurses are particularly suited to be case managers because of their ability to cross the various domains and roles.

Individual case management

In individual case management, the therapeutic relationship is a case manager/consumer dyad, although other staff may be involved. The approach differs from a traditional therapist in key ways. The case manager assists the client in obtaining whatever services and supports are needed for the best functioning possible, in addition to the supportive counselling that is the hallmark of traditional therapists. Case managers are also encouraged to see clients in their own environments rather than in an office.

Case management can be practised using a variety of therapeutic approaches including a brokerage model where the client is assessed and linked to the services needed to an inclusive model where the case manager provides: rehabilitation counselling; psychotherapy; assistance with symptoms and medications; crisis management; and basic life supports. The Hamilton Program for Schizophrenia emphasises the integration of treatment and rehabilitation to facilitate an individual's success and satisfaction (Dermer & Landeen, 1991). This community-based, long-term, case management program offers a comprehensive array of services, portions or all of which can be accessed to meet a particular client's needs and goals. Since its inception in 1972, this program continues to evolve and grow as advances are made in all areas of treatment and rehabilitation for individuals with schizophrenia. It must be emphasised that the need for staff to stay abreast of these changes and to assist their clients to make sense of the new opportunities is ongoing. The ability to shift between PSR and biological paradigms is essential to staff success in this program.

Team case management

The PACT model (Program for Assertive Community Treatment) is a team case management model. It has been widely evaluated and shown to be successful in using the community as its treatment arena and focusing on eliminating long-term hospital care. This model has been referred to as a hospital without walls because it offers services traditionally found only in hospitals. Critical elements of the PACT model include: a multidisciplinary team; round the clock support; small caseloads with a fixed client roster; services which are ongoing and unlimited in duration, assertive outreach; and treatment and rehabilitation occur *in vivo* in the client's natural environment (Lachance & Santos, 1995). The relationship is built with the team so there is availability over time. However, within the team there will be specific members who are more involved with a client. Assertive community treatment programs have long practised supported services, including supported education, supported employment and supported housing.

Implications for nursing

Keep abreast of rapidly changing knowledge
Given the unprecedented expanse of knowledge in brain functioning and effective biological and psychosocial approaches, it is imperative that nurses keep up to date. It is hard to predict how quickly new understandings will emerge. Nurses must be able to explain new interventions to better informed consumers and their families. In this age of specialisation in nursing it is critical for psychiatric nurses to become truly experts in their chosen field and that they can understand and interpret the new information as it is released in the press and scientific journals.

Develop new or adapted intervention combining knowledge from different fields
As discussed previously, psychosocial rehabilitation is most effective when it is combined with biological, cognitive, and other psychosocial approaches. By developing interventions that combine these bodies of knowledge, nurses can lead the way in providing excellent patient care and in bringing the profession into the twenty-first century.

Publicise nursing's areas of expertise so that the least well trained do not become the primary care givers for the most ill individuals
In other areas of nursing, for example in critical care units, leaving the most ill in the care of the least well trained is inconceivable. Unfortunately this has not been the case in psychiatry. There is the widely held belief that if an individual has a chronic illness, they no longer require expert nurses. However, it is precisely then that highly trained and skilled nursing is essential if the complexity of approaches and the unique needs of the client are to be integrated. Unless nursing articulates and proves this necessity through sound research for itself and for the various funders, the least well trained will be left caring for those with the most complex problems.

Advocate for necessary services in changing mental health delivery systems
Nursing has traditionally not been a strong advocate for consumers of its services, but has left the advocacy role mainly to others. If nurses want to influence health care systems so that they provide comprehensive, integrated services as described above, then they will need to serve on decision-making boards and committees. This inclusion will only occur through constant, effective lobbying. Only by maintaining a strong voice will nursing be viewed by others as having an important contribution to make in designing effective mental health delivery systems.

Maintain hopeful environments that allow clients to take full advantage of all that we now know

It is imperative that nurses maintain environments that nurture growth, for both clients and themselves. This is often difficult in the face of the slow rate of change in both clients and bureaucratic systems. However, it is both possible and essential if clients and their families are to benefit from current and emerging treatment approaches. Truly believing that change is possible for every individual and carrying this message of hope into all areas of practice is one of the most valuable contributions that nursing has to make.

Remember the person who has the illness and keep his or her strengths and needs as central in all approaches

We end at the beginning. It is the unique client before us who directs what we do. We can be most effective only by looking for and nurturing the person who is hidden by the symptoms of the illness. It is both humbling and personally rewarding to help the individual emerge again after an extended psychosis. The courage and endurance of the severely mentally ill can serve as the inspiration to nurses to bring their very best to each new client.

The following is one community nurse's story of working with a man who was basically institutionalised in the community. It demonstrates the integration of the biomedical and psychosocial approaches (see Fig. 2.5).

Roy was a very psychotic middle-aged man living in a supervised boarding home. A history of extremely aggressive behaviour had resulted in over two decades of institutionalisation. Large amounts of two antipsychotic medications controlled the aggression and allowed him to live outside of hospital, which he preferred, but left him marginalised while still psychotic. He lived in a four-bed room with virtually no privacy. I had two objectives:

- Develop a therapeutic relationship and provide some social support
- Manage a reduction in his psychotropic medication, and initiate an atypical anti-psychotic.

At first, Roy refused to speak with me, so I met with the boarding home staff. In a few weeks, we had our first visit. He declined to go out for coffee, but we sat and talked for 20 minutes. I listened to incredibly derailed thought processes, delusional ideas, watched him respond to auditory hallucinations. He was being tortured by his bizarre thought content, including visions of infants being smothered in blood and faeces, and wars inside his head. From that point on, I brought coffee for our visits and we sat and visited over coffee. As the Haloperidol was decreased, we noticed changes. Roy had fewer outbursts, less agitation and pacing (probably from decreased akathesia), was calmer in dealing with other people, and started looking after his personal hygiene with encouragement. And a relationship was forming between us – he recognised who I was, said thank you for the coffee. For a few moments we could sit and focus on realities, like his visit with his aunt – a real breakthrough. We increased our visits to twice weekly.

Within two months, we went out for lunch at his request. His behaviour indicated that it had been a really long time since he had been to a restaurant. He asked me to order his food. He responded to auditory hallucinations as he took great mouthfuls of food, swallowed almost without chewing it, had food all over his face, and belched loudly. He was not conscious of his behaviour, and was oblivious to the presence of others. However, he was really appreciative of going to the restaurant and told the house staff that I was the only person who cared about him.

As we decreased the medications we watched a person emerging and my dual role continued – monitoring the medication reduction and helping that person to emerge. In our conversations the balance between delusional conversation and reality orientated conversation was swinging toward reality orientated. We began talking about goals.

Not having akathesia was a great benefit and Roy could sit and have a conversation. But he remained incredibly psychotic and quite hostile to other people. We initiated an atypical antipsychotic while continuing to decrease his other medication. About a month later, there was a real change, he simply didn't respond to the voices anymore. Conversations were reality orientated.

When he complained of boredom, I got scared. His psychosis which had dominated his way of thinking and viewing the world for most of his adult life was disappearing. He was literally left with memories of being a teenager. I asked the house staff to watch for suicidal ideation and I did the same. I was concerned that his psychosis be replaced with something meaningful. I asked our program staff to become involved to give some structure and meaning to his day. I worked with him so he could begin to realise that there could be a new life and I would help him with it.

Over the next several months, he began advocating for himself, wanting to get new shoes, clean clothes, new glasses. The person was really beginning to emerge. He became aware of other people around him. His conversation was generally reality based and becoming purposeful. Goals were emerging: 'I need this', 'Can you do this for me?' or 'I'd like to go there', 'I'd like to get a job'. Then his conversation included social graces – please, thank you, hello, how are you? – patting me on the shoulder as a greeting, shaking my hand, taking notice of those around him. He started to show a sense of humour. He asked that his long and shaggy hair be cut and his beard be removed. His conversation shifted from himself to include my interests and how I was doing.

I now see Roy three times a week. It is nine months and today we took the bus for the first time. Although anxious, he did fine with support, he got on the bus, and got off at the right stop. It was a triumph. We went to the same restaurant. But today, instead of taking great gulps of food, he took smaller bites, he enjoyed the food, was conscious of other people. His conversation centred on the food, and included all the social graces.

My goal now is to help Roy develop and achieve goals for his new life. And we continue to adjust the medications.

Fig. 2.5   Working with Roy.

References

Anthony, W.A. (1993) Recovery from mental illness: The guiding vision of the mental health service system in the 1990s. *Psychosocial Rehabilitation Journal*, **16**(4), 10–23.

Anthony, W. (1996) Integrating psychiatric rehabilitation into managed care. *Psychiatric Rehabilitation Journal*, **20**(2), 39–44.

Anthony, W., Cohen, M., & Farkas, M. (1990) *Psychiatric Rehabilitation*. Centre for Psychiatric Rehabilitation: Boston University, Boston.

Awad, A.G. (1993) Subjective response to neuroleptics in schizophrenia. *Schizophrenia Bulletin*, **19**(3), 609–18.

Bachrach, L. (1992) Psychosocial rehabilitation and psychiatry in the care of long-term patients. *American Journal of Psychiatry*, **149**(11), 1455–63.

Boyd, M. (1994) Integration of psychosocial rehabilitation into psychiatric nursing practice. *Issues in Mental Health Nursing*, **15**, 13–26.

Braden, A. (1997) The question of our time. *Bulletin: Schizophrenia Society of Canada*,

6(2). (Available from the Schizophrenia Society of Canada, 75 The Donway West, Suite 814, Don Mills, Ontario, Canada, M3C 2E9.)

Buckley, P.F., Buchanan, R.W., Schulz, S.C. & Tanninga, C.A. (1996) Catching up on schizophrenia. *Archives of General Psychiatry*, **53**, 456–62.

Byrne, C., Woodside, H., Landeen, J., Kirkpatrick, H., Bernardo, A. & Pawlick, J. (1994) The importance of relationships in fostering hope. *Journal of Psychosocial Nursing*, **32**(9), 31–4.

Caldwell, C.B. & Gottesman, I.I. (1990) Schizophrenics kill themselves too: A review of risk factors for suicide. *Schizophrenia Bulletin*, **16**(4), 573–89.

Carling, P. (1996) Innovations in Mental Health Planning. Paper presented at *Systems Thinking and Innovations in Mental Health Programs*, St. Catharines, Ontario.

Cleghorn, J.M., Zipinsky, R.B. & List, S.J. (1991) Structural and functional brain imaging in schizophrenia. *Journal of Psychiatric Neuroscience*, **16**(2), 53–74.

Corrigan, P.W., Liberman, R.P. & Engel, J.D. (1990) From noncompliance to collaboration in the treatment of schizophrenia. *Hospital & Community Psychiatry*, **41**(11), 1203–10.

Deegan, P.E. (1988) Recovery: The lived experience of rehabilitation. *Psychosocial Rehabilitation Journal*, **11**(4), 11–19.

Deegan, P.E. (1992) Recovery, rehabilitation and the conspiracy of hope: A keynote address. Paper presented at the *8th Annual Garwood-Jones Lecture*, Hamilton, Ontario.

Dermer, S.W. & Landeen, J.L. (1991) Establishing a model for care in schizophrenia: One program's experience. *Canadian Journal of Psychiatry*, **36**, 588–93.

Dunn, J. (1993) Medical skills and knowledge: How necessary are they for psychiatric nurses? *Journal of Psychosocial Nursing*, **31**(12), 25–8.

Eckman, T.R., Liberman, R.P., Phipps, C.C. & Blair, K.E. (1990) Teaching medication management skills to schizophrenic patients. *Journal of Clinical Psychology*, **10**(1), 33–8.

Fogel, B.S. (1996) A neuropsychiatric approach to impairment of goal-directed behaviour. *Review of Psychiatry*, **15**, 163–73.

Furlong-Norman, K., Palmer-Erbs, V. & Jonikas, J. (1997) Strengthening psychiatric rehabilitation nursing practice with new information and ideas. *Journal of Psychosocial Nursing*, **35**(1), 35–7.

Gerlach, J. & Peacock, L. (1995) New antipsychotics: The present status. *International Clinical Psychopharmacology*, **10**(Suppl.3), 39–48.

Green, M.F. (1996) What are the functional consequences of neruocognitive deficits in schizophrenia? *American Journal of Psychiatry*, **153**(3), 321–30.

Harding, C. & Zahniser, J. (1994) Empirical correction of seven myths about schizophrenia with implications for treatment. *Acta Psychiatr Scand*, **90**(suppl. 384), 140–46.

Hayes, A. (1995) Psychiatric nursing: What does biology have to do with it? *Archives of Psychiatric Nursing*, **9**(4), 216–24.

Heinssen, R.K. (1996) The cognitive exoskeleton: Environmental interventions in cognitive rehabilitation. In: *Cognitive Rehabilitation and Neuropsychiatric Disorders* (eds P.S. Corrigan & S.C. Yudofsky), pp.395–423. American Psychiatric Press, Washington DC.

Herz, M.I., Glazer, W.M., Mostert, M.A., Sheard, M.A., Szymanski, H.V., Hafez, H., Mirza, M. & Vana, J. (1991) Intermittent vs. maintenance medication in schizophrenia. *Archives of General Psychiatry*, **48**, 333–9.

Hogarty, G. (1993) Prevention of relapse in chronic schizophrenic patients. *Journal of Clinical Psychiatry*, **54**(3, suppl), 18–22.

Hutchinson, D.S. (1996) Promoting wellness in rehabilitation and recovery – A call to action. *Community Support Network News*, **11**(2), 1–3.

Jevne, R. (1993) Enhancing hope in the chronically ill. *Humane Medicine*, **9**(2), 121–30.

Kirkpatrick, H., Landeen, J., Byrne, C., Woodside, H., Pawlick, J. & Bernardo, A. (1995) Hope and Schizophrenia: Clinicians Identify Hope-Instilling Strategies. *Journal of Psychosocial Nursing*, **33**(6), 15–19.

Kirkpatrick, H., Younger, J. & Links, P. (1995) Hospital-based schizophrenia program evaluates its supported housing project. *Leadership*, **4**(2), 27–32.

Kirkpatrick, H., Younger, J., Links, P. & Saunders, P. (1996). Life after years in hospital: What does it hold. *Psychiatric Rehabilitation Journal*, **19**(4), 75–8.

Krch-Cole, E., Lynch, P., Hughes, J. & Nakanishim D. (1997) Bridging the chasm: Incorporating the medically compromised patient into psychiatric practice. *Journal of Psychosocial Nursing*, **35**(5), 28–33.

Lachance, K. & Santos, A. (1995) Modifying the PACT model: Preserving critical elements. *Psychiatric Services*, **46**(6), 601–604.

Landeen, J., Kirkpatrick, H., Woodside, H., Byrne, C., Bernardo, A. & Pawlick, J. (1996) Factors influencing staff hopefulness in working with people with schizophrenia. *Issues in Mental Health Nursing*, **17**(5), 457–67.

Leete, E. (1987) The treatment of schizophrenia: A patient's perspective. *Hospital and Community Psychiatry*, **38**(5), 486–91.

Links, P., Kirkpatrick, H. & Whelton, C. (1994) Psychosocial rehabilitation and the role of psychiatrist. *Psychosocial Rehabilitation Journal*, **18**(1), 121–30.

Littrell, K.H., Herth, K.A. & Hinte, L.E. (1996) The experience of hope in adults with schizophrenia. *Psychiatric Rehabilitation Journal*, **19**(4), 61–5.

Lovejoy, M. (1984) Recovery from schizophrenia: A personal odyssey. *Hospital and Community Psychiatry*, **35**(8), 809–12.

Lowery, B. (1992) Psychiatric nursing in the 1990s & beyond. *Journal of Psychosocial Nursing*, **30**(1), 7–13.

McBride, A. (1990) Psychiatric nursing in the 1990s. *Archives of Psychiatric Nursing*, **4**(1), 21–8.

McFarlane, W.R. (ed.) (1983) *Family treatment in schizophrenia*. Guilford Press, New York.

McGlashan, T.H. (1994) What has become of the psychotherapy of schizophrenia? *Acta Psychiatr Scand*, **90** (Suppl. 384), 147–52.

Miller, J.F. (1992) *Coping with chronic illness: Overcoming powerlessness* 2nd edn. F.A. Davis Co, Philadelphia.

Ministry of Health of Ontario (1993) *Putting people first: The reform of mental health services in Ontario*. Queens Printer for Ontario, Toronto, Ontario.

Ministry of Health of Ontario (1995) *Implementation planning guidelines for mental health reform*. Queens Printer for Ontario, Toronto, Ontario.

Mound, B., Gyulay, R., Khan, P. & Goering, P. (1991) The expanded role of nurse case managers. *Journal of Psychosocial Nursing*, **29**(6), 18–22.

Mueser, K.T. & Gingerich, S. (1994) *Coping with schizophrenia: A guide for family*. New Harbinger Publications, Oakland, CA.

Munich, R.L. & Lang, E. (1993) The boundaries of psychiatric rehabilitation. *Hospital and Community Psychiatry*, **44**(7), 661–5.

O'Connor, F. & Eggert, L. (1994) Psychosocial assessment for treatment planning and evaluation. *Journal of Psychosocial Nursing*, **32**(5), 31–42.

Palmer-Erbs, V. (1996) Psychiatric rehabilitation: A breath of fresh air in a turbulent health-care environment. *Journal of Psychosocial Nursing*, **32**(9), 16–21.

Palmer-Erbs, V. & Anthony, W. (1995) Incorporating psychiatric rehabilitation principles into mental health nursing. *Journal of Psychosocial Nursing*, **33**(3), 36–44.

Pawlick, J., Woodside, H., Landeen, J., Kirkpatrick, H. & Byrne, C. (1997) *Hope and individuals with schizophrenia: A quantitative study*. Manuscript submitted for publication.

Remington, G. (1995) Understanding schizophrenia: The impact of novel anti-psychotics. *Canadian Journal of Psychiatry*, **40**(Suppl. 2), S29–S32.

Seeman, P. (1995) Dopamine receptors and psychosis. *Scientific American Science and Medicine*, **2**(5), 28–37.

Spitzer, M. (1995) Conceptual developments in the neurosciences relevant to psychiatry. *Current Opinion in Psychiatry*, **8**, 317–29.

Starkey, D., Glick, B., O'Donnell, C., Souze, A., Tarantino, S., Godin, P., Tierney, T. & Leadholm, B. (1997) Who's the patient here? In patient psychiatric rehabilitation in a state hospital setting. *Journal of Psychosocial Nursing*, **35**(1), 10–15.

Streicker, S.K., Amdur, M. & Dincin, J. (1986) Educating patients about psychiatric medications: Failure to enhance compliance. *Psychosocial Rehabilitation Journal*, **9**(4), 15–26.

Tanney, B.L. (1992). Mental disorders, psychiatric patients, and suicide. In: *Assessment and prediction of suicide* (eds R. Maris, A. Berman, J. Maltsberger & R. Yugit), pp. 277–320. The Guilford Press, New York.

Velligan, D.I., Mahurin, R.K., True, J.E., Lefton, R.S. & Flores, C.V. (1996) Preliminary evaluation of cognitive adaptation training to compensate for cognitive deficits in schizophrenia. *Psychiatric Services*, **47**(4), 415–17.

Wasylenki, D.A. (1992) Psychotherapy of schizophrenia revisited. *Hospital and Community Psychiatry*, **43**(2), 123–7.

Wilson, J.H. & Hobbs, J. (1995) Therapeutic partnership: A model for clinical practice. *Journal of Psychosocial Nursing*, **33**(2), 27–30.

Woodside, H., Landeen, J., Kirkpatrick, H., Byrne, C., Bernardo, A. & Pawlicki, J. (1994) Hope and schizophrenia: Exploring attitudes of clinicians. *Psychosocial Rehabilitation Journal*, **18** (1), 140–44.

Wyatt, R.J. (1991) Neuroleptic and the natural course of schizophrenia. *Schizophrenia Bulletin*, **17**, 325–51.

3 Social Skills and Social Networks: Making a Place for People with Serious Mental Illness

Catherine H. Stein

There is a growing consensus that mental health services should help people with serious mental illness* maximise their opportunities to live independent and meaningful lives. Yet, limited budgets for social services, shortage of staff, and the constant demand for mental health services make it difficult to implement even the most basic treatment programs. Moreover, many existing programs are structured in ways that perpetuate the segregation of people with mental illness, rather than their integration into the community. The short comings of the public mental health system can overwhelm even the most dedicated mental health professionals.

This chapter describes an action-research project centered around a university-based course on social relationships for people with serious mental illness and college undergraduates. Details of the project are presented to illustrate how community programs can be structured to promote valued social roles and community integration for people with serious mental illness. The university course was based on the premise that not only people with psychiatric disability can benefit from effective communication skills and satisfying social relationships. Using cooperative learning techniques, the course was structured to enhance the social skills and personal relationships of both clients and undergraduates.

Creating social settings: the power of a place

The importance of community integration for people with serious mental illness is evident in recent models of community mental health services for this population in the United States. For example, the Community Support System (CSS) model started in the late 1970s called for a comprehensive system of services that allowed people with serious mental illness to 'meet their needs and develop their potentials without being unnecessarily isolated or excluded from the community' (Turner & Shifren, 1979). In the

---

* A broad definition of serious mental illness is used in this chapter: 'A group of specific disorders which, although varying in cause, course and treatment, share common characteristics and produce long-term adverse effects or significant levels of impairment' (Clinton & Nelson, 1996, p.400).

1980s, psychiatric rehabilitation models emphasised the need for professionals to look beyond psychiatric symptoms to also assist people with mental illness in overcoming the social disadvantages which results from psychiatric disability (Anthony, 1982). Here again, the goal of rehabilitation services for people with serious mental illness is social acceptance and participation in community life. The 'recovery' movement of the late 1980s and 1990s expanded rehabilitation concepts. It argued that removing barriers so that people with psychiatric disability can participate in meaningful social roles in the community is an essential element of 'recovery-orientated' treatment services (Anthony, 1993).

Despite the aims of such service delivery models, many of the community programs offered for people with serious mental illness are provided within the confines of community mental health facilities. Community integration, although an admirable goal, has proven extremely difficult to implement in America over the past 20 years.

In his ecological view of social settings, Kelly (1987a; 1987b) provides some interesting observations about the role of the professional working in the community. In designing community interventions, Kelly contends that professionals can take explicit steps to create a 'social setting' that fosters support and collaboration among participants. The social environment can be structured in such a way as to allow participants to experience meaningful social roles, reciprocity of relationships and allow opportunities for problem solving. For Kelly, a social setting can provide participants with a personal sense of purpose and meaning.

While Kelly's description may initially appear rather abstract, it is not too difficult to think of 'social settings' that can foster such experiences for participants. For example, people who belong to civic and veterans organisations, church groups, and social clubs often engage in problem solving around such things as fund raising and charitable activities. Within such organisations, valued social roles such as president, treasurer, secretary, committee chairperson, are created and filled by members, often on a rotating basis. Members form friendships, as well as giving and receiving help and advice. Participation in these kinds of organisations often provides members with a sense of identity and purpose.

Moreover, Kelly's view assumes that a professional is capable of helping to construct a social setting that supports collaborative relationships among participants. The role of the professional is neither to teach specific skills to individuals nor to try to develop an equal relationship with participants. Rather, the goal is to create with participants a social setting or social environment where the expectations for social interactions are collaborative and personally meaningful. The professional's job is to alter the existing social structure and norms that have helped to keep people separate, isolated, or competitive with one another.

Kelly argues that participation in a newly created social setting can offset an individual's past experience of ineffectiveness. Collaborative social settings generate a shared belief that persons can give and receive support, take action and achieve something meaningful. The concept of 'small wins'

(Weick, 1984) applies to the process of creating a social setting as participants practice defining manageable goals, and recognising incremental steps toward their achievement. Kelly contends that a 'small wins' mindset that develops such a social setting often leads to rituals and celebrations that serve to validate the setting and its participants.

What are the implications of Kelly's approach for creating community programs for people with serious mental illness? His approach helps to articulate basic elements needed to create a social setting that 'makes a place' for people with serious mental illness. If we wish to foster community integration, the creation of the social setting needs to occur in the community, rather than within the confines of a mental health facility. The setting needs to have a diverse set of participants and include people who do not suffer from mental illness along with those who do. The circumstances of the social setting need to alter existing expectations and norms that keep people with serious mental illness socially isolated. To be successful, the social setting needs to foster valued social roles that are accessible to people with serious mental illness and allow them to collaborate with others as equals. The setting must not simply focus on differences or deficits of people with serious mental illness. Rather, the setting must foster appreciation for the similarities between people.

Social network ties: differences and similarities

Researchers have long recognised the importance of social networks for mental health and well-being (Mitchell & Tricket, 1980; Stein, *et al.*, 1992a). Network members such as family, friends, work associates and neighbours can provide individuals with emotional support, advice and assistance. Network ties have been found to be particularly important in helping individuals with serious mental illness remain in the community (Hammer, 1981; Morin & Seidman, 1986). Social network relationships can give an individual with mental illness chances to both give and receive information, help and support. Such social exchanges are seen as basic to community life (Grusky *et al.*, 1985).

Research on social networks finds differences in network characteristics between people with serious mental illness and nonpsychiatric control group members. Studies find that psychiatric patients' networks are characterised by fewer members, a larger proportion of kin, fewer intimate relationships, a greater number of asymmetrical relationships, and are perceived as less supportive than those of nonpsychiatric controls (Pattison, *et al.*, 1975; Sokolovsky, *et al.*, 1978; Tolsdorf, 1976). Network characteristics, such as size, role composition (number of relatives, friends, professionals) and network density (interconnectedness among members), have been associated with length of psychiatric hospitalization (Dozier, *et al.*, 1987; Holmes-Eber & Riger, 1990; Lipton *et al.*, 1981), and type of community treatment program made available to clients (Cutler, *et al.*, 1987).

Research suggests that social skills may play a role in the formation and use of social network ties. Using a college sample, Sarason *et al.* (1985) found that respondents who reported having supportive social networks also were rated as having better social skills by independent judges than respondents with less supportive social networks. Results also showed that respondents low in social support appeared to both themselves and to others to be less likeable and less interpersonally effective than other people.

In a study of psychiatric outpatients, Mitchell (1982) found that patients' problem solving abilities were positively related to the number of intimates in their networks. In other research, social competence was consistently found to have the strongest association with schizophrenic patients' network ties outside of residential facilities (Denoff & Pilkonis, 1987). Findings suggest that enhancing social competence can help individuals take an active role in creating and maintaining supportive social networks.

Social skills training

Since 1980 social skills training has emerged as a major form of intervention for people with serious mental illness. Social skills training programs assume that people with serious mental illness lack the cognitive and interpersonal skills that allow them to effectively interact with others. Such decreased 'social competence' limits an individual's ability to develop and maintain meaningful social relationships and to function effectively in the community. Proponents of social skills training assume that specific elements that enable a person to engage in 'successful' social exchanges can be identified, taught and learned. Social skills training programs also have been applied to nonclinical populations ranging from elementary school children (Spivack, *et al.*, 1976), to college students (Conger & Conger, 1982).

Definitions of social skills vary in their comprehensiveness. For example, early definitions view social skills as the 'skill to elicit social reinforcement from others' (Dorty 1975). More recent definitions describe social skills as 'those interpersonal behaviors needed to maintain independence and community living and to develop and deepen supportive personal relationships' (Liberman, *et al.*, 1986). However, as Wallace, *et al.* (1980) note, all of the conceptual definitions of social skills imply that the goal of training is to allow individuals to increase their level of social competence in a wide variety of interpersonal situations. Yet, training programs typically take place for specified time periods in treatment facilities and involve working in groups comprised of other people with serious mental illness. Role playing is used in skills training programs in an effort to broaden the exposure of program participants to various types of interpersonal situations.

In a typical training session, a patient is asked to role play an interpersonal situation with the 'trainer' (e.g. the mental health professional running the program) or with another patient in the program. The trainer then provides feedback to the patient about his or her performance and invites the patient to engage in another role play to incorporate feedback and improve skills. Modelling or coaching can also be used to help the patient learn particular skills. Typically, the focus of instruction and feedback is on the topological features of patients' interaction such as eye contact, nonverbals, speech duration and intensity. Content-related behaviours such as the degree of compliance, hostility, affection, and appreciation conveyed by the patient in the interaction are also reviewed. Recently, some social skills programs have increased their emphasis on patients' cognitive appraisals of interpersonal situations.

The unparallelled growth in the popularity of social skills training is not difficult to understand. Practically speaking, social skills training programs are relatively cost efficient and easy to administer. Social skills programs typically have a structured curriculum, do not require much training on the part of staff to administer and are run in groups. Conceptually, social skills training is consistent with current views of community treatment for serious mental illness.

The amount of empirical research conducted to evaluate social skills training also adds to its wide spread appeal. The structure and behavioural orientation of skills training lends itself to studies evaluating its efficacy resulting in numerous reviews of research conducted on training programs in the past twenty years (Bellack, *et al.*, 1984; Dion & Anthony, 1987; Wallace, *et al.*, 1980). In their meta-analysis of skills training research, Dilk and Bond (1996) find substantial evidence that social skills training is effective in teaching a variety of social and living skills to people with serious mental illness. Studies indicate that patients can learn interpersonal and assertiveness skills as measured by increases in the acquisition of skills being taught and by reduction in symptoms. These findings have been substantiated by an impressive number of rigorous experimental and quasi-experimental studies.

However, there is little empirical evidence that gains made by patients in social skills programs generalize to their social relationships in the community (Wallace, *et al.*, 1980; Dilk & Bond, 1996). This is particularly important since having patients use their newly acquired ways of relating to others outside of the treatment setting is the prime goal of social skills training. There can be no successful 'rehabilitation' of people with serious mental illness without the generalisation of social skills to everyday living.

Interpersonal situations are richly complex, and role play vignettes do not foster generalisation of social skills. Moreover, social skills programs typically require that patients conduct these scripted role plays with fellow patients in the program, who may not be as adept in interpersonal interactions as people that patients encounter in the community. The structure of many social skills training programs may also unwittingly serve to keep patients segregated in community treatment facilities and isolated from others. Applying social skills training to 'real life' may require planned opportunities for people with serious mental illness to interact with other people and the tailoring of training specifically to clients' network ties.

A closer look at social competence

The concept of social competence is at the heart of our discussion of social skills training and social network ties. As Schlundt and McFall (1985) described, social competence is a value-based judgement concerning the effectiveness of an individual's performance in an interpersonal context. Social competence is a judgement based on a set of behaviours within a social context and not a judgement about an enduring characteristic of the performer. The judge who evaluates the competence of a performance does so on the basis of certain implicit or explicit values about the nature of social interactions. In other words, social competence is a relativistic construct. Social competence is continually developing in the course of a person's life. The requirements for social competence change across the life course. What works for the child in interpersonal relationships does not work for the adult. Similarly, the passage of time within a given relationship impacts judgements of social competence. What creates a new friendship does not necessarily sustain it.

The relativistic nature of social competence has direct implications for working with people with serious mental illness. It suggests that there is no such thing as a 'socially competent' person who can deal effectively in any kind of social interaction. Rather, a person can be judged more or less 'competent' depending on the interpersonal context and our values about what makes an interpersonal exchange 'successful'. In other words, there is no single way to attain social competence. Social competence is not a static goal, but rather a dynamic feature of interpersonal relationships.

In fact, researchers and practitioners in the area of psychiatric rehabilitation tend to overlook evidence that social skills and supportive relationships are important in promoting mental health in general as well as treating mental illness (Durlak, 1983; Gottleib, 1988). For example, there is substantial research to indicate that college undergraduates can benefit from interpersonal skills training (Frosh & Summerfield, 1986) and that supportive network ties play an important role in the mental health of college students (Salzinger, *et al.*, 1988).

Such findings suggest that college undergraduates and people with mental illness might benefit from working together to enhance their own interpersonal skills and strengthen network ties. When undergraduates work with people with serious mental illness, it is typically in the role of nonprofessional helper. In this role, undergraduates generally assist people with serious mental illness in activities of daily living such as providing transportation, or helping with cooking and shopping. Although undergraduates can be effective helpers (Durlak, 1979; McVeigh, *et al.*, 1984), the helper role perpetuates an unequal relationship between undergraduates and clients where clients occupy the subordinate role. There is evidence to suggest that individuals with opportunities to both give and receive help feel better about themselves and others than those who are constantly either giving or receiving assistance. If college undergraduates are to be utilised as a community resource, new roles need to be created that emphasise the ability of both undergraduates and people with mental illness to be helpful and to learn from one another.

It is remarkably easy to consider new roles for people with mental illness and college undergraduates when we consider similarities between the two groups instead of their differences. Meaningful social relationships are important in the lives of most people. Studies suggest that both college undergraduates and people with serious mental illness can benefit from social skills training and supportive social networks. However, the diversity of backgrounds and abilities of undergraduates and people with mental illness may initially make them appear to be unlikely partners for a combined community program.

Cooperative learning and status equalisation techniques

Interestingly, educators have been grappling with similar issues in their search to promote equal classroom participation among students with diverse backgrounds and abilities. Disenchanted with traditional approaches of instruction, educators have developed 'cooperative learning models' that seek to create a classroom environment that fosters active student participation and peer learning. Cooperative learning approaches stress both social and academic development. It is assumed that learning how to work together and function as a member of a team is a valuable educational outcome. Classroom activities are designed to support both experiential and conceptual learning (Johnson, *et al.*, 1981; Slavin, 1990).

Active student participation is basic to cooperative learning approaches. However, research suggests that opportunities for students to participate in the classroom are not inherently equal. Investigators have found that participation in heterogeneous classrooms is often based on 'status characteristics' of the students such as their race, gender, reading or athletic ability (Rosenhotz, 1985). 'High status' students are more likely to participate in classroom discussions, take leadership roles in groups and be perceived as making better contributions to group performance than their 'low status' counterparts. This is typically independent of the relevance of the status characteristic to the classroom activity (Cohen, *et al.*, 1988). For example, the high school star basketball player may be seen as a person whose views are more valued than others, even if the classroom discussion is totally unrelated to basketball.

Intervention strategies designed to modify status effects among students in classroom settings include:

(1) The introduction of 'multiple abilities' expectations to the classroom
(2) The use of norms for equal participation
(3) The teacher as a source of expectations for competence (see Cohen, 1982 for a review).

Multiple abilities interventions involve the introduction of new status characteristics to the classroom that are inconsistent with those that previously differentiated students. For example, a group classroom activity that requires knowledge about people from different ethnic backgrounds to successfully complete, might be used to produce equal-status behaviour among a group of interracial students.

Norms for participation in the classroom can also be explicitly stated to promote equal participation of students in mixed status groups. Equal participation norms are often elaborated into a set of behavioural skills for classroom activities such as guidelines that students 'listen to others' and 'give everyone a chance to talk' (Cohen, 1982). The teacher, as a high status source, can model expectations for student competence that reduce the status advantage of high status students in the classroom.

Cooperative learning situations have been found to improve academic achievement (Johnson & Johnson, 1986; Slavin, 1990) and promote equal participation among diverse students (Cohen, *et al.*, 1988). Studies have also shown that cooperative learning approaches have increased interpersonal attraction and friendships among students (Cohen, *et al.*, 1990).

The university classroom as an innovative setting

What follows is an example of a community intervention for people with mental illness and college undergraduates that capitalises on the university classroom as an innovative social setting. The intervention project was developed at a midwestern university in United States, and has recently been implemented at an urban university in Australia. In each case, the goal of the project was to create a social setting that provided opportunities for both people with serious mental illness and college undergraduates to experience valued social roles, supportive others, and to enhance their interpersonal skills. Each project consisted of a university course for undergraduates and people with serious mental illness and evaluation research designed to examine its efficacy. Details of the structure and outcomes of the original project will be presented. Implementation of the course in Australia will then be discussed to illustrate ways that the project can be adapted to fit local needs and resources.

The context for the original project was a one semester (15 week) practicum course on social relationships offered at a midwestern university to 14 people with serious mental illness and 14 college undergraduates. The course combined social network techniques and social skills concepts to help both undergraduates and mental health centre clients enhance their interpersonal skills and social ties. Status equalisation techniques were used to promote collaboration between participants in the classroom. The practicum course was specifically structured to facilitate direct application of knowledge about social skills in the community. To evaluate the efficacy of the practicum course, the composition of participants' social networks, attitudes towards people with mental illness, interpersonal self-efficacy and social skills were assessed at two times of measurement and compared with a non-practicum control group.

Network connections practicum

A total of 14 clients receiving services at a community mental health center in Wood County, Ohio and 14 upper-level undergraduates attending Bowling Green State University (BGSU), a midwestern university, enrolled in the 15 week practicum course offered by the psychology department. Thirty-one undergraduates and 30 interested clients completed pre-registration interviews for the practicum. A total of 28 people (14 undergraduates and 14 clients) participated in the practicum and 28 people (14 undergraduates and 14 clients) served in the non-practicum control group. Procedures for enrolment for university courses did not permit random assignment of participants to practicum and control groups. Selection for the practicum or control group was based on the interest and time availability of applicants. Participants in the non-practicum control group completed interview and observational assessments at time intervals identical to the practicum participants, but did not complete the practicum course.

There were eight men and six women who were clients at the mental health centre who enrolled in the practicum course. Clients in the practicum, referred to in the course as 'community students', were an average of 35 years old (SD = 9.1). The majority of clients (64%) were single, and the rest were separated or divorced. About half of the clients had not completed high school. Of these practicum clients, over half had a psychiatric diagnosis of schizophrenia or schizoaffective disorder. The rest were diagnosed with bipolar disorder or a personality disorder. Over 80% of these individuals had been hospitalised at least once, and about 30% had been hospitalised in the preceding year. The majority of practicum clients (73%) reported being on psychiatric medication. Over 60% of practicum clients were not employed and 36% reported part-time employment.

All of the 14 undergraduates that enrolled in the course were women and were an average age of 21 years (SD = 1.1). A majority of undergraduates in the practicum, referred to in the course as 'BG students', were psychology majors (71%) in their junior and senior years of college (94%). Most undergraduates in the practicum were single (93%), 57% held part-time employment and 36% were not working. Data suggest that clients and undergraduates in the practicum did not significantly differ from their control group counterparts on demographic characteristics, hospitalisation history, reliance on psychiatric medication or psychiatric diagnosis.

Course structure and requirements
The practicum course met for 90 minutes twice a week for the 15 week semester. Clients and undergraduates in the practicum were paired as 'student partners' by having participants draw numbers from a paper bag. 'Student teams' consisting of four people (two pairs of student partners) were also randomly decided. Partners or teams were required to meet in the community for approximately three hours each week to complete homework assignments and to practise new material. Other requirements

for the course included keeping a class notebook to be evaluated during the semester and writing a final class paper.

A major aim of the practicum was to create a social environment that encouraged student collaboration and an appreciation of individual differences. Consistent with the idea of multiple abilities and equal student participation in the cooperative learning literature, the instructor emphasised that 'when it comes to social relationships, we are all "experts" by virtue of our experiences in the world' and that the practicum was set up so that 'everybody in the class has something to teach and something to learn'. The instructor emphasised the course goals of learning and applying class material to students' own personal relationships.

A typical class session began with the instructor presenting material about some aspect of social skills or social relationships. To facilitate note taking among both community and BG students, handouts were provided that required students to complete information about the topic being presented by the instructor. Students then were invited to work with their partners or in teams on group exercises designed to illustrate that day's topic. At the end of the class session, students were given homework assignments designed to help them practise material with their partners or apply skills to their network relationships. Alternatively, in some class sessions, students were invited to form larger groups and complete a brief class reading (read aloud by group members). Students then discussed their reactions to the reading and shared their experiences conducting homework assignments in the community.

The content of the course included material and techniques used in social skills training. Skills training materials were adapted from a model by Wallace, *et al.* (1980) and Liberman, *et al.* (1989) that classified interpersonal behaviours into receiving, processing and sending skills. Students in the course were asked to do role plays and provide feedback to classmates in an effort to learn and practice social skills.

However, course topics went beyond skills training to incorporate theory and research on social networks and personal relationships into the practicum. Topics such as self-disclosure, loneliness, social support, family ties, friendship networks and holiday stress were presented and applied in the practicum course. Both community and BG students appeared enthusiastic about studying material that had direct implications for their views about themselves and others. A fuller description of topics and source material can be found elsewhere (Stein, *et al.*, 1992c).

Throughout the semester, explicit expectations about the valued nature of social exchanges in the practicum were reinforced by the structure of classroom activities, small group discussions and community assignments. Instructional practices stressed norms for equal participation among students and recognised the importance of multiple abilities for successful completion of course material. Such classroom elements were thought to assist in creating a learning environment that personalised knowledge, stressed common inquiry and gave value to the ideas and contributions of participants.

Unlike many traditional university classroom experiences, a sense of cohesion and 'course identity' seemed to develop in the practicum course. In the classroom, informal 'celebrations' took place over time as individual events and achievements were recognised. Spontaneously celebrated in class were such accomplishments as good grades on 'tough' exams in other courses, temperamental automobiles that had successfully undergone repair, as well as birthdays, wedding engagements and anniversaries. In small group discussions, students often made 'progress reports' on their personal goals and group members applauded one another on their 'small wins'. A final class dinner, arranged by student volunteers, celebrated the successful completion of the course.

Assessing practicum outcomes

As previously mentioned, we obtained an equal number of clients and undergraduates to serve as a non-practicum control group in our research evaluation of the practicum project. Participants in both the practicum and control groups completed detailed interviews and observational assessments of social skills before and after the 15 week practicum. Results of the evaluation research are detailed elsewhere (Stein, *et al.*, 1992b). What follows is a discussion of the relationship between some of the major findings of the evaluation and the experience of the practicum as a social setting.

Positive change in social skills
Similar to other social skills programs, results of our evaluation showed positive changes in social skills for clients participating in the practicum relative to clients in the non-practicum control group. Before and after the 15 week practicum, participants in practicum and control conditions were asked to role play 6 standardised interpersonal situations adapted from the Behavioral Assertiveness Test – Revised (BAT-R) (Eisler, *et al.*, 1975), for a total of 12 role play situations across the two times of measurement. Performances were videotaped and later scored using a coding system described in Eisler, *et al.* (1975).

In general, results indicated that clients in the practicum exhibited more positive skills change over the 15 week period in their nonverbal behaviour, overall interpersonal assertiveness, and skills behaviours than did clients in the control condition. Undergraduates in the practicum also displayed more positive change in overall interpersonal assertiveness and skills behaviours than did their control group counterparts, although gains were generally less substantial than those made by clients.

Results of our evaluation are consistent with previous studies that conclude that specific social behaviours can be taught and successfully learned by people with serious mental illness. Unlike other studies, our data suggest that skills training can be successfully accomplished in a community setting working in groups with people not diagnosed with a serious mental illness. Our findings also indicate that positive changes in participants' social skills can be achieved using a broader and more varied curriculum than is typical for skills training programs with this population.

Perceptions of changes in social relationships

In the post-practicum assessment, practicum and control group participants were asked several global questions about their views regarding social skills and personal relationships. Participants in the practicum and control group conditions had similar views about the capacity of people in general to improve their skills and relationships. However, when asked about their own capacities, both clients and undergraduates in the practicum generally reported feeling significantly more capable of improving their skills and relationships than did their control group counterparts. Clients and undergraduates in the practicum saw themselves as equally capable of improving their own skills and relationships. Both clients and undergraduates in the practicum reported putting significantly more effort into their social relationships and reported greater improvement in their relationships than did those in the control group.

Interestingly, results do more than suggest that practicum participants had more positive perceptions of their social relationships than did those who had not been in the course. Findings suggest that undergraduates and clients did not significantly differ from one another in their perceptions of their capacity to improve their relationships, the effort they put into their relationships, and the amount of improvement they perceived in their relationships at the end of the practicum. In other words, despite the potential differences in their backgrounds, past interpersonal experiences or feelings of social effectiveness, clients and undergraduates were similar in their views of the overall impact of the course on their social relationships.

Interpersonal self-efficacy

As a part of the evaluation, practicum and control participants' perceptions of interpersonal self-efficacy were assessed using the Interpersonal Self-efficacy Scale (ISE) by Vitkus & Horowitz (1987). This 15 item questionnaire is designed to tap feelings of self-efficacy with respect to solving interpersonal problems. Results of pre- and post-practicum assessments reveal no significant changes in reports of interpersonal self-efficacy for members of the control group.

However, compared with their control group counterparts, clients in the practicum reported feeling more effective in their interpersonal relations after completing the course. Undergraduates in the practicum reported feeling less interpersonally effective after the course, relative to undergraduates in the control group.

How can we understand the differing effect of the practicum on undergraduates' and clients' perceptions of their interpersonal self-efficacy? Clients in the practicum had the opportunity to learn about social relationships and practice class material with people who listen and have few major difficulties in communicating. It appears that these opportunities for social interaction positively impacted clients' perceptions of their own interpersonal effectiveness. In other words, it seems that clients' experiences of successfully interacting with 'normal' college students in a college classroom helped them to feel more positively about their own interpersonal abilities.

In contrast, it is likely that undergraduates in the practicum had little previous exposure to people with whom they could not always make themselves understood. Initial self ratings of undergraduates' interpersonal effectiveness were high and experiences interacting with clients were sometimes challenging. It appears that class material and social interactions with people different than themselves helped undergraduates to recalibrate overall estimates of their interpersonal effectiveness.

Negative consequences of interconnected social networks

Research suggests that the social networks of adults with serious mental illness are smaller than those of adults who do not suffer from mental illness (Morin & Seidman, 1986; Tolsdorf, 1976). Indeed, results indicate that clients in both the practicum and control group conditions reported significantly smaller total and helping networks on average than did undergraduates in the two conditions. Undergraduates also averaged larger total and helping friend network sectors, more family helpers, and fewer professionals in their networks than did clients as a group. Interestingly, our data suggest that clients and undergraduates did not significantly differ in the overall interconnectedness of their networks (known as network density). Although clients networks were generally smaller, both clients and undergraduates generally had fairly dense networks, where the people in their networks were well acquainted with one another.

Unlike traditional university courses, what happened to students outside of class was uniquely relevant to what was happening in the classroom. The practicum highlighted some of the negative consequences of dense networks when coping with a mental illness. For example, a number of community students lived in the same subsidised housing complex, one which has a high concentration of mental health centre clients. In the course of the semester, a community student who lived in the housing complex began to experience a manic episode and was hospitalised.

Two other community students who lived in the same housing complex spoke privately with the instructor about the student's hospitalisation day after it happened. The incident had prompted the two students to question their own ability to stay out of the hospital. For both of these community students, the dates of their own hospitalisations were like personal 'milestones'. Similar to anniversaries, these individuals marked the time since their last hospitalisation as symbolic of their current degree of mental health. Both community students felt that they had made great strides since their last hospitalisation, yet their distress and identification with the hospitalised student was very strong.

In this example, the segregation of people with serious mental illness in subsidised housing had created a high degree of 'social interconnectedness' among members in the housing complex. Many of these residents interacted with one another in multiple roles such as clients at the mental health centre, participants in partial hospitalisation groups, people with the same case manager and so on. One individual in the network experiencing a crisis caused a substantial amount of stress to other network members.

This type of 'network crisis' has been thought of as a by-product of dense social networks and applies equally to people who are not experiencing a serious mental illness. Consider the impact on our own lives when a member of our network, such as a friend or family member, is diagnosed with cancer, has a heart attack or goes through a divorce. The impact of such an event is often substantial, compelling us to evaluate our own lives. Yet, we are not typically forced by circumstances to associate exclusively with individuals at high risk for heart attacks, cancer or divorce. People with mental illness who are segregated in the community do not typically have the same degree of choice about their social connections.

The community student who was in crisis spent a week in the hospital and contacted the instructor the day of his discharge to turn in previous class assignments. He returned to class the following day and successfully completed the course. When others in the practicum learned that the student was in the hospital, undergraduate students as well as community students were confronted with the sense of unpredictability that accompanies mental illness. The human context in which mental illness occurs became salient as undergraduates realised that some of their classmates, people with whom they had shared many things, were coping with problems of a magnitude beyond most of their experiences.

Attitudes to mental illness

To examine the possible impact of the practicum on participants' attitudes to mental illness, practicum and control group members were asked to complete the Social Response Questionnaire (SRQ) (Beiser, *et al.*, 1987) before and after the practicum. The SRQ is a measure of informal labelling of persons with mental illness and consists of 17 adjective descriptors. Respondents are asked to rate the degree to which each adjective described 'a person suffering from mental illness'. On a separate form, participants in practicum and control conditions were also asked to use the same set of adjective descriptors to rate themselves.

Clients in the practicum did not significantly differ from their control group counterparts in their overall attitudes about people with serious mental illness, nor did their views significantly change across time. However, compared with all other groups, undergraduates in the practicum reported a significant decrease in negative feelings about people with mental illness across the 15 week semester. Clients in the practicum reported a significant decrease in negative descriptors of themselves relative to the other groups. Self descriptor ratings for individuals in all other conditions did not significantly change across time. These results suggest that the practicum had a positive impact on undergraduates' overall views of people with serious mental illness and had a positive impact on clients' views of themselves.

Given that the practicum focused exclusively on personal relationships and interpersonal skills, these results may seem surprising. The course contained no objective material on mental illness, no information about psychiatric etiology, symptoms or treatment practices. Yet, it appears that the structure of the course allowed for shared personal experiences that provided powerful, experiential knowledge of issues faced by people suffering from serious mental illness.

Material presented in class was first applied in relationships with student partners and classmates. The development of relationships between student partners often served to dispel stereotypes about what 'people with mental illness' are like. For example, Susan is a 20 year old undergraduate student. In her final paper, Susan writes about Eric, her community student partner:

> 'Eric has taught me to enjoy life and to never take anything for granted. He has shown me how to gain a better appreciation for the little things in life. During every class meeting and in the community, Eric gave me his undivided attention, regardless. I feel I taught Eric how to laugh a little more and to not take everything so seriously.'

Eric is a 31 year old community student who suffers from schizophrenia. Here is his view of Susan:

> 'On meeting my partner in class, I was mostly afraid of being stereotyped, and in doing so, I was probably stereotyping her ... I have learned that the qualities my partner has – such as decisiveness and directness – are valuable assets in communication, and are things I can work towards – where before I have always tried to "work around" not having these. I don't know if my partner has learned anything from me, but it was encouraging that she was happy with our match-up.'

In her final paper for the course, 21 year old Mary Jo writes about her views regarding mental illness:

> 'When the subject of mental health comes up with my roommates, I find myself explaining the completely human aspects of people dealing with mental disorders and how these people are no different than us. They only have a different set of pressures.'

News from Australia: collaborative education in mental health

The practicum project has recently been undertaken by Michael Clinton, Sioban Nelson and their associates at Queensland University of Technology (QUT) in Brisbane, Australia. Known as *Collaborative Education in*

Mental Health, the practicum course was offered by the School of Nursing to 18 senior undergraduate students and 18 people with serious mental illness. The adaptation of the project for nursing students is particularly important as psychiatric nurses typically play a major role in delivering services to people with serious mental illness in Australia.

The Australian version of the practicum course consisted of 90 minute class sessions that met once a week for a total of 14 weeks. The course is described as an experiential learning program structured to assist participants in enhancing their communication skills. The structure of the QUT course is similar to the original practicum, using cooperative education techniques to present course material, experiential exercises to facilitate learning in the classroom, and structured homework assignments to help further integrate learning in the community.

The content of the collaborative education course has been adapted to focus on core communication skills such as empathy, active listening, assertiveness, individual qualities such as confidence, and strategies for personal change. Since there is no single 'curriculum' dictated for the practicum course, the focus of the course can be tailored to reflect the expertise of the instructors and their assessment of the educational needs of their students.

Preliminary results evaluating the collaborative education course are very encouraging. Clinton and Nelson report that feedback on the course has been universally positive and participants have recommended that it be undertaken by all senior undergraduate students. Preliminary data monitoring practicum participants' views of the group process indicate that participants gave positive ratings of their ability to get along with other group members, the usefulness of the sessions, and group cohesiveness and supportiveness. Community students and QUT undergraduates did not significantly differ in their overall ratings of these elements of the educational experience.

In written critiques of the collaborative education course, participants expressed how the course had helped them deepen their social network relationships and rethink aspects of their self-esteem. Community and undergraduate students wrote moving personal accounts of their experiences in the course. Undergraduate students described how their attitudes about people with mental illness had changed as a result of getting to know people with serious mental illness. Community students discussed how it felt to overcome fears about being stigmatised. Both community and undergraduate students wrote about how the course had challenged them to make changes in their lives.

Final thoughts

Our own experiences and preliminary findings from Australia suggest the usefulness of the university as a community resource for people with serious mental illness. The chance for people with serious mental illness to assume the valued social role of 'student' and the opportunity to interact with others in the community as equal participants appear to be key elements in the success of the program. All participants had a clear understanding of course expectations and the tasks that comprised the student role and patterned their behaviour accordingly. Moreover, many clients in the practicum demonstrated a deep sense of pride in their student status in the university classroom that undergraduates and faculty often take for granted.

For undergraduates, the course promoted an experiential knowledge and understanding of mental illness, quite distinct from that presented in most traditional college courses on 'abnormal behavior'. Undergraduates in the practicum learned about issues faced by people with psychiatric disabilities not from a textbook, but in the context of personal interactions with men and women who must daily cope with such problems in living. The practicum provided opportunities for people with mental illness and college undergraduates to share their common experiences and place their own life concerns in a larger developmental context. The practicum experience also highlighted some of the negative aspects of social connectedness in coping with mental illness as participants witnessed the unpredictability of mental illness in the lives of classmates. The practicum resulted in powerful lessons about mental illness learned in a context of personal relationships.

The practicum project also underscores the importance of social context in community interventions. There are an increasing number of programs for people with psychiatric disabilities that focus on social skills training. However, most programs are offered exclusively to people with mental illness in either in-patient or outpatient settings. The practicum course would have been fundamentally different had it been offered to only mental health center clients or had college undergraduates been invited to the mental health center to attend the practicum. We believe that the role of student in a legitimate student setting strongly influenced the behaviours of practicum members. We hope that our experiences stimulate further thinking about the ways that mental health professionals can foster meaningful social settings that support community integration for people with serious mental illness.

References

Anthony, W. (1982) Explaining 'psychiatric rehabilitation' by an analogy to 'physical rehabilitation'. *Psychosocial Rehabilitation Journal*, 5, 61–5.

Anthony, W. (1993) Recovery from mental illness: The guiding vision of the mental health service system in the 1990s. *Psychosocial Rehabilitation Journal*, 4, 11–24.

Beiser, M., Waxler-Morrison, N., Iacono, W.G., Lin, T., Fleming A.E. & Husted, J. (1987) A measure of the 'sick' label in psychiatric disorder and physical illness. *Social Science Medicine*, 25, 251–61.

Bellack, A.S., Turner, S.M., Hersen, M. & Luber, R.F. (1984) An evaluation of the efficacy of social skills training for chronic schizophrenic patients. *Hospital and Community Psychiatry*, 35, 1023–8.

Clinton, M. & Nelson, S. (1996) *Mental Health and Nursing Practice*. Prentice Hall, Sydney.

Cohen, E.G. (1982) Expectation states and interracial interaction in school settings. *Annual Review of Sociology*, **8**, 209–35.

Cohen, E G., Lotan, R. & Catanzarite, L. (1988) Can expectations for competence be altered in the classroom? In: *Status Generalization: New theory and research* (eds M. Webster & M. Foschi), pp. 29–54. Stanford University Press, Stanford CA.

Cohen, E., Lotan, R. & Catanzarite, L. (1990) Treating status problems in cooperative classrooms. In: *Cooperative learning: Theory and research* (ed. S. Sharan), pp. 203–30). Longman, New York.

Conger J.C. & Conger, A.J. (1982) Components of heterosocial competence. In: *Social skills training* (eds J.P. Curran & P.M. Monti). Guilford Press, New York.

Cutler, D.L., Tatum, E. & Shore, J. H. (1987) A comparison of schizophrenic patients in different community support treatment approaches. *Community Mental Health Journal*, **23**, 103–13.

Denoff, M.S. & Pilkonis, P.A. (1987) The social network of the schizophrenic: Patient and residential determinants. *Journal of Community Psychology*, **15**, 228–44.

Dilk, M.N. & Bond, G. R. (1996) Meta-analytic evaluation of skills training research for individuals with severe mental illness. *Journal of Consulting and Clinical Psychology*, **64**, 1337–46.

Dion, G.L. & Anthony, W.A. (1987) Research in psychiatric rehabilitation: A review of experimental and quasi-experimental studies. *Rehabilitation Counseling Bulletin*, **30**, 177–82.

Dorty, D.W. (1975) Role playing and incentives in the modification of the social interaction of chronic psychiatric patients. *Journal of Consulting and Clinical Psychology*, **43**, 676–82.

Dozier, M., Harris, M. & Bergman, H. (1987) Social network density and rehospitalization among young adult patients. *Hospital and Community Psychiatry*, **38**, 61–4.

Durlak, J.A. (1979) Comparative effectiveness of paraprofessional and professional helpers. *Psychological Bulletin*, **86**, 80–92.

Durlak, J.A. (1983) Social problem-solving as a primary prevention strategy. In: *Prevention psychology: Theory, research and practice* (eds R.D. Felner, L.A. Jason, J.N. Moritsugu & S.S. Farber). Pergamon Press, New York.

Eisler, R.M., Hersen, M., Miller, P.M. & Blanchard, J.P. (1975) Situational determinants of assertive behaviors. *Journal of Consulting and Clinical Psychology*, **43**, 330–40.

Frosh, S. & Summerfield, A.B. (1986) Social skills training with adults. In: *Handbook of social skills training* (eds C.R. Hollin & P. Trower). Pergamon Press, New York.

Gottlieb, B.H. (1988) *Marshalling social support: Formats, processes and effects*. Sage, Beverly Hills, CA.

Grusky, O., Tierney, K., Manderscheid, R.W. & Grusky, D.B. (1985) Social bonding and community adjustment of chronically mentally ill adults. *Journal of Health and Social Behavior*, **26**, 49–63.

Hammer, M. (1981) Social supports, social networks and schizophrenia. *Schizophrenia Bulletin*, **7**, 45–58.

Holmes-Eber, P. & Riger, S. (1990) Hospitalization and the composition of mental patients' social networks. *Schizophrenia Bulletin*, **16**, 157–64.

Johnson, D.W., Maruyama, G., Johnson, R., Nelson, D. & Skon, L. (1981) Effects of cooperative, competitive and individualistic goal structures on achievement: A meta-analysis. *Psychological Bulletin*, **89**, 47–62.

Johnson, D.W. & Johnson, R.T. (1986) *Learning together and alone*, 2nd edn. Prentice-Hall, Englewood Cliffs, NJ.

Kelly, J.G. (1987a) Beyond prevention techniques: Generating social settings for a publics health. *The Tenth Erich Lindemann Memorial Lecture*, Boston, Mass. April 24, 1987.

Kelly, J.G. (1987b). An ecological paradigm: Defining mental health consultation as a preventive service. In: *The Ecology of Prevention: Illustrating Mental Health Consultation* (eds J.G. Kelly & R.E. Hess). The Haworth Press, New York.

Liberman, R.P., Mueser, K.T., Wallace, C.J., Jacobs, H.E., Eckman, T. & Massel, H.K. (1986) Training skills in the psychiatrically disabled: Learning coping and competence. *Schizophrenia Bulletin*, **12**, 631–47.

Liberman, R.P., DeRisi, W.J. & Mueser, K.T. (1989) *Social skills training for psychiatric patients*. Pergamon Press, New York.

Lipton, F.R., Cohen, C.I., Fischer, E. & Katz, S.E. (1981) Schizophrenia: A network crisis. *Schizophrenia Bulletin*, **7**, 144–51.

McVeigh, J.S., Davidson, W.S. & Redner, R. (1984) The long-term impact of nonprofessional service experience on college students. *American Journal of Community Psychology*, **12**, 725–29.

Mitchell, R. (1982) Social networks and psychiatric clients: The personal and environmental context. *American Journal of Community Psychology*, **10**, 387–401.

Mitchell, R.E. & Tricket, E.J. (1980) Task force report: Social networks as mediators of social support. *Community Mental Health Journal*, **16**, 27–44.

Morin, R.C. & Seidman, E. (1986) A social network approach and the revolving door patient. *Schizophrenia Bulletin*, **12**, 262–73.

Pattison, E.M., DeFrancisco, D., Frazer, H., Wood, P.E. & Crowder, J. (1975) A psychosocial kinship model for family therapy. *American Journal of Psychiatry*, **132**, 1246–51.

Rosenhotz, S.J. (1985) Modifying status expectations in the traditional classroom. In: *Status, rewards and influence: How expectations organize behavior* (eds J. Berger & M. Zeldtich), pp. 445–70. Jossey-Bass, San Francisco.

Salzinger, S., Antrobus, J. & Hammer, M. (1988) The social networks of children, adolescents and college students. Lawrence Erbaum, New York.

Sarason, B.R., Sarason, I.G., Hacker, T.A. & Basham, R.B. (1985) Concominants of social support: Social skills, physical attractiveness and gender. *Journal of Personality and Social Psychology*, **49**, 469–80.

Schlundt, D.G. & McFall, R.M. (1985) New directions in the assessment of social competence and social skills. In: *Handbook of social skills training and research* (eds L. L'Abate and M.A. Milan), p. 22–49. Wiley, New York.

Slavin, R.E. (1990) *Cooperative learning theory: Theory, research and practice*. Prentice-Hall, Englewood Cliffs, NJ.

Sokolovsky, J., Cohen, C., Berger, D. & Geiger, J. (1978) Personal networks of ex-mental patients in a Manhattan hotel. *Human Organization*, **37**, 5–15.

Spivack, G., Platt, J.J. & Shure, M.B. (1976) *The problem-solving approach to adjustment*. Jossey-Bass, San Francisco.

Stein, C.H., Bush, E.G., Ross, R.R. & Ward, M. (1992a) Mine, yours and ours: A configural analysis of the networks of married couples in relation to marital satisfaction and individual well-being. *Journal of Social and Personal Relationships*, **9**, 365–83.

Stein, C.H., Cislo, D.A. & Ward, M. (1992b) Collaboration in the college classroom: Evaluation of a social network and social skills program for undergraduates and people with serious mental illness. *Psychosocial Rehabilitation Journal*, **18**, 13–33.

Stein, C.H., Ward, M. & Cislo, D.A. (1992c) The power of a place: Opening the college classroom to people with serious mental illness. *American Journal of Community Psychology*, **20**, 523–47.

Tolsdorf, C.C. (1976) Social networks, support, and coping: An exploratory study. *Family Process*, **15**, 407–18.

Turner, J.E. & Shifren, I. (1979) Community support systems: How comprehensive? *New Directions for Mental Health Services*, **2**, 1–23.

Vitkus, J & Horowitz, L.M. (1987) Poor social performance of lonely people: Lacking a skill or adopting a role? *Journal of Personality and Social Psychology*, **52**, 1266–73.

Wallace, C.J., Nelson, C.J., Liberman, R.P., Altchison, R.A., Lukoff, D., Elder, J.P. & Ferris, C. (1980) A review and critique of social skills training with schizophrenic patients. *Schizophrenia Bulletin*, **6**, 42–63.

Weick, K.E. (1984) Small wins: Redefining the scale of social problems. *American Psychologist*, **39**, 40–49.

4 The Therapeutic Alliance

Sandra Speedy

Introduction

A sense of continuing crisis permeates mental health care. In Australia, this crisis can be attributed to a range of factors, not the least being problems of recruitment and retention and the inadequate educational preparation of professional staff for the therapeutic role. There has long been a trend for psychiatrists and other mental health professionals, including nurses, to abandon the public sector and the treatment of patients with serious mental illness, thus creating a serious service gap. This gap is demonstrated in one study which found that 77% of mentally ill patients are in private care: 55% of these are diagnosed with neuroses or personality disorders, while 26% are diagnosed as psychotic (Andrews, 1989). The McKay Report (1996), in reviewing usage of psychiatric services, acknowledged that half of all people with severe mental illness (approximately 250 000 Australians), continue to have inadequate or no access to treatment services. Unfortunately, this state of affairs is not specific to Australia (see Chapters 5, 6).

Furthermore, this situation has contributed to the historical neglect and continuing stigmatisation of the mentally ill, and outmoded ideas for their care. For carers of the mentally ill, this neglect and stigmatisation has led to substandard education, lack of work satisfaction and unease in dealing with those in need of care. It can be argued that there is a strong connection between sub-standard care, communication difficulties and work satisfaction, impacting on the quality of the therapeutic alliance for patient and nurse. Under these conditions mental health professionals cannot develop meaningful relationships with patients in public or private sector mental health, an inequitable situation for people with a mental illness.

This chapter examines the nurse's therapeutic role and its underpinnings. It also explores the knowledge that is crucial to an understanding of the self and others. This knowledge includes the social construction of mental illness, discourses, the role of power and language, and features of the therapeutic relationship. The chapter then provides an example from psychiatric/mental health practice to demonstrate the contrasting perspectives of nurse and patient. Finally, it concludes with a brief examination of the context of mental health care delivery, including the role of consumers, and the questions these issues raise for practising nurses, educators, managers, and researchers.

The therapeutic alliance

Factors such as the structural, political, social and economic context of mental health care play a major role in the causation, development and continuation of mental illness. While this assertion is not intended to rule out biological and psychological causes, as Hopton (1997, p. 492) suggests, 'mental health nursing can never develop truly liberating approaches to care unless it widens its focus from purely interpersonal relationships and addresses historical, structural and ideological influences on both mental health services and the causation of mental distress'. Nevertheless, the therapeutic alliance developed between carers and their patients is fundamental to effective practice. It is assumed that appropriate caring for the mentally ill cannot occur in the absence of a therapeutic alliance or relationship. While the terms 'therapeutic alliance' and 'therapeutic relationship' convey a similar meaning, the former also includes an understanding of the meaning given *by the patient*, so that the nurse or carer understands what makes particular patient's behaviour seem reasonable given their definition of the situation. Without that alliance, nurses who care for the mentally ill have a custodial role. This custodial model of care is now entirely outmoded and inappropriate and inappropriate for mental health nurses (Hall, 1996).

The absence of a therapeutic alliance reduces mental health professionals to an unsatisfying and limited care-taking role that constrains their effective involvement in the lives of their patients. Mental health professionals thus need to reflect on their capacity for developing and sustaining, through their practice, therapeutic alliances with their patients. As a beginning, this means the practitioner examining the reasons for being in this nursing specialisation. Are we here because we are intent on playing 'rescuer', 'persecutor' or even 'victim'? What are our real motives? To further facilitate the development of therapeutic alliances we must ask: what meaning does the experience of mental illness have for the patient? What is going on in the patient's world? It may not be what we, as nurses, think is going on, or what our imposed meaning might be.

Because we all have idiosyncratic histories which determine our interpretation of the world, we potentially share, with each other and our patients, worlds of cooperation, collision, confusion and conflict. It would be rare indeed if we could accurately predict the patient's meaning and understanding of the world without considerable effort. To be effective however, we have to understand where patients are 'coming from', with an appreciation of the unique contextual factors operating in their lives.

This is the basic premise on which this chapter rests: that knowledge can provide the basis for insight into ourselves, our feelings, our thoughts, and our values. We must look at ourselves, explore our feelings, our thoughts and our actions. It must be acknowledged that knowledge itself is insufficient; openness to exploration and insights are also fundamental. Can we ever have therapeutic alliances with others when we do not know who we are?

Knowledge foundations

There is a range of theoretical knowledge that can be used to provide the foundation for understanding ourselves, as nurses and therapists, and our patients who are experiencing mental ill health.

Social construction of mental health and ill-health

Discourse analysis is a technique that has been used to demonstrate the social construction of mental illness by questioning the 'truths inherent in the dominant medical discourse' (Eade & Bradshaw, 1995, p. 61). Such analysis is usually followed by reconstruction of a more relevant and meaningful discourse to those who are providing the critical analysis. By describing and giving meaning to events, we create a reality. Obviously the dominant discourse will create this reality because by definition, it has constructed it.

In an effort to create alternative understandings of nursing and the settings in which nurses undertake their roles, some authors have focused on the construction of nursing from ideological, discourse and representational perspectives (Delacour, 1991; Delacour & Short, 1992). These authors suggest that psychiatric nurses explore their values, attitudes, beliefs, and ways of perceiving by deconstructing their social worlds (and those of their patients) and reconstructing them. This process involves examining the role that dominant discourses play in their lives; that is, how language is used to construct reality. They also suggest that because language is dominated by paternalism, the reality created is paternalistic. Meaning and value are expressed through language, and created by language. In addition, language is a version of meaning, and meaning is always political. The language of psychiatry (from which mental health nurses gain much of their knowledge and clinical experience) is medical, authoritative, male-identified and powerful. It is used to control and regulate women and men in ways that are required for social acceptability in our society. The history of psychiatric treatment modes is replete with illustrations that demonstrate how medical discourse legitimises political authority, maintains the status quo and constrains behaviour, attitudes and beliefs within defined, acceptable sex roles. This is achieved by the diagnostic process, the assertion of specific 'women's diseases', and the documented gendered discourse of madness that history provides. Diagnosis is a social act, occurring within a sociocultural context, and at a particular historical moment (Hall, 1996; Delacour & Short, 1992). As such, it is a social barometer, authoritatively and powerfully indicating the acceptability or otherwise of behaviours. As Sontag (1990) notes:

> 'Nothing is more punitive than to give a disease a meaning – that meaning being invariably a moralistic one'.

> (Sontag, 1990, p. 58)

The fact that mental health and illness is socially constructed has been the focus of a great deal of literature and research (see, for example, Chesler, 1972; Pugliesi, 1992; Horsfall, 1994; Russell, 1995; Hazelton, 1993, 1995). Various authors point out that definitions of illness vary over time, and that factors other than symptomatology must be taken into account. For example, Hazelton (1995) discerns a range of constructions of people with mental illness by examining Australian mental health policy discourse and concludes that there is a competing version of 'rights discourse'. Russell (1995) and Horsfall (1994) object to the overt sexism rampant in the psychiatry literature, suggesting that the biomedical model, with its 'scientific' approach, causes problems for women by its moral guardianship. Pugliesi (1992), in examining feminist scholarship in mental health, notes that conceptions of mental health and insanity are fundamentally gendered, which builds on the now classic work of Broverman, *et. al.* (1970).

Since its use reflects power, language is a primary factor. The language used by nurses can be oppressive or emancipating to recipients; unfortunately, care provided for the mentally ill has often been characterised by the former. In studies on nurses' language, it has been noted that various types of power have been used, including overt, persuasive, agenda controlling, and power that is couched in terms of endearment (Hewison, 1995).

It is important to acknowledge the reality that there is a power differential between psychiatrists, nurses and patients and that 'mentally distressed people are unambiguously located on the downside of sociopolitical power relations' (Hopton, 1997, p. 497). The moral and ethical dilemmas leading to abuse in the nurse–patient relationship are elaborated by Packard and Ferrara (1988), who see little hope for equity and justice given the conditions under which nurses work, and their conformity to the status quo. On the one hand, attempts to empower patients are viewed as an imperative but on the other it has been argued that treating patients as partners in an alliance is an unrealistic ideal, as well as inappropriate for the development of professionalism among nurses, since professionalism demands objectification of the patient at some level (Lupton, 1995; Van Hooft, 1987). Treating people as individuals does not necessarily avoid discrimination or dehumanisation, and in fact can result in 'an even greater extension of medical surveillance' and hence make them 'more vulnerable to the exercise of disciplinary, and possibly coercive, power' (Lupton, 1995, pp. 160–61). From the perspective of psychotherapeutic practice, critics call for recognition of 'the lies, the flaws, the harm ... the imbalance in power, the arrogance, the condescension, the pretensions' inherent in such practice, and call for its abolition (Masson, 1993, p. 299).

This is a vexed issue, as it must also be recognised that, while some patients prefer to be more participatory in their care, others find it stressful and intrusive. For Van Hooft (1987), compassion for patients must be based on a recognition of one's own power and good fortune, in contrast to that of the patient. This means that mutual growth and rapport, which seeks to place the relationship on an equal footing, is just not possible. The important issue is to approach the therapeutic role with a continuing and critical deconstruction and reconstruction of our world before and during the development of effective therapeutic alliances with our patients. Discovering the patient's meaning is one task, 'unpacking' our baggage prior to our involvement is another. This will provide the potential to transform our nursing practice by opening up the possibilities for alternative representations and meanings.

Meaning and the therapeutic role: historical developments

If it is true, as Frankl argues, that our lives constitute a search for meaning, then seeking the meaning that mental illness has for our patients is vital in the development of our therapeutic role. In 1959 Frankl developed a theory he called 'logotherapy', a word derived from the Greek word 'logos', denoting 'meaning'. It focuses on the meaning of human existence as well as on the search for meaning. According to Frankl, 'the striving to find a meaning in one's life is the primary motivational force in man' (*sic*) (p. 154). The task for Frankl was to assist patients to find meaning in their lives; it was 'therapy through meaning', rather than 'meaning through therapy' (or that 'therapy produces the meaning'). It was not concerned with the therapist's meaning, but that of the patient.

Other literature, traceable back to the 1960s, also makes similar propositions, but does not go this far. Howard and Orlinsky (1972), in a paper that examined therapeutic processes, cite Opler (1968) who proposed that the time had come when professional therapists should finally realise that they must learn to communicate effectively with different segments of the patient population, particularly those with different cultural and class orientations. Prior to this period, therapists were intent on helping patients see the error of their ways; to help them adjust to a world with which they (the patients) had difficulty. It was a period when the underlying premise for treatment was *blaming* patients for their problems and difficulties, rather than appreciating the role of social, cultural, economic and political factors in the development and continuation of their illness.

Some practitioners were proposing the importance of empathy, warmth and genuineness for effective psychotherapy. Others promoted 'accurate empathy' (Rogers & Truax, 1967) which focused on the therapist's sensitive grasp of the phenomenological meaning to the patient of events and experiences and the current experiential impact of the patient's feelings. Gurman (1977) maintained that it was the patient's perception of the quality of the therapeutic relationship that mediated therapeutic change, while noting that there was very little agreement between patients' and therapists' perceptions of the quality of the therapeutic relationship. This research established the principle of seeking and accepting the patient as a valid observer of, and contributor to, the existing scene.

The issue that nurses must confront is: whose questions are we asking? Are they those of the patient, or those we think we need the answers to? Questions we ask can effectively silence us and our patients, which is why an examination of the powerful and dominant discourse in psychiatry is an essential part of this exploration. Establishing the meaning of this experience of mental illness is difficult, even impossible if we do not stand back and consider what the questions might be, if asked by our patients. What is their perception of events?

Compliance and the therapeutic role

There is a considerable literature that addresses the therapeutic alliance, linking it with non-compliance and the controlling of those in care. Part of the process of critically analysing the social reality of mental illness and health care is to examine the ideological premises on which some of this literature is based. There may be a case for suggesting that patients are forced into non-compliance partly because we offer them unsatisfactory and ineffective therapeutic relationships. Accepting the patient as a human being with rights and responsibilities has challenged the traditional conception of the patient role. It has resulted in patients endeavouring to exert some measure of control, for which they have been historically condemned. Non-compliance can be viewed as one means by which patients endeavour to modify the treatment originally posited by the therapist. Determining the meaning of non-compliance to the patient, therefore, is critical. Failure to investigate this can result in the failure of bonding in a therapeutic alliance, and hence a totally negative experience. In a paper which examines 'motivation for treatment', Miller (1985) notes that patients are categorised as compliant when they accept the therapist's diagnosis and treatment, or as non-compliant when they disagree with the diagnosis, and do not accept the treatment suggested. Miller recognises the importance of shifting this type of victim-blaming from patients to examining patients' perceptions of therapeutic care.

In developing a deconstructive approach, it is instructive for nurses to critically examine literature that focuses on patients who seek to control situations, who are manipulative and disruptive because they do not agree with the therapist's views of reality (Hayes-Bautista, 1976); who are unwilling to cooperate or adapt to institutional demands and the authority of the mental health professional (Kelley & May, 1982); who sabotage treatment (Colson, *et al.*, 1985); who refuse, or are unable, to return the therapist's efforts on their behalf with improvement, compliance and gratification (Robbins, *et al.*, 1988).

In the 1980s there was a perceptible shift in the literature addressing this important area. The concept of 'therapeutic alliance' gained credence. In theory, the patient was to be given the opportunity to develop a sense of control, of being involved as an active participant, of having a positive relationship (including warmth, friendship, empathy, respect, concern) with the therapist, of receiving information and feedback, negotiating mutual expectations and clarifying rights and responsibilities of both parties. Human relationships are here placed at the centre of nursing work, with the patient viewed as 'not just ... the object of clinical practice and administrative procedure, but also as an *experiencing subject* (May & Purkis, 1995, p. 286, italics in original).

While the 'alliance' concept appears to have a greater acceptance of patients' enhanced involvement with therapy, and recognition of the fact that their perception of events is vital, there is little evidence that this actually occurs in practice. It is particularly difficult to dislodge ingrained attitudes of, and beliefs about, the role of health professionals and patients, particularly in the areas of compliance and appropriateness of behaviour. Carers quickly fall into making moralistic judgements and exerting control, which does not fit comfortably with shifting some of that control to our patients.

Enhancing the therapeutic role

While there are a number of concepts that effective communicators should be cognisant of, it is also important to be aware of the range of factors which militate against the development of an effective therapeutic alliance. These include, for example: lack of understanding of components of the relationship, such as self-disclosure (Crispin, 1993); failure to develop empathy (Olson, 1995) and 'positive connectedness' (Heifner, 1993); trust, and mutuality (Henson, 1997); decrease in openness and self-esteem; lack of privacy; environmental distractions; techno-worship; economic rationalism and structural factors, including contamination of role, as occurs in specific legal responsibilities, such as those required for nurses supervising home or community treatment orders (Street & Walsh, 1994).

A therapeutic alliance demands the involvement of both patient and nurse and requires a shared system of beliefs about the value of the individual, the meaning of health and illness and the required outcomes of intervening and interrelating. For Muetzel (1988) there are three elements essential to the therapeutic process, namely: partnership, intimacy and reciprocity. Partnership and intimacy include the qualities of security and freedom; partnership and reciprocity include the qualities of contact and control; while reciprocity and intimacy include the qualities of closeness and vulnerability. McMahon (1991, p. 8) notes that the ability of the nurse to participate in a therapeutic relationship is 'reliant on her first having developed as a person and as a member of the nursing team'. This means that 'reciprocity reflects the belief and value that the nurse–patient relationship may be healing for the nurse as well as the patient' ... and that without reciprocity, 'the nurse–patient relationship almost certainly lacks balance and depth' (p. 8). These views are reinforced by Walsh (1994) who examines the nurse–patient relationship from ontological perspectives (defined as what it means to 'Be').

In considering the definition of Being, Walsh (1994) notes that inauthenticity occurs when we fail to ask ourselves who we are. He addresses the important issue of 'over-involvement' and a 'less than professional attitude' which is often suggested as a defect in those who take this line of approach. He believes that it is over-involvement that is inauthentic, because 'becoming the other' cannot be therapeutic, since it leads to objectification of the patient. Benner and Wrubel (1989) suggest that over-involvement may be a strategy which aims for greater control of the patient, and hence diminishes the vulnerability that accompanies the caring response of the nurse. Van Hooft (1987) suggests that nurses should not be responsible for the patient's growth in a holistic sense, nor should they be expected to share 'the most intimate levels of existence' (p. 33), since this makes for an impossible professional life. The question that this raises, of course, is whether this further objectifies the patient, rather than facilitating the relationship and enhancing the alliance. Furthermore, it demands an analysis and critique of the literature addressing caring in nursing, in all its forms (see, for example, MacDougall, 1997; Hopton, 1997; Barker & Reynolds, 1994; Walters, 1994; Dunlop, 1986; Campbell, 1984; Griffin, 1983). Caring involves a broad, global human concept of investing the self in the experiences of patients to the extent that we become parti-cipants in our patients' lives. Being a participant demands establishing the meaning of the patient's experiences. An exploration of this literature can therefore assist in enlarging the knowledge base of the nurse therapist in establishing meaning, and understanding the meanings of others.

The practice context: perspectives of patient and nurse

One example of psychiatric practice that exemplifies the lack of congruence between the perspectives of nurses and patients, is that of placement in seclusion. There is a continuing debate surrounding the necessity for seclusion in any circumstances, and under what conditions it might be necessary. The research remains equivocal, as will be noted below. What is important is that nurses critically review their past and current practice, understand what seclusion means to the patient, their own motives for adopting this line of intervention, and what alternatives there may be, either for avoiding the need to seclude, or providing a process that is fully cognisant of the impact it has on patients' future relationship with them. This means, in essence, questioning the therapeutic value of seclusion, and considering whether security is actually compromised when seclusion practices are reduced (Farrell & Dares 1996).

The experience of seclusion for patient and nurse

Implicit in the argument presented in this chapter is that nurses must recognise and acknowledge the realities of their patients. As Norris and Kennedy (1992) point out:

> 'Perceptions influence feelings and feelings influence behaviour. Whatever the patients' perceptions, it is that reality with which staff must work ... (a)ppre-ciating the uniqueness of individual perceptions allows staff to respond sensi-tively to each patient in the most therapeutic manner'.

> (Norris & Kennedy, 1992, p. 7, p. 13).

Nowhere is this more pertinent than in the experience of seclusion. Considerable research attention has been paid to seclusion and the factors that increase or decrease its likelihood. Researchers also investigated the degree to which a secure environment enhances therapeutic care, including staffing levels, gender mix and level of experience (Morrison 1990; 1995); the 'social climate' and general influence of physical surroundings (Morrison, *et al.*, 1997b).

From the point of view of developing a therapeutic alliance, the most useful research studies have examined the differing perceptions that patients and staff have of this form of 'treatment'. Overall, these studies suggest that patients have more dissimilar views than do nurses about the value and impact of the seclusion process. For example, patients perceive seclusion in a negative way, whereas nursing staff do not (Soliday 1985); patients view seclusion as harmful to patients, while nursing staff believe it to be therapeutic (Cashin, 1996; Human Rights and Equal Opportunities Commission, 1993; Tooke & Brown, 1992; Richardson, 1987); patients and staff have differing perceptions about why seclusion and restraint needs to be used (Outlaw & Lowery, 1994); and who is benefiting most from seclusion (Outlaw & Lowery, 1992). These studies also found that: seclusion is sometimes used by staff to effect smooth functioning of the ward, and thus has a controlling function (Fisher, 1994; Tooke & Brown, 1992); some patients believed that seclusion is a punitive act on the part of some staff who use it to demonstrate their power over patients (Hewison, 1995; Morrison, 1994; Stilling, 1992; Topping-Morris, 1992); seclusion has also been defined as criminal assault perpetrated on patients (Hopton, 1995). Other research suggests various ways of improving the seclusion process (Tooke & Brown, 1992; Soliday, 1985); alternatives to it (Morales, 1995; Craig, *et al.*, 1989); or additional, complementary strategies (Maier, *et al.*, 1994).

The overwhelming message in this research is that there is a considerable gap in the understandings between patients and nurses about the need for seclusion and process by which it is enacted. Nurses do not perceive that patients feel powerless, fearful, humiliated, deprived, lonely and resentful, which raises a question about the value of seclusion as a 'therapeutic' act. It is quite conceivable that the negative feelings generated in patients who are secluded make it impossible for a future therapeutic relationship with the nurse or nurses involved. This is particularly the case if patients view seclusion as an act of violence against them, and then retaliate with aggression, further escalating the situation (Morrison, 1994). Seclusion, therefore, in these cases, has further jeopardised the mental health of the patient.

The present day commitment to consultation and negotiation between consumers and carers regarding the quality and type of services provided will bring the process and necessity for seclusion under even closer scrutiny (Farrell & Dares, 1996). Such consultation should result in a shift in the locus of power and control in favour of consumers, and be more congruent with stated institutional and treatment objectives (Morrison, *et al.*,

1997a); it may also result in decreased frequency of assaultive behaviours (Morrison, *et al.*, 1997b). The focus on consumers brings into sharp relief the issue of 'the ethical nature of constraining practices which persist in psychiatric settings' (Muir-Cochrane, 1995). This latter author points out the impact of institutional ideology '... and a medical model of care which encourages the relinquishing of autonomy and responsibility in a paternalistic fashion' (Muir-Cochrane, 1995, p. 19), and calls for a sustained, critical review of this practice.

Contextual factors influencing Australian mental health practice

Government policy

In line with international trends the Report of the Mental Health Consumer Outcomes Task Force produced a Statement of Rights and Responsibilities which was adopted by the Australian Health Ministers in 1991. It was primarily concerned with the rights of the mentally ill, and the responsibilities of society in the provision of services for the mentally disturbed. It did not explicitly address the ethics of care, but was premised on the principles of equity, access and social justice. Mental health reform as part of the movement to establish people-focussed services explicitly supports the concepts of social justice, citizen integrity, social policy and citizen participation.

Professional standards

On a professional level the Standards of Mental Health Nursing Practice developed by the Australian Congress of Mental Health Nurses in 1985 and updated in 1995, provided principles and rationales for care, levels of acceptable practice and attributes of the practitioner (knowledge, skills, attitudes and outcomes) that should be held and met by practising mental health nurses. This document is premised on an ethic of caring and concern, since each Standard has caring as a component (ANZCMHN Inc, 1995). It is quite clear that these Standards include a therapeutic domain and use of the self in interpersonal relationships with patients in nursing care.

Consumer perspectives

Consideration of the views of consumers and acting on their input was formally acknowledged with the inclusion of consumer participation in the Australian National Mental Health Policy and Plan (1992). This signalled a change from the paternalistic view that the mentally ill are incapable of expressing valid opinions about their care, to a more enlightened view that consumers have clear understandings of their needs. This new policy development includes the perspectives of those who are or have been mentally ill, as well as those who undertake a carer's role.

The therapeutic alliance in practice

Mental health nursing practice, be it clinical, education, management or research, occurs in a range of situations and contexts. In recognition of this diversity, this section can only provide general comments that may be adapted to the readers' specific situation.

Nurses and nurse therapists

Mental health nursing practice can be complex, confusing and dangerous – which raises a host of moral and ethical issues for practitioners. A recent study identified three major ethical problems encountered in day-to-day practice:

• The need to balance support for patient autonomy with the need to maintain control
• The need to distance oneself with the desire to establish therapeutic relationships, and
• The desire to 'do the right thing' for the patient, with the need to gain acceptance by colleagues.

(Fisher, 1995)

It is clear that nursing practice must address the struggle that occurs in relationships between patient and nurse, nurse and nurse, and with other significant persons in the specific context of practice.

Some of the nursing literature suggests that it is naive to believe that nurses can be ethical and moral in their practice. It has been argued that nurses cannot be moral and ethical persons because the existing social and structural constraints of the institutions in which they provide care militate against it (Yarling & McElmurry, 1986). Furthermore, nursing's generally apolitical posture, and its emphasis of the personal, has militated against active reform of institutions and their structures. Nurses have tended to identify with 'the interests of powerful others' and adapted to the existing social order (Packard & Ferrara, 1988, p. 65). A more optimistic view is provided by Cooper (1988), who suggests that effective therapeutic alliances are possible if premised on discovering the patient's meaning. Only then can a moral and ethical basis for care be established. Thus:

'interaction within this [covenantal] relationship is ultimately dependent, not on the degree of restraint within the institution or the cooperative spirit of the health care team, but on the *willingness of the nurse and patient to become so engaged.*'

(Cooper 1988 p. 49, *italics added*)

Parker (1991) contributes to this argument in asserting that nurses must develop a wider and deeper understanding of the issues at stake here, noting the importance of

'an ethical stance of responsibility towards the socio-cultural environment ... directed towards scholarly and political activities by nurses ... [which] will facilitate the laying open of oppressive structures of meaning that constrain the coming into being of fuller expressions of possibility.'

(Parker, 1991, p. 306)

As was noted earlier, the more recent acceptance of consumer consultation and participation demonstrates an attempt to invoke moral concepts such as justice, freedom and equality in the delivery of care.

There are a number of strategies that can be used to move from providing therapeutic care which pays lip-service to 'understanding the patient' to developing meanings. Two of these, phenomenology and story telling, will be briefly described below.

Phenomenology provides a way of 'capturing the human meanings of the lived-experience of patients in a language essential for social change shaped according to the values of the recipient of health care' (Bartjes, 1991, p. 261).

One person with mental illness describes how she made sense of her lived-experience:

'I found the treatment in the institutions humiliating. I was consistently patronised, as was everyone else there. I had no compassion for anyone else. As far as I was concerned, all other inmates were really mad but I was just sick. It took me years to discover, after meeting many people who'd spent years in mental institutions, that it's a conviction that first strikes every patient – that everybody else is mad but somehow you're just sick.

By and large the professionals do try to help. I guess what hurts is that they really don't know how to help and I find them now resisting the knowledge that it really is simple – not easy, by no means easy, but definitely simple'.

(quoted in Bartjes, 1991, p. 260)

This patient adds that the major problem for the mentally ill is 'the agonising loss of personal value, *of living without a sense of worth and meaning*' (Bartjes, 1991, p. 260, italics added).

This observation of mental illness as a loss of value returns us to the question of whether nurses see their patients as they really are, and know them for their own reality and with their own meanings. Without the capacity to take this perspective, 'nurses can only stand on one side of the chasm, forever unable to get to the other side and forever separated from the human being as he or she authentically is' (Bartjes, 1991, p. 261).

Another technique for developing an understanding of patients, situations and relationships is that of story telling. Underpinned by hermeneutics whose primary concern is interpretation and understanding, it seeks to uncover the hidden meanings of experience. A recent study examined transactions between nurses and those in their care, for interpretation and theme development. The aim of the study was to reveal knowledge about mental health nursing and test nursing theory, in particular, theory relating to nurse-client relationships (Geanellos, 1995). Major themes arising from the knowledge this evoked included: guiding the potential for change; therapeutic use of self; and mobilising the community as a resource, all of which are critical to the delivery of therapeutic care. While there are additional ways of establishing meaning, strategies based on phenomenology and story telling will also provide a basis for confirming mental health nursing knowledge, and contribute to development of the discipline.

Research

In keeping with the ideas presented in this chapter, it is appropriate that nurse researchers critically review and analyse long-held assumptions and 'facts'. What is proposed is that mental health nurses no longer accept the world view that is fed them by those whose interests are served in doing so. Nurses have to consider, given an awakening critical awareness, what it is that they want to achieve, and whether what they are currently doing is likely to culminate in these achievements. It means that nurses consider the contradictions, the incongruities and the so-called 'realities' of life. This approach is clearly in support of *the search for meaning* that has been central to this chapter.

In terms of specific areas for nursing research, there are some areas that are immediately apparent for examination. For example, what is the meaning and lived experience of those who experience mental illness? What are the models of care that can provide the best outcomes for our patients? Answers to the unresolved questions involved in seclusion are also needed. Additional research that focuses on the nurse includes: What type of people decide to become psychiatric and/or mental health nurses? What motivates them? What are their personality characteristics, their needs, their beliefs, their attitudes and values, their hopes and dreams? What is the lived experience of caring for mental health nurses? Can nursing research help to determine what preparation nurses need to uncover their clients' meanings and work therapeutically? Most importantly, nurse researchers should collaborate with practitioners and patients in defining the meanings of their experiences; practitioners can assist nurse researchers with respect to relevance and appropriateness of research questions, and the conduct of such research.

Conclusion

This chapter has described a range of concepts that are components of knowledge essential in the development of a therapeutic alliance. To demonstrate the differing meanings attached to specific experiences, it also provides examples of ways in which the experiences of patients are perceived, often in contrast to those of nurses. This demonstrates the multiple meanings which arise from the histories and contexts in which nurses and their patients exist.

The chapter suggests a range of ways to extend the value of nursing practice. Fundamental to this approach is a consideration of meaning, both for patient and nurse, and of each other, within socio-cultural and political contexts. To do less is to deprive mental health nurses, their patients and other carers of deriving meanings, thus reducing their capacity for growth and extension. By accepting the underlying premise of this chapter, that mental health nurses need to understand themselves and what their meanings are, the process described by Baldwin (1961) is begun: and the 'questions which one asks oneself begin, at last, to illuminate the world, and become one's key to the experience of others' (Baldwin, 1961).

In the final analysis:

> 'The remarkable thing is that we really love our neighbour as ourselves; we do unto others as we do unto ourselves. We hate others when we hate ourselves. We are tolerant towards others when we tolerate ourselves.

> (Hoffer, 1954, p. 100)

In essence, we understand others when we understand ourselves.

References

Andrews, G. (1989) Public and private psychiatry: a comparison of two health care systems. *American Journal of Psychiatry,* **146**, (7), 881–6.

Australian & New Zealand College of Mental Health Nurses (ANZCMHN) Inc. (1995) *Standards of Practice for Mental Health Nursing in Australia.* ANZCMHN, South Australia.

Australian Health Ministers (1992) *National Mental Health Policy.* Australian Government Publishing Service, Canberra.

Baldwin, J. (1961) Nobody Knows My Name. Quoted in *The International Thesaurus of Quotations* (1976) (ed. R.T. Tripp), Penguin.

Bartjes, A. (1991) Phenomenology in Clinical Practice. In: *Towards a Discipline of Nursing* (eds G. Gray & R. Pratt), Churchill Livingstone, Melbourne.

Barker, P. & Reynolds, W. (1994) A critique: Watson's caring ideology, the proper focus of psychiatric nursing. *Journal of Psychosocial Nursing and Mental Health Services,* **32** (5), 17–22.

Benner, P. & Wrubel, J. (1989) *The Primacy of Caring: Stress and Coping in Health and Illness.* Addison-Wesley, Menlo Park.

Broverman, I.K., Broverman, D.M., Clarkson, F.E., Rosenkrantz, F.S. & Vogel, S.R. (1970) Sex-role Stereotypes and Clinical Judgements of Mental Health. *Journal of Consulting and Clinical Psychology,* **34**, 1–7.

Campbell, A.V. (1984) *Moderated Love: A Theology of Professional Care.* SPCK, London.

Cashin, A. (1996) Seclusion: the quest to determine effectiveness. *Journal of Psychosocial Nursing,* **34** (11), 17–23.

Chesler, P. (1972) *Women and Madness,* Avon, New York.

Colson, D.B., Allen, J.G. & Coyne, L. (1985) Patterns of Staff Perception of Difficult Patients in a Long-term Psychiatric Hospital. *Hospital Community Psychiatry,* **36**, 168–72.

Cooper, M.C. (1988) Covenantal Relationships: Grounding for the Nursing Ethic. *Advances in Nursing Science,* **10** (4), 48–59.

Cotton, P. (1997) Psychological health on the level playing field. *Psych,* **19** (2), 12–14.

Craig, C., Ray, F. & Hix, C. (1989) Seclusion and Restraint: Decreasing the Discomfort. *Journal of Psychosocial Nursing,* **27** (7), 16–19.

Crispin, W. (1993) Self-disclosure as a Facilitative Function of the Mental Health Nursing. *Australian Journal of Mental Health Nursing.* **2** (7), 299–305.

Delacour, S. (1991) The Construction of Nursing: Ideology, Discourse, and Representation. In: *Towards a Discipline of Nursing.* (eds G. Gray & R. Pratt), Churchill Livingstone, Melbourne.

Delacour, S. & Short, S.D. (1992) Nursing, Medicine and Women's Health: A Discourse Analysis. *Issues in Nursing 3* (eds G. Gray & R. Pratt), Churchill Livingstone, Melbourne.

Dunlop, M. (1986) Is a Science of Caring Possible? *Journal of Advanced Nursing,* **11**, 661–70.

Eade, G. & Bradshaw, J. (1995) Understanding Discourses of the Worried Well. *Australian and New Zealand Journal of Mental Health Nursing,* **4** (2), 61–9.

Farrell, G. & Dares, G. (1996) Seclusion or solitary confinement: therapeutic or punitive treatment? *Australian and New Zealand Journal of Mental Health Nursing,* **5** (4), 171–9.

Fisher, A. (1995) The ethical problems encountered in psychiatric nursing practice with dangerous mentally ill persons. *Scholarly Inquiry for Nursing Practice: An International Journal,* **9** (2), 193–208.

Fisher, W.A. (1994) Restraint and seclusion: a review of the literature. *American Journal of Psychiatry,* **15**, 1584–91.

Frankl, V.E. (1959) *Man's Search for Meaning.* Washington Square Press, New York.

Gaskill, D. & Cooney, H. (1991) Coping With Schizophrenia: What Does the Spouse Need to Know? *Australian Journal of Advanced Nursing,* **9** (2), 10–15.

Geanellos, R. (1995) Story-telling: What Can it Reveal About the Knowledge of Mental Health Nursing? *Australian and New Zealand Journal of Mental Health Nursing,* **4** (2), 87–94.

Griffin, A. (1983) A Philosophical Analysis of Caring in Nursing. *Journal of Advanced Nursing,* **8**, 289–95.

Gurman, A.S. (1977) The Patient's Perception of the Therapeutic Relationship. In: *Effective Psychotherapy: A Handbook of Research* (eds A.S. Gurman & A.M. Razin), Pergamon Press, Oxford.

Hall, B.A. (1996) The psychiatric medical model: a critical analysis of its undermining effects on nursing in chronic mental illness. *Advances in Nursing Science,* **18** (3), 16–26.

Hayes-Bautista, D.E. (1976) Modifying the Treatment: Patient Compliance, Patient Control and Medical Care. *Social Science and Medicine,* **10**, 233–8.

Hazelton, M. (1993) The Discourse of Mental Health Reform: A Critical Analysis. *Australian Journal of Mental Health Nursing,* **2** (4), 141–54.

Hazelton, M. (1995) Mental Health, Deinstitutionalization, and the Problem of Citizenship. *Australian and New Zealand Journal of Mental Health Nursing,* **4** (3), 103–14.

Heifner, C. (1993) Positive connectedness in the psychiatric nurse-patient relationship. *Archives of Psychiatric Nursing,* **VII** (1), 11–15.

Henson, R.H. (1997) Analysis of the concept of mutuality. *Image: Journal of Nursing Scholarship,* **29** (1), 77–81.

Hewison, A. (1995) Nurses' Power in Interactions with Patients. *Journal of Advanced Nursing,* **21**, 75–82.

Hoffer, E. (1954) The Passionate State of Mind. Quoted in *The International Thesaurus of Quotations* (1976) (ed. R.T.Tripp), Penguin.

Hopton, J. (1997) Towards a critical theory of mental health nursing. *Journal of Advanced Nursing,* **25** (3), 492–500.

Hopton, J. (1995) Control and restraint in contemporary psychiatric nursing: some ethical considerations. *Journal of Advanced Nursing*, **22**, 110–15.

Horsfall, J. (1994) *Social Constructions in Women's Mental Health*. University of New England Press, Armidale.

Howard, K.I. & Orlinsky, D.E. (1972). Psychotherapeutic Processes. *Annual Review of Psychology*, **23**, 615–68.

Human Rights and Equal Opportunity Commission (1993) *Human Rights and Mental Illness. Report of the National Inquiry into the Human Rights of People with Mental Illness* (The Burdekin Report). Vols. 1 and 2, Australian Government Publishing Service, Canberra.

Jewell, K. & Posner, N. (1996) A Consumer Focus. In: *Mental Health and Nursing Practice* (eds M. Clinton & S. Nelson), Prentice Hall, Sydney.

Kelley, M.P. & May, D. (1982). Good and Bad Patients: A Review of the Literature and a Theoretical Critique. *Journal of Advanced Nursing*, **7**, 147–56.

Lupton, D. (1995) Perspectives on Power, Communication and the Medical Encounter: Implications for Nursing Theory and Practice. *Nursing Inquiry*, **2** (3), 157–63.

MacDougall, G. (1997) Caring – a masculine perspective. *Journal of Advanced Nursing*, **25** (4), 809–13.

Maier, G.J., van Rybroek, G.J. & Mays, D.V. (1994) A report on staff injuries and ambulatory restraints. *Journal of Psychosocial Nursing and Mental Health Services*, **32** (11), 23–30.

McKay, B. (1996) *Proposals for change: optimum supply and effective use of psychiatrists*. Department of Human Services and Health, Canberra.

McMahon, R. (1991) Therapeutic Nursing: Theory, Issues and Practice. In: *Nursing As Therapy* (eds R. McMahon & A. Pearson). Chapman & Hall, London.

Masson, J. (1993) *Against Therapy*. HarperCollins, London.

May, C.R. & Purkis, M.E. (1995). The configuration of nurse-patient relationships: a critical review. *Scholarly Inquiry for Nursing Practice*, **9** (4), 283–95.

Miller, W.R. (1985) Motivation for Treatment: A Review With Special Emphasis on Alcoholism. *Psychological Bulletin*, **98** (1), 84–107.

Morales, E. (1995) Least restrictive measures: alternatives to four-point restraints and seclusion. *Journal of Psychosocial Nursing*, **33** (10), 13–16.

Morrison, E. (1994) The evolution of a concept: aggression and violence in psychiatric settings. *Archives of Psychiatric Nursing*, **VIII** (4), 245–53.

Morrison, P., Lehane, M., Palmer, C. & Meehan, T. (1997a) The use of behavioural mapping in a study of seclusion. *Australian and New Zealand Journal of Mental Health Nursing*, **6** (1), 11–18.

Morrison, P., Burnard, P. & Phillips, C. (1997b) Nurses' and patients' perceptions of the social climate in a forensic unit in Wales. *International Journal of Offender Therapy and Comparative Criminology*, **41** (1), 65–78.

Morrison, P., Burnard, P. & Philips, C. (1996) Patient satisfaction in a forensic unit. *Journal of Mental Health*, **5** (4), 369–77.

Morrison, P. (1995) Staffing levels and seclusion use. *Journal of Advanced Nursing*, **22**, 1193–202.

Morrison, P. (1990) The use of environmental seclusion in psychiatric settings: a multidimensional scalogram analysis. *Journal of Environmental Psychology*, **10**, 353–62.

Muetzel, P. (1988) Therapeutic Nursing. In: *Primary Nursing: Nursing in the Burford and Oxford Nursing Development Units* (ed. A. Pearson), Croon Helm, London.

Muir-Cochrane, E. (1995) An Exploration of Ethical Issues Associated with the Seclusion of Psychiatric Patients. *Collegian*, **2** (3), 14–19.

National Mental Health Report Overview 1994 (1995) Second Annual Report. *Changes in Australia's Mental Health Services in Year Two of the National Mental Health Strategy*. Australian Government Publishing Service, Canberra.

National Mental Health Policy and Plan (1992) Australian Government Publishing Service, Canberra.

Norris, M.K. & Kennedy, C.W. (1992) How Patients Perceive the Seclusion Process. *Journal of Psychosocial Nursing and Mental Health Services*, **30** (3), 7–13.

Olson, J.K. (1995) Relationships between nurse expressed empathy, patient-perceived empathy and patient distress. *Image: Journal of Nursing Scholarship*, **27** (4), 317–22.

Opler, M.K. (1968) The Social and Cultural Nature of Mental Illness and Its Treatment. In: *Psychotherapeutic Processes* (1972) (eds K.I. Howard & D.E. Orlinsky), *Annual Review of Psychology*, **23**, 615–68.

Outlaw, F.H. & Lowery, B.J. (1994) An attributional study of seclusion and restraint in psychiatric patients. *Archives of Psychiatric Nursing*, **VIII** (2), 69–77.

Outlaw, F.H. & Lowery, B.J. (1992) Seclusion: the nursing challenge. *Journal of Psychosocial Nursing and Mental Health Services*, **30** (4), 13–17.

Packard, J.S. & Ferrara, M. (1988) In search of the moral foundation of nursing. *Advances in Nursing Science*, **90** (4), 60–71.

Parker, J. (1991) Being and Nature: An Interpretation of Person and Environment. In: *Towards a Discipline of Nursing* (eds G. Gray & R. Pratt), Churchill Livingstone, Melbourne.

Pugliesi, K. (1992) Women and Mental Health: Two Traditions of Feminist Research. *Women and Health*, **19** (2/3), 43–68.

Richardson, B. (1987) Psychiatric Inpatients' Perceptions of the Seclusion-room Experience. *Nursing Research*, **36**, 224–38.

Rich, D. (1994) Measuring Client Satisfaction with Psychiatric Treatment. Development of an Objective, Criterion Referenced Scale. *Australian and New Zealand Journal of Mental Health Nursing*, **3** (3), 91–4.

Robbins, J.M., Beck, P.R., Mueller, D.P. & Mizener, D.A. (1988) Therapists' Perceptions of Difficult Psychiatric Patients. *Journal of Nervous and Mental Disease*, **176** (8), 490–97.

Rogers, C.R. & Truax, C.B. (1967) The Therapeutic Conditions Antecedent to Change: A Theoretical View. In: *The Therapeutic Relationship and Its Impact: A Study of Psychotherapy with Schizophrenics* (ed. C.R. Rogers), University of Wisconsin Press, Madison, Wis.

Rudge, T. & Gerschwitz, M. (1995) Validation of Cues for Competencies of beginning Level Mental Health Nurses: An Exploratory Study in South Australian Mental Health Agencies. *Australian and New Zealand Journal of Mental Health Nursing*, **4** (1), 31–41.

Russell, D. (1995) *Women, Madness and Medicine*, Polity Press, Cambridge.

Sebastian, L. (1987) Psychiatric Hospital Admissions: Assessing Patients' Perceptions. *Journal of Psychosocial Nursing*. **25** (6), 25–8.

Soliday, S.M. (1985) A Comparison of Patient and Staff Attitudes Towards Seclusion. *Journal of Nervous and Mental Diseases*, **173**, 282–6.

Sontag, S. (1990) *Illness as Metaphor*. Anchor, New York.

Stilling, L. (1992) The pros and cons of physical restraints and behaviour controls. *Journal of Psychosocial Nursing and Mental Health Services*, **30** (3), 18–20.

Street, A. & Walsh, C. (1994) The legalisation of a therapeutic role: implications for the practice of community mental health nurses using the New Zealand Mental Health (Compulsory Assessment and Treatment) Act of 1992. *Australian and New Zealand Journal of Mental Health Nursing,* **3** (2), 39–44.

Tooke, S.K. & Brown, J.S. (1992) Perceptions of Seclusion: Comparing Patient and Staff Reactions. *Journal of Psychosocial Nursing,* **30** (8), 23–6.

Topping-Morris, B. (1992) Prisoners of the System. *Nursing Times,* **88** (24), 39–41.

Van Hooft, S. (1987) Caring and Professional Commitment. *Australian Journal of Advanced Nursing,* **4** (4), 29–38.

Walsh, K. (1994) Ontology and the Nurse-patient Relationship in Psychiatric Nursing. *Australian and New Zealand Journal of Mental Health Nursing,* **3** (4), 113–18.

Walters, A.J. (1994) *Caring as a Theoretical Construct,* University of New England Press, Armidale.

Yarling, R.R. & McElmurry, B.J. (1986) The Moral Foundation of Nursing. *Advances in Nursing Science,* **8** (2), 63–73.

5 Community Services and Supports

Jennifer Pyke

This chapter uses an inclusive concept of community to provide an overview of the catalysts and needs involved in shifting from an institutionally focused to a community-focused mental health system. The implications for nursing activities and roles in a reformed mental health system will be discussed, as will how nurses and nursing might meet these challenges. Throughout the chapter, the consumer population discussed refers to people with serious and persistent mental illnesses who experience significant problems in community living.

Mental health services in Canada: an historical overview

Deinstitutionalisation realised the goal of moving people into community settings. However, the failure to simultaneously re-allocate human and fiscal resources resulted in significant problems. Patients, moved into a largely unprepared 'community' and unable to meet their own needs, too often ended up living in sub-standard housing, roaming the streets or incarcerated (Toews & Barnes, 1986). With fewer beds hospital stays became much shorter. But the lack of supports in the community created a new phenomenon, the aptly named *revolving door syndrome*, in which people had brief but frequent stays in hospital, often returning to the same problematic situations time and time again.

Increasing dissatisfaction with a disconnected non-system coupled with steadily rising health care costs provided the impetus for a more systematic reform of the mental health system. All ten Canadian provinces now have plans in place to reform their mental health systems. Consistent themes in the provincial planning process have been:

- Priority setting (the most seriously mentally ill)
- (Re)allocation of resources from institutions to community (see Table 5.1 for Ontario's plan)
- Coordination
- Regionalisation/decentralisation (to allow for locally identified needs)
- Individualisation of service delivery
- Increased opportunities for self-help/mutual aid, and
- Consumer and family participation in the mental health system (Mcnaughton, 1992).

Table 5.1   Re-allocation of resources in Ontario.

	Mental health dollar		Psychiatric beds
	Community Services	Institution	(per 100 000 pop'n)
1993	21%	79%	58
2003	60%	40%	30

Ministry of Health, 1993

Common goals are to:

- Reduce psychiatric beds
- Increase community-based services
- Include all stake holders in planning
- Develop regional authorities, and
- Establish evaluation and monitoring mechanisms

In a parallel process, professional associations also reviewed mental health issues and needs. The Canadian Nurses Association (CNA) developed a discussion paper on shortfalls in mental health care delivery in Canada with recommendations for mental health reform (Canadian Nurses Association, 1991). The CNA (1991) advocated an integrated community-based system of service delivery with a single entry point to ensure referral to the most appropriate service, and the shifting of resources from institution-based services to community-based alternatives.

Unfortunately, governments, while swift and decisive in reducing funding to hospitals, have been slow to re-allocate these savings to much needed community services and supports. When governments reduce the number of hospital beds without adequate community supports in place, they would do well to recall Santanya's words, that, 'Those who cannot remember the past are condemned to repeat it', a caveat repeated by Talbott (1979) when describing the disaster of deinstitutionalisation a few decades ago. In Canada, no less than throughout the rest of the world, change is occurring rapidly and at many levels – federal, provincial, regional, local, and in the day-to-day work of mental health services. Change brings threat, opportunities and challenge.

The challenge of change

Not so very long ago we were talking about 'ex-psychiatric patients' or 'chronic patients' or 'schizophrenics' receiving 'aftercare'. These labels infer that someone becomes their illness and is forever labelled as the result of being hospitalised for a psychiatric illness (unlike other illnesses or conditions). Moreover, it is implied that care really happens in institutions, and anything that happens in the community is essentially a 'follow-up' to inpatient care. Thankfully, such labels and beliefs have to a great extent been abandoned. Now, 'consumers', 'clients', 'consumer/survivors', 'members', are terms more commonly used to describe a service user's relationship with a service (Mueser, *et al.*, 1996). In their discussion paper on nursing and mental health care reform, the Canadian Nurses Association (1991) uses the term 'consumer', as it 'suggests a reciprocal relationship between the individual and the caregiver' (p.viii) (see Chapter 1).

While language is important, real reform starts by creating a mechanism for consumers/survivors and family members to participate in the mental health planning process (Lord & Hutchison, 1993; Pyke, *et al.*, 1991; Vandergang, 1996). The challenge for nurses then lies in our willingness to listen and to re-conceptualise what constitutes services and supports (Trainor, *et al.*, 1996; White, 1992). Although we already have some indication of what is likely to be helpful to this reconceptualisation, issues of power and control within and between professional, consumer and family groups (Reissman, 1990; Trainor, *et al.*, 1996) continue to impede the change process. Service providers have to accept, as Anthony declares, that: 'There are many paths to recovery, including choosing not to be part of the mental health system' (Anthony, 1993, p. 18).

From hospital to community

Anthony's (1993) seminal paper on recovery from mental illness noted that recovery does not mean that a person is 'cured' of their illness, but that they can have, '... a satisfying, hopeful, and contributing life even with limitations caused by illness', (p. 15). This section will discuss key components of a recovery-orientated system, namely:

- A community-focused mental health system
- Less reliance on formal services and better use of community resources and informal supports, and
- Greater involvement by service users and their families in planning, developing and delivering services

Until relatively recently, people with mental health problems had their service needs met by institutions or by community-based agencies which were specifically mandated (and limited) to serve that population. We know now that for real community integration to occur 'community' must be viewed in a broad non-segregated perspective. In this broad perspective, 'community' is a place that contains a variety of resources, for a variety of needs, for a variety of people. In the context of rehabilitation, Anthony, *et al.* (1990, p. 77) define resources as those, 'people, places, things and activities necessary for the client to be successful in (his or her) chosen environment.'

As Capponi (1993) noted in recounting her life as a psychiatric survivor, family members, friends, neighbours, other people with mental health problems, and mental health service providers contribute helpful support at different times and for various reasons. Importantly, Anthony emphasises that 'People who are recovering talk about the people who believed in them when they did not believe in themselves, who encouraged their recovery but did not force it...' (Anthony, 1993, p. 18).

To provide a more individualised service and to facilitate community integration, many services are moving from a 'supported' approach to a 'supportive' approach. In a 'supported' approach, clients receive services in a program specifically designed for, and limited to, people with serious mental health problems. In the 'supportive' approach, clients are assisted to use a range of community services and supports. Housing services in particular are shifting from a site-focused to a client-focused service model, and incorporating a number of case management activities to do so (Pyke & Lowe, 1996).

An individualised approach enables clients to select from a broad array of potential resources, whereas a program-dominated approach tends to utilise 'in-house' resources and to limit other possibilities. Access to a range of resources increases the capacity to develop and strengthen social networks and, crucially, reduces the iatrogenic potential of restricted environments (White, 1992). For instance it has been found that high-staffed group homes provide an environment that can limit social network opportunities (Goering, *et al.*, 1992).

Significantly, the benefits of support from consumer/survivor operated initiatives are often underestimated or unacknowledged, especially by professionals. In a survey undertaken in Ontario, users of consumer controlled services were asked to rank the relative helpfulness and/or harmfulness of various components of the mental health system (see Table 5.2). Users were also asked to rate various groups of individuals. The respondents scored consumers as the most helpful and psychiatrists as the least helpful groups or individuals. Nurses were ranked near the top in helpfulness in the service provider group; however, the site of nursing practice was not noted. In neither of the ratings were any of the supports or components seen as not helpful (Trainor, *et al.*, 1996). This survey supports findings of the social network literature that emphasises that what is helpful or not helpful is determined by the recipient and not the provider (see Chapter 3). Service providers need to assist clients to develop, re-build, mend and maintain their social networks, using informal supports to the greatest degree possible (Biegel, *et al.*, 1994; Walsh, 1994). Furthermore, the mental health system must recognise, support and utilise the too often neglected strengths and benefits of family, friends and neighbours.

Table 5.2 Rank order of consumers' perceptions of relative helpfulness of various components of the mental health system.

Consumer/survivor development initiatives

Other self-help groups

Community mental health agencies

General hospital psychiatric units

Psychiatric hospitals

Trainor, *et al.*, 1996

Some service and systems approaches to community-focused care

In a community-focused system, services that were once institutionally based will be available in community settings, including clients' homes. The following are examples of services that have made the transition.

Home Treatment

Home treatment of acute illness provides an alternative to hospital admission or a means to reduce the length of stay in hospital for people who require less than 24-hour nursing care. In Toronto, a community nursing service contracts directly with community mental health organisations to provide home treatment for clients who meet the specified criteria. Home treatment can be used in any instance where it would not pose a risk, does not require an involuntary admission to hospital because of serious risk to the person or others, and the person consents to the sharing of information between service providers (e.g. nurse and physician).

The client receives nursing care similar to that provided in a hospital – medication and symptom management, assistance with self-care, health care teaching, and supportive counselling. The nurse also offers education and support to family members or significant others, and liaises with other health care workers, including case managers. In addition, depending on the support network, the nurse may assist the client with household and time management activities. The amount of direct nursing care is dependent on the client's needs and support systems: a nurse is available by phone to the client 24 hours a day. The client is discharged from home treatment using similar criteria to that for discharge from hospital. Although the benefits of home treatment have been well described (Dykes, *et al.*, 1990; Wasylenki, *et al.*, 1997), it has not been widely practiced. It may well take a reduction in hospital beds to make this a more used alternative to hospitalisation.

Program for Assertive Community Treatment (PACT)

This is based on the Training in Community Living program, one of the first attempts in North America to provide community-based treatment to severely ill people (Stein & Test, 1980). The key elements of the PACT approach are a comprehensive range of treatment, rehabilitation and support services all provided by a community-based multidisciplinary team. Nurses, psychiatrists, social workers, and vocational specialists provide services based on their particular knowledge and skill base; nursing specific tasks usually relate to medication management. While some see the benefit of having resources located within one program, others view it as an institutional model delivered in the community that limits clients' choices and options. The PACT approach is prevalent in the USA. Modified versions, referred to as Assertive Community Treatment (ACT), are also provided in some parts of the USA and Canada. Some ACT models resemble the Full Support model of case management, which will be described later.

Crisis services

These are often limited to the emergency department of hospitals or distress centre phone lines, but there are a number of other ways to provide these services. In Toronto services range from a pre-crisis 'warm-line' for people who need someone to talk to (Habel-Brosek, 1995) to a comprehensive mobile psychosocial crisis service. It is of particular note that both of these services emphasise the involvement of consumer/survivors. In the clubhouse 'warm-line' model, all the telephone support is provided by trained consumer/survivors. The crisis centre provides comprehensive training for consumer/survivors with particular language skills or cultural backgrounds to prepare them to be service providers. In this way the centre makes its service more accessible to Toronto's diverse ethno-racial community.

Systems initiatives

People who have serious mental health problems can be found in many settings outside the hospital. As with other community members, people with mental illness live in various situations in the community: by themselves or with others, in correctional facilities, in nursing homes, using shelters or living on the streets. Their situations are often complex, and in addition to serious mental health problems there may be co-existing substance abuse, a developmental disability, or physical health problems. Language and culture, social isolation, poverty, abuse and racism may also be issues and pose barriers to service.

Partnerships and alliances can reduce overlap and more effectively utilise limited resources for under-served people or unmet needs. For example, in Ontario the Ministry of the Attorney General and the Ministry of Health are working together to develop mental health court support services, a service that is already well-established in Vancouver (Wilson, *et al.*, 1995). In this scheme mental health workers (funded by the Ministry of Health) are situated in the criminal courts and work with the justice system to divert mentally disordered low-risk offenders to community supports. A brokerage model of case management is used to link people to a range of short-term and long-term supports and services.

Thus services can be provided in a variety of locations and in many different ways, and partnership and collaboration can enhance and expand service capability. The next segment of this chapter deals with a proliferating model of community-based service, case management.

Case management

Since case management is such a critical piece of a community-focused system it will be addressed in some detail. The term 'case management' is used because it has some universal understanding. However, it should be noted that many services elect to use a term more in keeping with a client-directed approach, such as 'community support'. Case management has been described as,

> 'a service that encompasses a continuum of flexible, comprehensive interventions to coordinate a fragmented system for persons with disabilities. The relationship between practitioner and client is core to case management. This relationship emphasises a client-directed partnership, maintained over time in order to provide continuity of care'.
>
> (Gehrs, 1993, p. 4)

Case management offers an effective approach for people with long-term serious mental health problems, as well as others whose needs are multiple, complex and ongoing and who require support to live in the community, such as people who have a developmental disability. In the 1970s case management was seen as a way to assist people with serious mental health problems who had spent lengthy periods in psychiatric institutions acquire mandated services from a fragmented system (Intagliata, 1982). With an early emphasis on brokerage functions, case managers initially paid little attention to their relationship with the client. It is now understood that to enable real change or recovery to occur the case manager must develop and maintain a strong working relationship which emphasises the client's potential for change (Anthony, 1993; Gehrs & Goering, 1994; Goering & Stylianos, 1988).

Still useful as a service model for people who have experienced lengthy or frequent psychiatric hospitalisations, case management has also been demonstrated to be effective with other mental health populations. These populations include mentally disordered offenders (Cooke, *et al.*, 1994; Dvoskin & Steadman, 1994; Solomon & Draine, 1995; Wilson, *et al.*, 1995), homeless mentally ill people (Wasylenki, *et al.*, 1993), and people with a dual diagnosis of mental illness and substance abuse (Drake, 1994).

While there have been significant changes, namely the emphasis on the relationship and less reliance on the use of formal mental health resources, the fundamental objectives of case management are unchanged. These objectives are:

- *Efficiency* – services are received when and where they are needed, with no gaps or overlaps
- *Effectiveness* – the goals and outcomes of the service are met
- *Accountability* – one person or agency is responsible
- *Accessibility* – the client is assisted to access services
- *Comprehensiveness* – assessment and interventions address all the client's needs
- *Continuity* – the client's needs are met in a comprehensive, coordinated and integrated way at any given time and over time, as needs change

The original core functions of case management: assessment, planning, linking, monitoring, and evaluation (Intagliata, 1982) and advocacy, now constitute the minimal or basic functions. Other functions have been added as service models evolved: assertive outreach, client identification (case finding), forming therapeutic relationships in the context of case management, system advocacy and resource development, skills development, crisis prevention and intervention, assistance with symptom/behaviour management, supportive counselling, family support and education, and public and professional education. A possible result of the emphasis on a non-threatening supportive relationship has been the increase in client report of childhood sexual abuse to case managers (Rose, 1991).

Each case management function is carried out through several activities, each of which is determined by the unique needs and situation of each client. For example, the function of linking may include any or all of the activities of making a referral, discussion with the client about how to get to the resource, arranging bus fares, ensuring adequate clothing, assisting the client in preparing a lunch to take to the resource, accompanying the client, introducing the client to others, staying with the client at the resource for a period of time for support. The case manager may seek supports to carry out many of these activities from the client's informal support system. If there are no available informal supports, the case manager will either find a formal support or perform the task herself or himself. The case manager's responsibility is to ensure that all the activities needed to effectively link the client to a resource are carried out.

Case managers require a sound working knowledge of a range of resources (formal and informal, general and specific, available and potential), and the ability to establish strong working relationships with resources. In some instances, formal agreements may be required to work effectively with some settings. An example of a formal arrangement at a service level would be a written agreement between a community-based case management service and a hospital which clearly lays out each other's roles and expectations (Pyke, *et al.*, 1993).

'Functional equivalence' is a case management approach that cobbles together two or more resources to meet a client's need. Rural and small urban areas often use this approach and they can serve as a model in the use of natural resources and supports. For example, if a client requires a supportive living arrangement, the rural case manager might find a room in a private home and arrange for interpersonal support through a church or service organisation. While smaller areas are likely to see themselves as under-resourced (and may well be), they are also more likely to see and use the potential of the larger community.

In order to effect change a certain number of contacts between the case manager and the client are needed (Dixon, *et al.*, 1993). However, Sands and Cnaan (1994) found no discernible improvement in outcome above a certain frequency, and there is some indication that extensive 'monitoring' may be detrimental (Corrigan & Kayton-Wellberg, 1993; Solomon & Draine, 1995).

Models of case management

The following description of models of case management shows how additional functions have become incorporated as 'essential' functions.

Rehabilitation, Personal Strengths and *Full Support* are the principal models described in the mental health literature in North America (Robinson, 1991). The experience of 'Joseph', a hypothetical 'typical' client, will be used to briefly illustrate key differences between these models.

Joseph is in his early 30s, he is unemployed and shares a room with two other men in a boarding house. Joseph has a diagnosis of schizophrenia, and has had several admissions to psychiatric facilities. He has been referred for case management services by an out-patient nurse who has agreed to coordinate his medical/therapeutic services.

In the *Rehabilitation model* the client's goals and needs, rather than pre-established system goals, dictate the response and services. The overall goal is to enable the client to be successful and satisfied in his or her chosen work, education, housing and social environments, relying as little as possible on resources from the formal mental health system. In this model skill training is important as it assists the client to function in these environments.

Over several meetings in a coffee shop, Shaheen, the case manager, takes time to understand from Joseph how his basic needs are being met, what his supports are, and what he likes or dislikes about his current situation and environments. One of the things she learns is that Joseph dislikes his present housing situation. Shaheen assists Joseph to identify what is important to him in housing, and learns that he values privacy and wants a room of his own, that he wants to be close to public transport and stores, and to be able to prepare his own meals.

Once they have a good understanding of what to look for, they identify the skills and resources required for Joseph to be successful and satisfied in his housing of choice. Skills would include being able to cook, to shop, to budget and to pay the rent, etc. Resources would include adequate income and some furnishings. Joseph and Shaheen review which of the skills and resources Joseph has, and which he needs to acquire. Skills can be identified through 'show or tell', and strategies devised to get resources. For example, while Joseph wants to be able to cook in his own place, he doesn't know how. He and Shaheen talk about who might teach him to cook, and discover that his sister would do this.

The *Personal Strengths model* is based on the assumption that people need assistance to get the resources that will support and develop their potential. The community is viewed as a network of resources (individuals, groups and organisations) which can improve the person's situation. Mentorship and advocacy are significant components of this model.

Ken meets with Joseph in a community setting and learns during the course of several meetings how Joseph is managing his needs and what supports he has. He learns early on in the relationship that Joseph has always wanted his own place. He also learns that Joseph has been told repeatedly by hospital staff that he could never manage by himself, and so he is returned to the boarding house after each hospitalisation. At each of their meetings, Ken identifies and reinforces Joseph's strengths, and emphasises the positive - that he could in fact learn how to live more independently. Ken and Joseph agree that he will need some support to achieve his goal, and Ken offers to talk with his colleagues about what might be helpful for Joseph. He learns about a new volunteer centre and goes with Joseph to meet the staff. They ask for a volunteer who could spend time with Joseph and assist him to find housing. After a few meetings the volunteer agrees to help Joseph find a place of his own, and later offers to introduce Joseph to other community services and supports such as the recreation centre and church groups.

The *Full Support model* combines the teaching of coping skills with clinical management and environmental support. The service is mainly provided through a multidisciplinary treatment team whose members perform specialised functions as well as general case management functions.

Pavel's role is as both a nurse and a generic case manager. When he meets with Joseph it is to assess his current situation and to review his medical/therapeutic status. A detailed history is obtained, and Pavel takes this information back to a team meeting. Pavel notes that Joseph is somewhat symptomatic and may be experiencing auditory hallucinations. Team members discuss Joseph's situation and how best his needs can be addressed by the team, including medication management and money management. It is decided that the emphasis of inter-vention at this time will be to stabilise Joseph on his medication. To do this, Pavel will arrange for Joseph's psychiatric care to be transferred to the Full Support Team. Pavel will take Joseph's medications to him every day, and monitor his response. The team discusses Joseph's expressed interest in more independent living. It is decided to assess his independent living skills once he is less symp-tomatic.

While a program may have an affinity for a particular model, most not only incorporate components of other models but also make other modi-fications. Since what works in one place is not necessarily going to be effective in another (Bachrach, 1988; Cnaan, 1994), the model needs adaptation to suit the program's particular environment, culture, economic or other situation. Case management is not any easy job, and case managers need a strong support system, adequate resources, competent supervision and opportunities for ongoing training and education.

Strengths and limitations of case management

Case management can reduce hospital days (Bigelow & Young, 1991; Holloway, *et al.*, 1995), identify and meet service needs (Goering, *et al.*, 1998), improve quality of life (Bigelow & Young, 1991), reduce family burden (Pyke & Apa, 1994), and increase the likelihood of people staying connected to mental health services (Blank, *et al.*, 1996; Harris & Bergman, 1988; Holloway, *et al.*, 1995). Because of its outreach component it is, to date, still the most effective way to connect with and serve traditionally hard-to-serve populations such as homeless and socially isolated people ((Pyke, *et al.*, 1991; Wasylenki, *et al.*, 1993).

Unfortunately there is little consistency across studies. Quality of life and functional abilities are often conceptualised differently and a variety of instruments used to measure outcomes. As well, the field continues to be confounded by the lack of a standard definition of case management, and by variances in the role description and activities of the case manager

(Bachrach, 1992; Rubin, 1992; Scott & Dixon, 1995). Despite the many methodological problems in case management research, almost all studies report the relative effectiveness of this approach.

Service outcomes reported in the literature tend to be service provider or system determined, and until relatively recently consumers were not involved in establishing service outcomes or in evaluation activities (Morrell-Belai & Boydell, 1994). The trend to more participatory research should increase the likelihood that outcomes will also reflect what service users feel are important – decent housing, a job, family and friends, happiness, health, choice, privacy and freedom (Campbell & Schraiber, 1989).

Team models and one-to-one approaches in delivering case management services each have their benefits and limitations. Case load sizes in a full support team model may be as low as 8 clients per full time equivalent (fte) staff; in a one-to-one model, 15–20 clients per fte case manager is more common. The one-to-one model is obviously more practical for areas with limited staff resources. Its primary limitations are potential difficulties for client coverage (for example during staff vacations or illness), and for stress on the case manager who at times may be the only support in a client's life. Limitations of the team model rest in the potential for over-serving the client, and the consequent limiting of use of a broader range of resources. Regardless of the model or framework of practice, the service must ensure it is serving those for whom it is intended in a way that stresses client involvement, choice and growth (Cnaan, 1994). For, while case management is an important component of an individualised and community-focused system, it is not a panacea for a disjointed mental health system, and cannot replace other resources (Baldwin & Woods, 1994).

Nursing

The challenge of change for nurses:

> The licensing body for nurses in Ontario reported that in 1995, of registered nurses in Ontario who practise mental health/psychiatric nursing, approximately 3800 work in hospitals and only 146 in community settings.
>
> (College of Nurses, 1996)

Implications for hospital-based practice

Inpatient nursing
All too often nursing attention on inpatients is focused on assessment and immediate treatment and neglects the critical area of discharge planning. Yet discharge planning is still 'one of the most important ways in which hospital settings can influence post-hospital course' (Wasylenki, *et al.*, 1981, p. 672). Discharge planning activities can range from identifying the patient's community support and resource needs and assigning staff responsibility to make sure those will be met, to direct skills teaching (Sood, Baker & Bledin, 1996).

Out-patient nursing

Hospitals may consider re-allocating staff to provide case management services. If that is so, institutional practices and commitment must be carefully considered and addressed if such a change is to be effective, integrated and maintained (Krupa, *et al.*, 1992; Pyke, 1996). A community-focused proactive approach enables nurses to identify clients' changing needs and situations, to make sure that individualised plans are developed with each client and that support is provided in a manner and environment that facilitates the client's personal growth and satisfaction. Since institutionalisation does not only occur with inpatients, the importance of supports being provided to the greatest extent possible in the community cannot be over-emphasised.

Nurses and community-based services

In the community, nurses may work for nursing organisations, for agencies that use a multidisciplinary approach, or for agencies which employ people from a range of backgrounds to perform generic functions. Regardless of the setting, nurses are likely to experience some degree of 'culture shock'. For example, hospital nurses may feel a sense of isolation when they move into community practice and may miss the easy accessibility and teamwork of institutional work (Gehrs, *et al.*, in press). In hospital settings, care and support come from service providers, each of whom, including the nurse, has a clearly defined role. By contrast in community settings, roles are much more likely to be blurred, and tasks are determined by the needs of the client and resource accessibility (including family members). Community work is also more permeable – that is, the nurse may move in and out of roles and tasks through negotiation with others as determined by the client's unique needs and situation. Also, staff in institutional settings tend to use medicalised jargon which supposedly facilitates communication, but often serves to exclude 'outsiders'. Since most community services deal less with illness and more with functioning and day to day hassles in community living, language tends to be simpler and understandable by more people, including service recipients and family members.

Short-term community support is particularly well suited to people who, while not needing the intensity of case management, might benefit from community visits for a period of time. This is often most needed after a hospital admission. People who live on their own or have few friends comment on the sense of isolation they experience upon discharge. Short-term community support can assist the person to once again establish and carry out daily activities, and assist in linking them to other services and supports.

People who need *long-term community support* are those whose serious mental health problems affect their ability to get their basic needs met and to live successfully in the community. Non-intensive support or case coordination is appropriate for people who have a range of supports and resources in place, but need someone to coordinate services, and provide continuity and accountability. More intensive long-term support is provided by services such as case management or assertive community treatment teams.

In this section the changing roles of nurses have been briefly reviewed. Regardless of the site of practice, nurses need to incorporate a community focus in their work. To assist nurses to achieve the necessary skills to work in a reformed mental health system, education and training endeavours also need to be adapted to meet these new challenges.

Nursing education, training and re-training

Some needs and issues

For some nurses, the opportunity to develop additional skills and to work in less traditional settings will be a welcome challenge. For others, change may be perceived as threatening. Experienced managers are aware that change is not an event but a process, and that staff need opportunities to express their concerns as well as their enthusiasm. The more nurses are supported to participate in the change process, the more likely they are to buy into change.

Moving from a hospital setting to other locations requires nurses to build upon what they already know (knowledge) and can do (skills). Gournay (1995) found that community mental health nurses who did not have specialised skills, who were limited in the range of services they could provide and in their understanding and use of other relevant systems such as social services, failed to have an impact on clients. Interpersonal skills, such as empathy, genuineness and openness not only seem fundamental to the establishment of a working relationship, but have been demonstrated to be clearly related to mental health clients satisfaction with service (Sheppard, 1993).

An often overlooked but critical issue is the attitudinal shift that must occur if nurses are to work with all people with serious mental health problems. Chafetz (1990) describes how the absence of a sound philosophical belief that all people have the right to service and a better life can contribute to the inability of nurses to serve some populations – for instance homeless people.

Some responses

A changing mental health system requires re-thinking the process of nursing education, theoretical orientation and interventions (Betrus & Hoffman, 1992; Bodley, 1991; Carson & Arnold, 1996; Goering, 1993). Nursing models, such as the Neuman Systems Model (Neuman, 1989), incorporate a perspective which enables the nurse to view the client within the context of a broader community. Like case management models, nursing models may also need to be adapted to suit a particular locus of practice (Davies, 1989). While the nursing literature provides useful information, nurses need to go beyond the nursing field if they are to be fully informed. Literature and publications by and about consumers and family members, the psychosocial rehabilitation literature, and systems information can all contribute to informed nursing practice. For example, as more services move into the community the ethical issues and the boundaries that define community work become critically important (Curtis & Hodge, 1994).

Meanwhile, consumers and family members remain a largely untapped resource, an issue beginning to be acknowledged in mental health nursing (Britnell & Yonge, 1996). Educational facilities might consider ways to utilise their respective experience and expertise in curriculum development and in teaching activities. Very little information is currently available on the topic of consumer involvement in staff training (Pyke, *et al.*, in press), and none was found pertaining to educational facilities. Surely, if consumer involvement is important to the development of relevant services, then consumer involvement also has value in preparing people to work in these services.

The Ontario Chapter of the International Association of Psychosocial Rehabilitation Services (IAPSRS) has been active for a number of years in promoting the principles of psychosocial rehabilitation through education and training initiatives. In 1990, the IAPSRS, Ontario Chapter, in conjunction with a community college in Toronto, developed the curriculum for a Psychosocial Rehabilitation Certificate program. This program is currently available as a continuing education program in several community colleges, offering courses in psychosocial rehabilitation, functional assessment, skills training and case management. Courses are taught by a variety of mental health practitioners and consumers. Several nurses working in community settings are involved in both curriculum development and teaching. A number of nurses, especially those working in the psychiatric units of general hospitals, have enrolled in the program.

A more recent training initiative was undertaken in south-western Ontario to prepare staff of two provincial psychiatric hospitals which were being down-sized, to work in a reformed mental health system. Nurses played a key role in developing and delivering training which would build on the existing skills of trainees, many of whom were nurses, to enable them to provide case management services. Training modules were developed for each core function of case management using the respective skill and knowledge requirements and resources listed in the Mental Health Case Management Training Resource Guide (Gehrs, 1993). Nurses, other service providers (particularly from community-based services), consumers and family members participated in developing and delivering the training.

These two training initiatives, described in a report entitled, *Case management training initiatives in Ontario: two model programs* (International Association of Psychosocial Rehabilitation Services/Mental Health Case Management Association of Ontario, 1995), have the following important features.

- The curricula were developed by service providers and consumers and based on the principles and direction of mental health reform
- The curricula recognised and built upon the skills and experience of the learners
- The training was delivered by both consumers and service providers

Another innovation was an on-the-job training project to meet the learning needs and expand the professional roles of both institution-based and community-based nurses. In this instance, a three month job-exchange project was jointly designed by a psychiatric research institute and a community-based nursing organisation, for psychiatric nurses with little community experience and community nurses with little mental health experience. The intent of this project was to enable community nurses to gain skills in order to provide home treatment for people with acute mental illness, and to better prepare hospital-based psychiatric nurses for community roles. Hospital-based nurses selected learning goals which would enhance their knowledge of community resources, lead to a better understanding of what contributes to family burden, learn how to adapt client and family interventions in the home, and deal with crises in a community setting. Each participating nurse was a learner, a teacher and a resource. The project was highly successful from both a participant and organizational perspective (Gehrs, *et al.*, in press).

Future directions for research

Several areas warranting research have been touched upon in this chapter, for example, models of service delivery and service outcomes, staff training and education. Two major areas that nursing might focus on are, cost-effective ways to train and re-train nurses to work in a reformed mental health system; and secondly, the impact of creative nursing care in a reformed mental health system. A recommended sub-set for research is the impact of the involvement of consumers in developing and delivering training, and in research and education activities.

To facilitate practice-based research, formal linkages could be established between community practice settings and educational institutions. Such linkages commonly exist between teaching hospitals and academic settings, but are less commonly seen in community settings. Since community settings rarely have any resources for research and evaluation, graduate schools might approach community mental health agencies to enquire about research needs and opportunities.

Summary

This chapter reviewed the reform process of the mental health system in Canada, particularly the province of Ontario. Mental health reform, driven as it is by fiscal restraint, will increasingly emphasise collaboration, partnerships and outcomes. Since many countries share similar struggles and have like needs, it is hoped that the service and training examples provided in this chapter will also have relevance elsewhere. Nurses can continue to make a difference in the lives of people with serious mental health problems and their families in this changing landscape. With change comes both opportunities and challenge – how nurses and nursing respond will be critical.

References

Anthony, W.A. (1993) Recovery from mental illness: the guiding vision of the mental health service system in the 1990s. *Psychosocial Rehabilitation Journal*, **16**(4), 11–23.

Anthony, W., Cohen, M. & Farkas, M. (1990). *Psychiatric Rehabilitation*. Boston: Center for Psychiatric Rehabilitation, Boston University.

Bachrach, L.L. (1988) On exporting and importing model programs. *Hospital & Community Psychiatry*, **39**(12), 1257–8.

Bachrach, L. (1992) Case management revisited. *Hospital & Community Psychiatry*, **43**(3), 209–10.

Baldwin, S. & Woods, P.A. (1994) Case management and needs assessment: some issues of concern for the caring professions. *Journal of Mental Health*, **3**(3), 311–22.

Betrus, P.A. & Hoffman, A. (1992) Psychiatric-mental health nursing: career characteristics, professional activities, and client attributes of members of the American Nurses Association Council of Psychiatric Nurses. *Issues in Mental Health Nursing*, **13**, 39–50.

Biegel, D.E., Tracy, E.M. & Corvo, K.N. (1994) Strengthening social networks: intervention strategies for mental health case managers. *Health & Social Work*, **19**(3), 206–16.

Bigelow, D.A. & Young, D.J. (1991) Effectiveness of a case management program. *Community Mental Health Journal*, **27**(2), 115–23.

Blank, M.B., Chang, M.T., Fox, J.C., Lawson, C.A. & Modlinski, J. (1996) Case manager follow-up to failed appointments and subsequent service utilization. *Community Mental Health Journal*, **32**(1), 23–31.

Bodley, D.E. (1991) Adapting supervision strategies to meet the challenges of future mental health nursing practice. *Nurse Education Today*, **11**(5), 378–86.

Britnell, J. & Yonge, O. (1996) *Position paper on mental health/psychiatric nursing*. Canadian Federation of Mental Health Nurses. (Unpublished manuscript.)

Campbell, J. & Schraiber, R. (1989) *The well-being project: mental health clients speak for themselves*. California Department of Mental Health, Sacramento.

CFMHN (1995) *Canadian Standards of Psychiatric and Mental Health Nursing Practice* 2nd ed. Canadian Federation of Mental Health Nurses.

CNA (1991) *Mental health care reform: a priority for nurses. A discussion paper on mental health care*. Canadian Nurses Association, Ottawa.

Capponi, P. (1993) *Upstairs in the crazy house. The life of a psychiatric survivor*. Viking, Toronto.

Carson, V.B. & Arnold, E.N. (1996) *Mental health nursing. The nurse-patient journey*. Saunders, Philadelphia.

Chafetz, L. (1990) Withdrawal from the homeless mentally ill. *Community Mental Health Journal*, **26**(5), 449–61.

Cnaan, R.A. (1994) The new American social work gospel: case management of the chronically mentally ill. *British Journal of Social Work*, **24**(5), 533–57.

College of Nurses (1996). Membership statistics for Ontario registered nurses in 1995. Toronto.

Cooke, A., Ford, R., Thompson, T. & Wharne, S. (1994). 'Something to lose': case management for mentally disordered offenders. *Journal of Mental Health*, **3**(1), 59–67.

Corrigan, P.W. & Kayton-Wellberg, D. (1993). 'Aggressive' and 'problem-focused' models of case management for the severely mentally ill. *Community Mental Health Journal*, **29**(5), 449–58.

Curtis, L.C. & Hodge, M. (1994) Old standards, new dilemmas: ethics and boundaries in community support services. *Psychosocial Rehabilitation Journal*, **18**(2), 13–33.

Davies, P. (1989) In Wales: Use of the Neuman Systems Model by community psychiatric nurses. In: *The Neuman Systems Model* (ed. B. Neuman). Appleton & Lange, Connecticut.

Dixon, L., Friedman, N. & Lehman, A. (1993) Housing patterns of mentally ill persons receiving assertive treatment services. *Hospital & Community Psychiatry*, **44**(3), 286–8.

Drake, R.E. (1994) Case management for people with co-existing severe mental disorder and substance abuse disorder. *Psychiatric Annals*, **24**(8), 427–31.

Dvoskin, J.A. & Steadman, H.J. (1994) Using intensive case management to reduce violence by mentally ill persons in the community. *Hospital & Community Psychiatry*, **45**(7), 679–84.

Dykes, S., Patton, M. & Tinling, P. (1990) Community treatment: An alternative to hospitalization. *Community Mental Health in New Zealand*, **5**(2), 64–76.

Gehrs, M. (Ed.). (1993) *Mental Health Case Management Training Resource Guide*. Mental Health Case Management Association of Ontario, Ontario.

Gehrs, M. & Goering, P. (1994) The relationship between the working alliance and the rehabilitation outcomes of schizophrenia. *Psychosocial Rehabilitation Journal*, **18**(2), 43–54.

Gehrs, M., Johnston, N., Chavez, F., Malone, P. & Lefebre, N. (in press) Hospital-community job exchange: an innovative nursing staff development experiment. *Journal of Nursing Staff Development*.

Goering, P. (1993) Psychiatric nursing and the context of care. In: *A Nursing Perspective on Severe Mental Illness* (ed. L. Chafetz), pp. 3–12. *New Directions for Mental Health Services*, **58**. Jossey-Bass Publishers, San Francisco.

Goering, P, Durbin, J, Foster, R., Boyles, S., Babiak, T. & Lancee, B. (1992) Social networks of residents in supportive housing. *Community Mental Health Journal*, **28**(3), 199–214.

Goering, P.N. & Stylianos, S.K. (1988) Exploring the relationship between the schizophrenic client and the rehabilitation therapist. *American Journal of Orthopsychiatry*, **58**, 271–80.

Goering, P.N., Wasylenki, D.A., Farkas, M., Lancee, W.J. & Ballantyne, R. (1998) What difference does case management make? *Hospital & Community Psychiatry*, **39**(3), 272–6.

Gournay, K. (1995) Mental health nurses working purposefully with people with serious and enduring mental illness: An international perspective. Special issue: Mental Health Nursing. *International Journal of Nursing Studies*, **32**(4), 341–52.

Habal-Brosek, C. (1995) Warmline/Hotline: Being there for those in need. Paper presented at the *International Clubhouse Conference*, Salt Lake City, Utah.

Harris, M. & Bergman, H.C. (1988) Misconceptions about use of case management services by the chronically mentally ill: a utilization analysis. *Hospital & Community Psychiatry*, **39**(12), 1276–80.

Holloway, F., Oliver, N., Collins, E. & Carson, J. (1995). Case management: a critical review of the literature. *European Psychiatry*, **10**(3), 113–28.

Intagliata, J. (1982) Improving the quality of community care for the chronically mentally disabled: the role of case management. *Schizophrenia Bulletin*, **8**(4), 655–74.

International Association of Psychosocial Rehabilitation Services, Ontario Chapter & Mental Health Case Management Association of Ontario. (1995). *Case management training initiatives in Ontario: two model programs.* IAPSRS/MHCMAO, Ontario.

Krupa, T., Eastabrook, S., Blake, P. & Goering, P. (1992) Lessons learned: introducing psychiatric rehabilitation in a multi-disciplinary hospital setting. *Psychosocial Rehabilitation Journal*, **15**(3), 29–36.

Lord, J. & Hutchison, P. (1993) The process of empowerment: implications for theory and practice. *Canadian Journal of Community Mental Health*, **12**(1), 5–22.

Mcnaughton, E. (1992) Canadian mental health policy: the emergent picture. *Canada's Mental Health*, **40**(1), 3–10.

Morrell-Belai, T. & Boydell, K. (1994) The experience of mental health consumers as researchers. *Canadian Journal of Community Mental Health*, **13**(1), 97–108.

Mueser, K.T., Glynn, S.M., Corrigan, P.W. & Baber, W. (1996) A survey of preferred terms for users of mental health services. *Psychiatric Services*, **47**(7), 760–61.

Neuman, B. (1989) *The Neuman Systems Model*, 2nd ed. Appleton & Lange, Connecticut.

Pyke, J. (1996) Case management and mental health services. *The Canadian Nurse*, **92**(7), 31–5.

Pyke, J. & Apa, J. (1994) Evaluating a case management service: a family perspective. *Journal of Case Management*, **3**(1), 21–6.

Pyke, J., Bezzina, A., Robinson, M. & Wagner, A. (1993) Reaching in, reaching out: making the connection. In: *What works! Innovation in community mental health and addiction treatment programs.* Canadian Scholars' Press Inc., Toronto.

Pyke, J., Lancaster, J. & Pritchard, J. (in press) Training for partnership. *Psychiatric Rehabilitation Journal*.

Pyke, J. & Lowe, J. (1996) Supporting people, not structures: changes in the provision of housing support. *Psychiatric Rehabilitation Journal*, **19**(3), 5–12.

Pyke, J., Samuelson, G., Shepard, M. & Brown, N, (1991) Shaping mental health services. *The Canadian Nurse*, **87**(5), 17–19.

Reissman, F. (1990) Restructuring help: a human service paradigm for the 1990s. *American Journal of Community Psychology*, **18**(2), 221–30.

Robinson, G. (1991) Choices in case management. *Community Support Network News*, **7**(3), 1, 11–12.

Rose, S.M. (1991) Acknowledging abuse backgrounds of intensive case management clients. *Community Mental Health Journal*, **27**(4), 255–63.

Rubin, A. (1992) Is case management effective for people with serious mental illness? A research review. *Health & Social Work*, **17**(2), 138–50.

Sands, R.G., & Cnaan, R.A. (1994) Two modes of case management: assessing their impact. *Community Mental Health Journal*, **30**(5), 441–57.

Scott, J.E. & Dixon, L.B. (1995) Assertive Community Treatment and case management for schizophrenia. *Schizophrenia Bulletin*, **21**(4), 657–66.

Sheppard, M. (1993) Client satisfaction, extended intervention and interpersonal skills in community mental health. *Journal of Advanced Nursing*, **18**(2), 246–59.

Solomon, P. & Draine, J. (1995) One-year outcomes of a randomized trial of case management with seriously mentally ill clients leaving jail. *Evaluation review*, **19**(3), 256.

Sood, S., Baker, M., & Bledin, K. (1996) Social and living skills of new long-stay hospital patients and new long-term community patients. *Psychiatric Services,* **47**(6), 619–22.

Stein. L.I. & Test, M.A. (1980) Alternative to mental hospital treatment: I. Conceptual model, treatment program, and clinical evaluation. *Archives of General Psychiatry,* **37**(4), 392–7.

Talbott, J.A. (1979) Deinstitutionalization: avoiding the disasters of the past. *Hospital & Community Psychiatry,* **30**(9), 621–4.

Thornicroft, G. (1991) The concept of case management for long-term patients. *International Review of Psychiatry,* **3**, 125–32.

Toews, J. & Barnes, G. (1986) The chronic mental patient and community psychiatry: a system in trouble. *Canada's Mental Health,* **34**(2), 2–7.

Trainor, J., Shepherd, M., Boydell, K.M., Leff, A. & Crawford, E. (1997). Consumer/survivor initiatives: a case study. *Psychiatric Rehabilitation Journal,* **21**(2), 132–40.

Vandergang, A. (1996) Consumer/survivor participation in the operation of community mental health programs: input or impact? *Canadian Journal of Community Mental Health.* Special Edition on Power and Oppression, **15**(2), 153–70.

Walsh, J. (1994) The social networks of seriously mentally ill persons receiving case management services. *Journal of Case Management,* **3**(1), 27–35.

Wasylenki, D, Gehrs, M., Goering, P. & Toner, B. (1997) A home-based program for the treatment of acute psychosis. *Community Mental Health Journal,* **33**(2), 151–62.

Wasylenki, D.A., Goering, P., Lancee, W, Fischer, L. & Freeman, S.J.J. (1981) Psychiatric aftercare: identified needs versus referral patterns. *American Journal of Psychiatry,* **138**(9), 1228–31.

Wasylenki, D.A, Goering, P.N., Lemire, D., Lindsay, S. & Lancee, W.J. (1993) The Hostel Outreach program: assertive case management for homeless mentally ill persons. *Hospital & Community Psychiatry,* **44**(9), 848–53.

White, D. (1992) (De)-constructing continuity of care: the deinstitutionalization of support services for people with mental health problems. *Canadian Journal of Community Mental Health,* **11**(1), 85–99.

Wilson, D., Tien, G. & Eaves, D. (1995) Increasing the community tenure of mentally disordered offenders: an assertive case management program. Special issue: International perspectives on mental health issues in the criminal justice system. *International Journal of Law and Psychiatry,* **18**(1), 61–9.

6 Mental Health Workers

Kevin Gournay

Introduction

Throughout the developed world the clinical roles and professional preparation for all professions in the field of mental health have been undergoing major transformation. In the United Kingdom a review of workforce issues was undertaken in 1997. A major issue identified in this review is the problem associated with a workforce that has, by and large, been trained for work in hospitals and institutions, who are now expected to carry out tasks in the community. Moreover, these very tasks entail working across the traditional professional boundaries. The approach taken in this chapter argues that in order to consider workforce issues, one needs to consider the context in which various mental health workers exist. In this regard there are five essential elements:

- The nature of mental illness (and how it is viewed by various professional groups)
- The location of treatment
- The method of service delivery
- The evidence base for treatment and care
- The various current roles of professional mental health workers and others.

This chapter, then, explores workforce issues in mental health across these five domains.

One approach to mental health worker training in the United Kingdom discussed here is known as the Thorn Initiative. Based upon the modules of clinical case management, psychological interventions and family work, the Thorn approach sets out to provide a contemporary solution to improving the skill base of nurse practitioners in the mental health field as they undertake their work across diverse social and professional settings.

The context of mental health practice

Nature of mental illness

There is no doubt that although the precise aetiology of various mental illnesses is still elusive, we are beginning to understand a great deal more about the respective roles of biological, psychological and social variables. A great deal of the research effort in mental illness in the last decade has been directed towards schizophrenia. Advances in brain imaging and molecular genetics have provided definitive evidence that schizophrenia is a group of diseases with a clear underlying neuropathology (Gournay, 1996). Indeed we are beginning to realise that many other mental illnesses have a central organic cause (see for example the case of obsessive compulsive disorder (McGuire, *et al.*, 1994). However we also now know that psychological and social factors may trigger episodes of schizophrenic illness and long term social recovery is strongly influenced by a number of complex variables (Warner 1995).

A detailed review of the literature is obviously out of place in this chapter, however it is worth noting that we have to recognise that there is no universally accepted model of mental illness and various professional groups are educated from widely differing theoretical standpoints. There is little doubt that these differences have practical consequences in the way that people are cared for. For example, although there is considerable evidence that educational programs for people with schizophrenia that include material on biological causation lead to greater satisfaction with mental health services (e.g. Posner, *et al.*, 1992), it is likely that many professionals, including nurses and social workers, would be uneasy about providing such educational material.

With the likelihood that both undergraduate and postgraduate education for mental health professionals will become much more unified with different professional groups sharing the same educational programmes (see below) one must hope for a less fragmented approach. For the time being most mental health professional groups have reached a compromise, accepting that all mental health problems are a mixture of the biological, the psychological and the social. In this regard models of stress vulnerability advocated by Zubin and Spring (1977) may be very helpful. This model proposes that the underlying genetic susceptibility to mental illness may be triggered by various stresses, either alone or in combination, and that these stresses may include both social and psychological factors. In turn, the illness is maintained by the interaction of biological, social and psychological factors and relapse may be produced by stress.

The location of mental health services

The deinstitutionalisation that has taken place across the world has led to a great emphasis on community care and home based treatment. Nevertheless, despite the very laudable intent that lay behind moving persons with mental illness from almost medieval conditions in the large asylums to programs of care in the community, there have been a number of very negative consequences of this relocation. For example, many American authors have described a process called transinstitutionalisation, wherein the mentally ill have moved from asylum type institutions via the community and then into prisons and poor quality (for profit) nursing homes. Although the situation in the United States is most often cited, wherein a prison population of more than 1.4 million contains tens of thousands of persons with a serious mental illness, the same phenomenon undoubtedly exists in other countries. Evidence for transinstitutionalisation in cities across the western world is found in the burgeoning business of diversion from custody schemes. Such schemes can be found not only in large cities such as London and Sydney, but in many small towns and cities. In England in 1997 more than 100 such programmes existed.

Another aspect of de-institutionalisation is homelessness and this is now being studied carefully and systematically in several cities, including Sydney (Teesson, 1996) and London (Merson, *et al.*, 1992). Thus mental health workers now need to work in a variety of community settings, including the patient's home, community mental health centres, Salvation Army hostels, and jails. This of course requires staff to work much more flexibly. The demands of working with staff from other agencies may be considerable and nurses who have spent many years working in hospitals may find the transition very difficult. However, it is now known that some patients will always require 24 hour care and although in the last 20 years the tendency has been to provide new psychiatric facilities in general hospitals, mental health workers are now finding themselves working in a number of alternative residential facilities. Experience from the United States shows that high quality care can be provided in community houses and that hospital facilities are, apart from being expensive, often viewed by users as uncomfortable and stigmatising.

An example of the way forward may be found in Boulder, Colorado USA where residential care for acutely ill patients is provided in a large house in the middle of the community. This facility has a very high staff–patient ratio, with medical cover available on a 24 hour basis and a doctor always available to attend an emergency within a few minutes. The accommodation provided is much more comfortable than one would find in a hospital setting and the cost to the mental health service is less than half of traditional hospital care. Such community houses, like many other residential facilities in the United States, are staffed by well-trained workers who are usually educated to a least first degree level. However, only a minority of these personnel have a nursing background. Some are social work graduates, while others have a degree in a relevant social science such as psychology or sociology and receive a considerable amount of in-service training in relevant skills. As we will see below, the future may well see many traditional nursing roles being undertaken by people from other professional backgrounds. Indeed, in residential facilities where the level of supervision required is not so intensive, many States in the USA now employ case manager aides who may have themselves suffered from a severe and enduring mental illness. Again, this topic will be explored in more detail below.

Service delivery

The method of delivering our services has changed significantly and in the last 25 years. Case management has become the overall method of organising the delivery of care (see Chapter 5). This development, when it is applied in optimal fashion, prevents the fragmentation of services. However a recent Cochrane review – see below (Marshall, *et al.*, 1996) highlighted the fact that case management may be applied in an ineffective way by some providers. Effective models usually comprise approaches that come under the umbrella title of Assertive Community Treatment (Santos, *et al.*, 1995). In unified case management approaches mental health workers from various professional backgrounds will realise that there is considerable overlap in their core tasks. It is interesting that in Australia and the United Kingdom, a majority of case managers have a nursing background, while, as mentioned above, in the United States the majority of case managers will come from a social work or non-professional background.

Key elements of assertive community treatment

- Use of multidisciplinary working rather than key working
- Interventions all delivered by the team rather than by others
- Interventions delivered in the community and the patient's home
- Teams work with low staff patient ratios 1: 10/15

(Marshall, *et al.*, 1996)

Evidence base

The move to providing care and treatment based in evidence from clinical trials may well provide one of the biggest challenges for mental health nursing in the next few years. World-wide, medicine is now being guided by systematic reviews of evidence. The person we have to thank for this development is Archie Cochrane, whose influential book published in 1972 *Effectiveness and Efficiency: Random Reflections on Health Services* set out some simple but very important principles. Cochrane suggested that because resources would always be limited, they should be used to provide equitably those forms of health care that have been shown to be effective in properly designed evaluations. In particular he stressed the importance of using evidence from randomised controlled trials, because these were likely to provide much more reliable information than other sources of evidence. There is now an international network of Cochrane Centres. The Australasian Centre was established at the inception of this Initiative and is based at Flinders University. The Canadian Centre is based at the McMaster University in Hamilton, Ontario and the USA has three centres in Baltimore, San Antonio and San Francisco. The United Kingdom Cochrane Centre is based in Oxford.

We are beginning to accumulate evidence on effective methods of providing care and treatment for people with various mental illnesses. However, well designed randomised controlled trials in psychiatric nursing are rare, although the future should see an increase in this method as purchasers of mental health care are increasingly asking for evidence. We must remind ourselves that medicine in general, and mental health care in particular, has been bedevilled by the use of treatments which confer no benefit whatsoever over a placebo effect but which continue to be used. A classic example in mental health is the use of counselling in primary health care. Despite numerous studies (e.g. Balestrieri, *et al.*, 1988) which show that this intervention yields no overall benefit for people with anxiety depression and adjustment disorders in primary care, it continues to be delivered. It is particularly popular with psychiatric nurses, although a large randomised controlled trial (Gournay & Brooking, 1994) showed that it is not only ineffective, but very expensive.

The Thorn Initiative

The United Kingdom program, the Thorn Initiative, was originally funded by the Sir Jules Thorn Charitable Trust to train nurses in effective interventions in schizophrenia. The first program commenced in 1992 and the funding enabled the delivery of three one-year part-time courses at two bases, the Institute of Psychiatry and the University of Manchester. In addition, the program included an evaluation component (see below). In early 1997 several other centres in the United Kingdom were set up. The program is opening its doors to members of other professions and Thorn has now become the model around which training for mental health professionals in the UK is based. Initially the idea was to focus on training in family work in schizophrenia, but as the program has developed, three core modules of training based on research outcomes have developed. These are:

- Clinical case management
- Psychological interventions
- Family work

Clinical case management

Clinical case management incorporates the principles of assertive community treatment and home based care which seem to be effective in producing clinical, social and quality of life gains (Santos, *et al.*, 1995; Andrews & Teesson 1994). Students are trained in skills using various assessment protocols so that they can reliably rate symptoms and social functioning. They are also trained in the use of standardised measures of need (e.g. the Camberwell Assessment of Need, Phelan, *et al.*, 1995). Skill training involves considerable workshop activity and the use of exercises, such as videotapes of patient interviews to assist students become more proficient at identifying specific symptoms. Our experience so far shows that trainees can achieve levels of reliability which are very similar to those attained by psychiatrists in training.

Trainees are also provided with training in medication management, including the following core components:

- Education regarding the nature and action of psychotropic drugs
- Use of educational methods for patients and families
- Use of valid and reliable scales and checklists to measure side-effects
- Use of motivational interviewing techniques (Rollnick & Miller, 1995) in dealing with treatment non-adherence

Students are also taught theory and skills regarding other aspects of clinical case management including brokering, networking and collaborative engagement with other agencies involved in the patient's care. Inter-agency working is of course an essential ingredient in clinical case management and such activities have not traditionally been the focus for nurse education. Furthermore, considerable attention is given to the issue of teamworking and this is particularly important given the difficulties which are so evident in developing community mental health teams. A recent survey of the UK's 512 community mental health teams carried out by Onyett, *et al.*, 1995 showed that staff from various professional backgrounds still have considerable difficulties in working together as a team. There is also no doubt that teamwork brings with it issues of role overlap and blurring which may be difficult for some staff to deal with. This issue was examined recently by Filson and Kendrick (1997) who showed that community occupational therapists had very similar roles to community psychiatric nurses.

As the Thorn course is part time and spread over one year, with students attending one day per week, they have ample opportunity to use their clinical experience as a method of learning. Assessment of student skill includes the use of audio-tapes of clinical contact. Students bring back examples of their patient assessments and interventions so that their teachers can provide supervision based on this material. The model of clinical supervision used on Thorn places a great deal of emphasis on a review of direct clinical work by such methods, rather than the abstract model of supervision that is used by some mental health professionals.

Psychological interventions

Effective psychological interventions are, of course, not at all new in the treatment of schizophrenia. More than 30 years ago Ayllon and Azrin (1968) showed that operant conditioning techniques based on token reinforcement could dramatically modify the behaviour of people with schizophrenia. However, token economies were beset by two major problems, the first being the high input of suitably trained staff to achieve change and second, the difficulty of generalising from the very specific laboratory-like token economy unit to the more general world. Having said that, there is no doubt that the token economy represented the first systematic attempts to develop research based psychological intervention in schizophrenia. Today's cognitive behavioural procedures all have roots in this pioneering work.

In fact, there is an array of behavioural, cognitive and cognitive behavioural techniques which can do much to ameliorate the distress suffered by those with serious and enduring mental illness. However, it must be emphasised that these procedures will only have impact if they are used in the context of a comprehensive program of care and treatment which generally includes the use of an appropriate medication.

Thorn students receive basic training in the principles of psychological intervention and by the end of the course they are able to deliver a range of treatment, with the proviso that they are in receipt of supervision from a skilled practitioner. The central elements of training are:

- Acquisition of skills in functional analysis
- The use of behavioural strategies
- The use of social skills training
- Cognitive techniques
- The principles of measurement

These elements of the training will now be examined in turn.

Functional analysis

Functional analysis underpins all effective psychological treatment and students are trained to examine specific behaviours and symptoms, within the context of various cues and triggers and consequences. Thus, for example, they are able to examine a chain of events from factors that can make a behaviour more likely, trigger a symptom, or reinforce a particular behaviour. Using a building block approach, trainees are taught to examine the whole range of symptoms and behaviours to develop a picture of how particular states may be maintained. Functional analysis skills of course include the use of behavioural observations, but students become increasingly aware that they need to listen to the patient's own story in order to understand how the particular individual experiences their illness. One particular example is that of the hallucinatory experience. The individual account of what may be a very distressing and frightening experience will tell the observer much about what makes the symptom better or worse and this will thus lead the case manager to develop various coping strategies tailored to the individual.

Behavioural techniques

Serious mental illnesses such as schizophrenia have a major effect on behaviour, not least in the common manifestation of apathy and poor motivation. Simple behavioural techniques such as reinforcement may be used to great effect, and work with families often highlights the need to examine behavioural patterns within family systems. It is often the case that families and carers need particular help in identifying behavioural goals and to be given advice regarding the use of appropriate methods of reinforcement. For many patients with schizophrenia, simple activity schedules and timetables may be very helpful and training both patient and family in the use of behavioural diaries may give the team considerable information about the patient's condition.

Social skills training

Social skills deficits are extremely common in schizophrenia and either may be caused by the illness itself or arise as a consequence of inability to practise certain behaviours because of long periods of institutionalisation (Brady, 1984). With many patients social skills deficits may be a combination of both of these factors. Social skills training comprises a number of techniques, central of which are:

- Role play of specific behaviours by the patient
- Feedback (preferably using videotape) from therapist and other patients
- Modelling (by the therapist or another patient)
- Repeat of the role play (following feedback and modelling)
- Real life practice
- Feedback of real life experience
- More role play ... and so on.

Social skills training is often given in groups; this is obviously cost effective for the therapist's time but positive group effects, such as modelling support from peers may enhance effectiveness (see Chapter 3). Social skills training in serious and enduring mental illness has been tested within a number of randomised controlled trials over the past two decades. It has been shown to produce significant clinical and social improvement. For an excellent review see Smith, *et al.* (1996). The only criticism one can justifiably level at the technique is that it needs a considerable amount of therapeutic input, often amounting to more than 100 hours of treatment time to achieve clinically significant effects.

Cognitive behavioural techniques

A number of specific cognitive behavioural strategies have been developed in the past ten years, principally targeted at reducing the distress caused by hallucinations and delusions. However, it is worth noting that people with schizophrenia also suffer from general anxiety, phobias and depression and therefore one should not overlook the usefulness of techniques such as exposure therapy or cognitive re-structuring in helping with symptoms which may cause the patient considerable distress and handicap.

Many of the techniques used for hallucinations and delusions are simple and involve the use of distraction and alternative activities. Trainees are taught to undertake a careful functional analysis of patients' symptoms and, as previously mentioned, this can become the basis for developing strategic approaches to reduce the impact of these problems. The cognitive behavioural framework is also useful in identifying relapse patterns – i.e. the 'relapse signature' which is individual to each patient. Careful identification of this pattern can allow relatives, carers and the patient themselves to become aware at a much earlier point of relapse and this allows for remedial action by the patient's case manager or psychiatrist. For a full discussion of cognitive behavioural approaches, the reader is referred to Birchwood and Tarrier (1994), or Haddock and Slade (1996) – these texts provide a comprehensive account of not only the cognitive behavioural techniques available, but also detail of the assessment methods used.

Measurement

All Thorn trainees are helped to develop skills in evaluation and, in particular to use several valid and reliable methods to monitor progress. Trainees quickly realise that measurement packages should be individualised for each patient to reflect the unique expression of symptom and handicap. In cognitive behavioural work measurement is of course integral to the total approach. The student uses the selected measures to evaluate the effectiveness of various interventions. Central to all measurement is the principle that each patient should work collaboratively with their case manager to define treatment targets.

Family work

Initially the Thorn Initiative was greatly influenced by the work on expressed emotion, e.g. Leff, *et al.* (1982). However, a more behaviourally based approach (Tarrier, *et al.*, 1988) is used in the Manchester Centre. A recent systematic review of family intervention in schizophrenia (Mari, *et al.*, 1996) concluded that family intervention reduced the rate of relapse and hospital admission as well as improving compliance with medication. However the review also showed that family burden and expressed emotion status were unchanged. It must also be said that although the review examined a group of twelve studies of family intervention, there were some differences between the interventions used in the various trials. This area perhaps exemplifies the need to continue examining the evidence and to refine methods of treatment. For example, Solomon (1996) in her own literature review of family interventions has argued that treatments based on an expressed emotion paradigm may have a limited range of applicability. Conversely, she argues that brief focused family education might actually be a much more effective strategy, reaching much larger populations and producing a greater overall return for investment.

There has been some systematic evaluation of the Thorn training. Although the programe has yet to be tested by randomised controlled trial, these preliminary data are very encouraging. All trainees are required to identify four patients with serious mental illness on their caseload and for the first three years of the Thorn Initiative (1992–95) an independent evaluator measured symptoms and social functioning on all these patients at the beginning of the student's training and at the end. Students also collected data on their patients using measures of symptom and social functioning. By the summer of 1996, 101 students had entered the Thorn Programme and 85 had completed training. Early analysis of the data shows that there are improvements in positive, negative and affective symptoms and social functioning. Other measures also show that trainees acquire both skill and knowledge as a result of attending the Thorn Programme.

Nurse behaviour therapy

The psychiatrist Professor Isaac Marks is perhaps the most important individual in the development of advanced clinical roles for nurses in mental health in Britain. In 1972 he started a pilot course to train nurses in behavioural psychotherapy at the Maudsley Hospital, London. Five registered mental nurses undertook the full time program in behavioural psychotherapy for severe neurotic disorders between 1972 and 1975. These nurses developed skills in behavioural assessment and intervention for people with agoraphobia, obsessive compulsive disorders, specific and social phobias, social skills problems and various habit disorders such as tics, stammering and enuresis. In addition nurses were also provided with training in the management of sexual dysfunction (e.g. premature ejaculation, vaginismus and dyspareunia) and the management of other problem sexual behaviours such as exhibitionism and paedophilia. This programme, which was based on principles of intensive apprenticeship, focused on the acquisition of skills by a process of modelling, video feedback and real life practice. The course emphasised the use of tried and tested interventions such as exposure in vivo and response prevention within the setting of rigorous evaluation. Nurse therapists were trained in the use of valid and reliable measures of change, but also, then as now, each case treated involved a careful functional behavioural analysis that led to the definition of individual problems and target behaviours.

Problems targeted by nurse therapists

- Agoraphobia
- Obsessive compulsive disorder
- Specific phobias
- Social phobias
- Social skills problems
- Habit disorders
- Sexual dysfunctions
- Problem sexual behaviours

After this initial piloting the program became established in 1975 as an 18 month full-time training and continues to run at the Maudsley Hospital/ Institute of Psychiatry. In addition, the program has also been run at several other training centres across the UK and approximately 300 nurses have undergone this training between 1972 and 1996. Newell and Gournay (1994) conducted a 20-year follow up study of nurse therapists in the UK and obtained data on 113 of 142 eligible respondents. This survey found that the majority of nurse behaviour therapists remain in clinical practice after training and continue to further their education and develop clinical expertise. The study showed that over the years there has been a general shift towards the use of cognitive and short term interventions and towards practice based in primary care with general practitioners providing nurse therapists with most of their referrals.

Two decades ago Marks and colleagues (1977) showed that nurse therapists were as effective as experienced psychiatrists and psychologists and Marks (1985) went on to test the training within the context of a randomised controlled trial and economic analysis. This study showed that nurse therapists' treatment leads to very substantial clinical gains for patients in terms of symptom reduction and also increases social and occupational functioning. At the same time the economic analysis showed very substantial gains for both the patient and the health care system.

Given the very large numbers of people with conditions which have been shown to be responsive to behavioural psychotherapy (Marks, 1987; Gournay, 1995; Goldberg & Gournay, 1997) it is easy to see how much greater numbers of nurse therapists could be fully occupied in treating people with these conditions. However there are only small numbers of nurse therapists available and this situation is likely to maintain for the foreseeable future. There are major arguments for suggesting that nurse behaviour therapists should not restrict themselves to solely providing a direct treatment service. There are three key areas where nurse therapists can ensure that their behavioural skills are put to the greatest effect:

- The training of practice nurses and other general nurses in the treatment of anxiety disorders
- The dissemination of computer based approaches
- The use of other self help methods, including working with the various self help organisations

Expansion into these areas will, of course, require training to be given to nurse therapists in addition to that which they received in clinical skills. For example, the training of practice nurses obviously means that nurse therapists will have to acquire teaching skills and while this should present no real problems for most therapists, there is still a real training requirement in terms of the time and resource that needs consideration. Similarly, with the growth of computerised self help programs and the use of virtual reality approaches many nurse therapists will need fairly considerable training input concerning the use of information technology.

Outcomes of training

The nurse behaviour therapy program mentioned above stands out as an exception in that its trainees have been subject to careful controlled evaluation. Nevertheless, even this well researched program has very little data on the acquisition of skill per se and we can only speculate about what particular clinical skills are more or less important in determining patient outcomes. In the area of serious mental illness there is little well-controlled evidence regarding training outcomes. Brooker, *et al.*, 1994 showed that CPNs can be trained to deliver family interventions in schizophrenia. However it must be said that overall the gains from this intervention are arguably modest compared with the gains achieved by nurse behaviour therapists with neurotic populations. However, even if one accepts that family intervention with schizophrenia is an effective treatment, there is some research that shows that the central problem is that the treatment is not being applied after training. David Kavanagh and colleagues (1993) followed up a group of mental health professionals who had received training in family interventions in New South Wales. Rather depressingly they found that in the period after the training course graduates were either carrying out very little of the interventions in which they were trained, or only using the interventions in an altered form.

Now that clinical effectiveness has been rightly raised in its importance, surely we must also apply the same rules to training programmes that we apply to interventions. One difficulty is that the research outcome studies on interventions usually report an ideal situation wherein the intervention is delivered by highly trained workers who have been specially selected and prepared within the context of the research project. Furthermore, research studies usually have detailed treatment protocols that help to ensure that the intervention is effectively delivered. Of course the vast majority of clinical interventions given in services are not provided in this ideal way and therefore one needs to consider the differences which may exist between the research and clinical settings. Ideally, evaluations of training should use the randomised controlled trial as the ultimate test, randomising trainees into either the training intervention or a wait list control and then using both measures of skill on the trainees themselves and outcomes measures on the patients they are allocated to. Within such a design it then becomes possible to use the trainees who have been on a waiting list to serve as their own controls and for outcomes to be compared within this group between the period prior to training and then in the period after training. Clearly such evaluations are expensive and are not presently budgeted for within the research resource of any country in the world. However, it could be argued that if more attention was given to the efficacy, or otherwise, of training programmes there would, in the long run be a substantial cost benefit for the health care system. Moreover, such investment would ultimately lead to a great improvement in the lives of patients by ensuring that they receive the best of interventions.

Training for user case managers

For more than a decade case manager aides, who have themselves had a history of a mental health problem, have been trained within a number of programs in the USA. This initiative started in Denver, Colorado and research on this innovation was first reported by Sherman and Porter (1991). This team have developed a comprehensive program that includes the careful analysis of the prospective user case manager aides' own learning needs. The student then embarks on a comprehensive course which includes both theory and skills input. Students are provided with a range of knowledge concerning mental health problems and their mani- festations, drug treatments, legal aspects and so on. However, the success of the program probably rests on the tremendous effort put into proper preparation of the workplace and ongoing supervision. The Denver team recognised, quite rightly, that one of the major problems for user case manager aides would be resistance from other mental health workers and the setting up of various obstacles within the workplace. The trainers, therefore, took great pains to spend time in the workplace so that they could deal with problems first hand and prepare the environment prior to the user case manager being allocated to that setting for experience. The Denver program lasts one year and the data from the aforementioned 1991 paper and unpublished results (Porter, *personal communication*) are most encouraging. Overall these results show that user case management aides enhanced the benefits of the service given to clients, while at the same time the mental health status of the user case management aides themselves improved with little evidence of effects of stress or burnout on these personnel. The United States is obviously ahead of the rest of the world in these developments, but it is true to say that the user movement worldwide is a growing phenomenon. Hopefully, developments such as the Colorado Project, which can be seen in 30 of the states of the USA, will now spread to the rest of the world.

Future priorities for training

Future areas for training will to some extent be dictated by the accumulation of evidence of efficacy for various treatments. Thus, for example, the recent innovative work by Kemp, *et al.* (1996) in the use of treatment packages to enhance medication compliance in schizophrenia, should lead to greater numbers of nurses being trained in the various skills which make up this package (i.e. family education and the use of motivational interviewing). Given that non-compliance rates with medication have been estimated at between 50% and 80% (Bebbington, 1995) there is without doubt a priority for training as many mental health workers as possible in these strategies.

Another very important area is that of dual diagnosis, i.e. people with serious mental illness with a drug or alcohol problem. Recent research in the UK has suggested that up to 40% of people with schizophrenia in communities also have a drug and alcohol problem (Menezes, *et al.*, 1996). Furthermore, we are aware that this rising tide is something for which our services are not prepared (Gournay, *et al.*, 1997). However, there is some evidence that properly trained and prepared teams may have an impact on this population (Drake, *et al.*, 1993; Bartels, *et al.*, 1995). Although this work has been mainly carried out in the USA, some training initiatives are being developed (e.g. the University of Woolongong in New South Wales and the Institute of Psychiatry in London). These training programs emphasise the need to target both the serious mental illness and the substance abuse problem within the same service, rather than the traditional approach of separating out the two parts of the problem and subjecting the person to interventions by different therapists or treatment teams. The approach of dual diagnosis treatment is based on non-confrontational methods, emphasising the probability that the process of engagement with the patient may take many months. Workers with this population will need to be trained to a high level of skill and given the very large numbers of patients with a dual diagnosis the implications for workforce planning are considerable.

Conclusion – the future

This chapter is being completed at the time when a national review of roles and training for all the mental health professions in the UK is being published. This document *Pulling Together* (Sainsbury Centre for Mental Health, 1997) was the result of 18 months' work of a steering group of which the author was a member. This group commissioned several pieces of research and obtained written and oral evidence from a wide array of professional organisations and other interested parties. The implications of this review will not be restricted to the United Kingdom, as the work defines various difficulties associated with community care which are present across the whole world. These problems include the problems associated with a workforce which has, by and large, been trained for work in hospitals and institutions, who are now expected to carry out tasks in the community. Furthermore, these tasks involve working across the traditional boundaries that have, until now, demarcated professional roles. It is now true that nurses are now carrying out clinical tasks which were previously the responsibility of clinical psychologists, and are engaged in the assessment of mental health problems using the same procedures that were once the sole province of psychiatrists. At the same time, many of the caring duties, which were once seen as synonymous with nursing are carried out by non-nurses, including health care assistants, occupational therapists and social workers. *Pulling Together* showed that all professions have their own problems with education and training. For example, social work, across the world, has struggled with its philosophical roots; however, thankfully, the rhetoric of R.D.Laing is being replaced by that of evidence based case management.

All countries in the Western world have realised that the separation of health and social care for those with serious and enduring illness, is an artificial divide and boundaries between professions need to be softened and then dissolved. In some of the model services of the United States, all professions work harmoniously together in community mental health teams. However, in a great majority of services, the story is a familiar mixture of case management delivered cheaply by under-trained staff, or of office based psychiatry funded by insurance policies or cash, highlighting the divide between 'haves and have-nots'. In the United Kingdom and Australia the polarisation evident in the United States is not so extreme, nevertheless across the Western world community care faces the challenge of shrinking resources. Despite the depressing backdrop of shrinking resources, there are certainly some beacons of light. Initiatives such as the Thorn program offer fresh hope to sufferers and this model may well be adopted more widely. However, such developments will surely lead to a re-definition of professional roles and perhaps the generic mental health worker will eventually emerge as a replacement for many of today's mental health workers.

References

Ayllon, T. & Azrin, N. (1968) *The Token Economy: A Motivational System for Therapy and Rehabilitation*. Appleton-Century-Crofts, New York.

Andrews, G. & Teesson, M. (1994) Smart versus dumb treatment: services for mental disorders. *Current Opinion in Psychiatry*, **7**, 181–5.

Balestrieri, N., Williams, P. & Wilkinson, G. (1988) Specialist Mental Health treatment in general practice: a meta analysis. *Psychological Medicine*, **18**, 711–17.

Bartels, S., Drake, R. & Wallach, M. (1995) Long term course for substance misuse disorder among patients with severe mental illness. *Psychiatric Services*, **46**, 3, 248–51.

Bebbington, P. (1995) The content and context of compliance. *International Clinical Psychopharmicology*, **9**, 5, 41–50.

Birchwood, M. & Tarrier, N. (1994) *Psychological management of schizophrenia*. John Wylie, London.

Brady, J. (1984) Social skills training for psychiatric patients, I: concepts, methods and clinical results. *American Journal of Psychiatry*, **141**, 333–40.

Brooker, C., Fulloon, I., Butterworth, A. *et al.* (1994) The outcome of training of community psychiatric nurses to deliver psychosocial intervention. *British Journal of Psychiatry*, **165**, 222–30.

Cochrane, A. (1972) *Effectiveness and Efficiency: Random Reflections on Health Services*. Nuffield Provincial Hospitals Trust, London.

Drake, R., Bartels S. & Teague, G. (1993) Treatment of substance misuse in severely mentally ill patients. *Journal of Nervous and Mental Disorder*, **181**, 606–11.

Filson, P. & Kendrick, T. (1997) Survey of roles of community psychiatric nurses and occupational therapists. *Psychiatric Bulletin*, **21**, 2, 70–73.

Goldberg, D. & Gournay, K. (1997) The GP the Psychiatrist and the burden of Mental Health care. *Maudsley Discussion Paper*, Institute of Psychiatry/Maudsley Publications, London.

Gournay, K., Sandford, T., Johnson, S. & Thornicroft, G. (1997) Dual diagnosis of severe mental health problems. *Journal of Psychiatric and Mental Health Nursing*, **4**, 89–95.

Gournay, K.J.M. (1995) Management of anxiety states. *Nursing Times*, **91**, 45, 29–31.

Gournay, K.J.M. (1996) Schizophrenia: a review of the contemporary literature and implications for mental health nursing theory practice and education. *Journal of Psychiatric and Mental Health Nursing*, **3**, 1, 7–12.

Gournay, K. & Brooking, J. (1994) Community Psychiatric Nurses in Primary Health Care. *British Journal of Psychiatry*, **165**, 231–8.

Haddock, G. & Slade, P. (1996) *Cognitive Behavioural Interventions with Psychotic Disorders*. Routledge, London.

Kavanagh, D., Clark, D., Piatkowska, O., *et al.* (1993) Application of cognitive behavioural interventions for schizophrenia: what can the matter be? *Australian Psychologist*, **28**, 1–8.

Kemp, R., Hayward, P., Applewhaite, G., *et al.* (1996) Compliance, therapy and psychotic patients: a randomised controlled trial. *British Medical Journal*, **312**, 345–9.

Leff, J., Kuipers, L., Berkowitz, R., *et al.* (1982) A controlled trial of intervention in the families of schizophrenic patients. *British Journal of Psychiatry*, **141**, 121–34.

Marks, I., Connolly, J., Hallam, R. & Philpott, R. (1977) *Nursing in Behavioural Psychotherapy*. RCN Publications, London.

Marks, I. (1985) *Nurse Therapists in Primary Care*. RCN Publications, London.

Marks, I. (1987) *Fears, Phobias and Rituals*. Oxford Publications, London.

Mari, J., Adams, C., Streiner, D. (1996) *Family Intervention for those with Schizophrenia*. The Cochrane Library, BMJ Publications, 23 February 1996.

Marshall, N., Gray, A., Lockwood, A. & Green, R. (1996) *Case Management for People with Severe Mental Disorders* The Cochrane Library, issue 3, updated 26 February 1996.

McGuire, P., Bench, C., Frith, C., *et al.* (1994) Functional anatomy of obsessive compulsive disorder. *British Journal of Psychiatry*, **164**, 459–68.

Menezes, P., Johnson, S., Thornicroft, G., *et al.* (1996) Drug and alcohol problems among individuals with severe mental illness in South London. *British Journal of Psychiatry*, **168**, 612–19.

Merson, S., Tyrer, P., Onyett, S., *et al.* (1992) Early intervention in psychiatric emergencies: a controlled trial. *Lancet*, **339**, 1311–14.

Newell, R. & Gournay, K. (1994) British nurses in behavioural psychotherapy: a 20 year follow up. *Journal of Advanced Nursing*, **20**, 53–60.

Onyett, S., Pillinger, T. & Muijen, M. (1995) *Making Community Mental Health Teams Work*. Sainsbury Centre Publications, London.

Phelan, M., Slade, M., Thornicroft, G., *et al.* (1995) The Camberwell Assessment of Need. *British Journal of Psychiatry*, **167**, 589–95.

Posner, C., Wilson, K. & Kralm (1992) Family Psycho-education support groups in schizophrenia. *American Journal of Orthopsychiatry*, **62**, 206–18.

Rollnick, S. & Miller, W. (1995) What is motivational interviewing? *Behavioural Psychotherapy*, **23**, 4, 325–34.

Sainsbury Centre for Mental Health (1997) *Pulling Together*. Sainsbury Centre Publications, London.

Santos, A., Scott, W., Burns, B., *et al.* (1995) Research on field based services: models for reform. *American Journal of Psychiatry*, **152**, 8, 1111–23.

Sherman, P. & Porter, R. (1991) Mental health consumers as case manager aides. *Hospital and Community Psychiatry*, **42**, 5, 494–8.

Smith, T., Bellack, A. & Lieberman, R. (1996) Social skills training for schizophrenia: review and future directions. *Clinical Psychological Review*, **16**, 7, 599–617.

Solomon, P. (1996) Moving from psycho-education to family education for families of adults with serious mental illness. *Psychiatric Services*, **47**, 12, 1364–70.

Tarrier, N., Barraclough, C., Vaughn, C., *et al.* (1988) The Community Management of Schizophrenia: a controlled trial of a behavioural intervention with families to reduce relapse. *British Journal of Psychiatry*, **153**, 532–42.

Teesson, M. (1996) *An Evaluation of Mental Health Service Delivery in an Inner City Area*. Thesis, School of Psychiatry, University of New South Wales, Sydney.

Warner, R. (1995) *Recovery from Schizophrenia*. Routledge, London.

Zubin, J. & Spring, B. (1977) Vulnerability: a new view of schizophrenia. *Journal of Abnormal Psychology*, **86**, 260–66.

7 Nursing Care for Children and Adolescents with Mental Health Disorders, and their Families

Mary E. Evans

Nurses must be able to tolerate a considerable amount of ambiguity and change when caring for children and adolescents with mental health disorders and supporting their families. Like the children themselves, mental health services is a developing field. Uncertainty exists, for instance, in the number of children and adolescents with mental health disorders. In the United States, a study funded by the National Institute of Mental Health (NIMH) is currently being planned to determine the prevalence and incidence of child mental health disorders, the use of mental health services, and the costs associated with service use (Hoagwood, 1995). This study is expected to be a companion to the Epidemiological Catchment Area study conducted a number of years ago that provided systematic information on adult mental disorders (Robins & Regier, 1991). Until the NIMH study is completed, the field of child and adolescent mental health will continue to work with rough estimates. Among these are data from eight community studies in various countries that indicate 14% to 20% of children have moderate to severe mental health disorders (Brandenburg, *et al.*, 1990). A review of nine population surveys conducted in the 1980s and reviewed by Rog (1995) indicates that 14% to 26% of children and young people less than 18 years of age have some type of behavioural, emotional or developmental problem. Friedman, *et al.* (1996) reviewed the extant literature on estimating the size of the population of children with serious emotional disturbance. They concluded that between 9% and 19% of children meet the criteria for this designation. Despite the apparent need for mental health services, it is estimated that only 20% to 30% of children who have been identified as in need of services actually receive them (Office of Technology Assessment, 1986). Cox (1993) notes that in developed countries 80% to 90% of children with emotional and behavioural disorders do not receive speciality mental health services.

There is also considerable ambiguity regarding the causes of childhood mental disorder, and the contributions made by physical, environmental and societal factors, and their appropriate remediation. Not so ambiguous, however, is the significant minority of children experiencing emotional or behavioural disorders that respond to mental health interventions. Also apparent, as noted by the popular and professional press, is the increasing saliency of these disorders and their impact on public mental health and society. Societal issues under discussion, for example, include the number of children with learning disabilities and the cause of these disabilities, the effects of violence and socially toxic environments on children, possible overmedicalisation of acting-out behaviours, post-traumatic stress disorder following sexual abuse, and dual substance abuse and mental health disorders.

Few persons interested in the health and well-being of children would dispute the importance of preventing mental health disorders when possible and making available high quality, effective interventions for children who do develop emotional or behavioural disorders. Nurses, because of their focus on health promotion and family-focused care in diverse settings represent an important resource in providing effective care to children and their families. Nursing research is critical in determining the effectiveness of interventions and the quality of care provided to children and their families.

Historical context

An emergent understanding of the identification and treatment of mental disorders in children and adolescents is derived from the changing role of the child in developed countries. In the United States, for example, until the late 1800s and early 1900s, children were viewed primarily in economic terms. They contributed to the family income and well-being as they were able by working in the fields or sweat shops. Many were apprenticed at young ages to learn trades such as butchering, sewing, or metal working. Children with significant disabilities were viewed as burdens to their families because they failed to contribute economically, while continuing to consume family resources. With the development of institutions for poor and disabled children, these children were often placed out-of-home where they could receive treatment and/or custodial care at state or philanthropic organisation expense.

The late 1800s saw an increase in immigration, providing cheap labour, which, when coupled with the use of machinery and improved production methods led to material goods being produced more efficiently than with child labour. Concomitant with the declining need for child labour, secondary schools were being developed at public expense. A rise in the number of secondary schools was associated with the prolongation of childhood into adolescence and an increase in leisure time for young people. Thus, the major role of the child changed from that of an economically contributing member of the family to that of the student. A child's job then was to become educated and to make a socioemotional rather than economic contribution to the family. Accordingly, early in the 1920s the worth of children who were injured or killed in accidents shifted from lost earnings to pain and suffering experienced by their families (Zelizer, 1994).

Because of the increasing emphasis on the socioemotional role of children in the family in the 1920s and 1930s, more attention was paid to their emotional well-being and behaviour. Child guidance clinics were developed to foster children's mental health and the parenting abilities of their caregivers. Children with more disabling mental health problems were institutionalised or received inadequate care in the community. It was not until 1912 that the Boston Psychopathic Hospital, now the Massachusetts Mental Health Center, became the first hospital in the United States to accept children into their outpatient clinic (Taylor, 1982). The first article on childhood schizophrenia, published in 1933, was followed by a slow recognition, yet inadequate response, to the seriousness of childhood mental disorders. The Post-World War II baby boom produced a large number of children and adolescents, which resulted in increased attention to the mental health of these children.

For decades following World War II, however, society failed to recognise that children with the most severe disorders received the most inadequate care. A number of national conferences that focused on the mental health needs of children were held and recommendations derived from these meetings were made, but little action was taken. This changed when Jane Knitzer (1982) wrote *Unclaimed Children*, which described the inadequacy of the care provided to children who could be identified as having serious emotional disorders and the unwillingness of society to claim these children and to provide adequate care for them. As a consequence of her work, in 1984 the US Congress provided funds to establish the Child and Adolescent Service System Program (CASSP). This program permitted each of the states to acquire a small amount of money to hire a staff member to plan a coordinated multiagency approach to providing care for children with serious emotional disturbances. In the United States, CASSP has changed the way many providers organise and deliver their services. The guiding principles of this program are listed and discussed later in this chapter (see Fig. 7.1 System of care philosophy).

Changes in nursing practice

According to Finke (1994), the importance of quality psychiatric nursing care was recognised and supported by federal funding as early as the 1940s. Such funding was targeted primarily toward including principles of psychiatric care into nursing curricula. In general, however, recognition of the field of child and adolescent mental health nursing lagged behind that of adult mental health nursing. The first graduate program in child psychiatric nursing in the United States was opened in 1954 at Boston University (Yorker, 1994). Mereness (1982), in the foreword to the 11th Edition of her classic and widely used text (*Mereness' Essentials of Psychiatric Nursing*), notes that a chapter on children and adolescents was not added to the text until the 8th Edition, published in 1970, at which time the text was 30 years old.

Although the field of children's mental health lacks a critical analysis such as that done by Morrissey and Goldman (1984) in tracking the cycles of reform in the care of adults with chronic mental illness, it can be safely assumed that nurses were providing care for children in hospitals, clinics and other institutions before the movement to develop intensive community services for children and their families. Since CASSP in the United States and community service programs in other countries, psychiatric nurses have been wherever the children are: in schools, homes, camps, clinics, hospitals, group homes, residential treatment facilities, and other living and learning environments for children. The focus of their interventions has changed over time from being child-centered to family-centered, recognising that children are usually embedded within the context of a family and that the caregivers are partners in providing treatment and support to children and adolescents with mental disorders.

While the use of psychotropic drugs has increased over time and the popularity of particular therapeutic interventions has waxed and waned, the roles of the nurse have shown stability. Nursing's language has changed from identifying problems to making diagnoses and from the child's needs to the child's and family's strengths. McBride's (1986) assessment is that psychosocial nursing has played a major role in encouraging nursing as a profession to make the conceptual shift from a focus on the individual to family-centered care and that this shift may become one of the distinguishing characteristics of the profession.

Intervention frameworks

Three primary frameworks prove useful for guiding nursing interventions directed toward children and adolescents with mental disorders and their families. These are the nursing process, the use of self through multiple roles, and multidisciplinary, cross-system collaborations, such as those comprising CASSP. Each of these is discussed below and the reader is referred to other sources of information about each.

The nursing process

As within other nursing specialities, the nursing process guides the approach to identifying and meeting the therapeutic and life goals of the child and family. The steps of this process – assessment, diagnosis, planning, intervention, and evaluation – are described in greater detail elsewhere (Alfaro-LeFevre, 1994; Carpenito, 1995; Gettrust & Brabec, 1992). When applied to the care of children and adolescents with emotional and behavioural problems, particularly when the child and caregiver are active partners, the nursing process can be a powerful tool for identifying goals and diagnoses and intervening successfully.

In working with children and families, it is important to remember that interventions often require participation by persons from child-serving agencies other than mental health, such as schools or social services. Many interventions are family and/or environmentally focused to establish a supportive context for the child. The selection of interventions also offers the opportunity to individualise care, including the use of flexible service money to meet particular child and family needs (Dollard, *et al.*, 1994).

Role utilisation

In implementing a nursing care plan, the nurse functions in a number of roles, often several simultaneously. These may include: creator of a therapeutic environment, socialising agent, counsellor, parent surrogate, technician, therapist, case manager and advocate. Many of these roles have particular saliency when caring for children and families and all must be implemented based on an understanding of the child's developmental stage and the cultural background of the child and family.

Creator of a therapeutic environment

The creation of a therapeutic environment is particularly challenging in settings over which the nurse has little control, for example in schools and at home. Increasingly, however, children are receiving care in these settings rather than in more structured therapeutic settings such as hospitals and residential schools. Much of the nurse's work in establishing and maintaining the therapeutic environment occurs with caregivers and teachers. A basic requirement of a therapeutic environment for children and adolescents is one in which they feel safe and are safe from abuse and neglect. Establishment of such an environment may require teaching behaviour management and homemaking skills to the primary caregiver, using respite care, being a role model for the caregiver, and providing support by a parent advocate or mentor who has raised a child with an emotional or behavioral problem. Parent advocates or mentors provide support, role modelling and information to caregivers of children with emotional and behavioural disorders (Evans, *et al.*, 1994).

Socializing agent

Learning social skills, having opportunities for socialisation and having prosocial functioning fostered are particularly important for children. Nurses often function as role models and teachers and help to create situations in which children can practice skills and experience success. Meal times and other structured events, for instance, provide opportunities to impart social skills and to provide role modelling. Learning to interact socially and modifying behaviour to meet clearly defined limits are critical skills for children and adolescents to develop.

Counsellor, parent surrogate and therapist

Functioning as a counsellor and parent surrogate who provides affection and guidance are fundamental skills in caring for all children. Research by Weissman and Appleton (1995) indicates that hospitalised adolescents saw nurses as persons who provided comfort and nurturing. Functioning as a therapist is a frequent role for nurses caring for children and adolescents with emotional or behavioural problems. Nurses provide individual, group, family and milieu therapy in a variety of settings including private practice.

Technician

Technical nursing skills include administration of medications and other treatments. These are fundamental nursing skills, but they may require modification because of the emotional and physical needs of the child with a mental health problem, for example children with diabetes mellitus and a mental disorder are more challenging to care for than if either of these conditions existed alone. As in other areas involving nursing of children, implementation of the technical aspects of care requires knowledge of child growth and development.

Case manager

Case management is a role of increasing importance with the move toward managed care (see Chapter 5). Historically, nurses have seldom seen case management as their primary role except in community health nursing settings. Such a role was most often carried out by the social worker and involved obtaining and coordinating services for individuals. With the current emphasis on community-based care and the necessity to coordinate such care, case management may represent an emergent role for the nurse (Evans, *et al.*, 1993). Thus, as nurses continue to move into this evolving role, a number of models of case management will likely guide their actions (see Chapter 5). The use of case management models and the extension of nursing services to children with serious emotional disorders in the community could be expected to improve the continuity of care. Moreover, because of nursing's holistic perspective, it will function to shift the focus of intervention from a child to the family in its social and environmental context.

Advocacy

Advocacy at multiple levels, from case-specific to all children with emotional and behavioural problems, is strongly linked with case management. Nurses may also be members of child advocacy organisations and may be actively involved in political action to improve care and quality of life for children with special needs.

Multidisciplinary, cross-system collaborations: nursing in a system of care

It is generally recognised by those providing services to children with emotional and behavioural disorders and their families, that children are embedded within families, attend schools, often in special education programs, and may have contact with juvenile justice, social service agencies, recreational services, substance abuse services, and general health care practitioners. To meet the needs of children and adolescents, particularly those with serious emotional disturbance, a system of care approach is required to offer comprehensive care in an efficient manner. In the United States the principles and values of such a system of care were first articulated by Stroul and Friedman (1986). These values and principles, which continue to guide the development and evaluation of systems of care today, appear in Fig. 7.1.

Core values

1. The system of care should be child-centered and family focused, with the needs of the child and family dictating the types and mix of services provided.
2. The system of care should be community based, with the locus of services, as well as management and decision-making responsibility, resting at the community level.
3. The system of care should be culturally competent, with agencies, programs, and services being responsive to the cultural, racial and ethnic differences of the population they serve.

Guiding Principles

1. Children with emotional disturbances should have access to a comprehensive array of services that addresses their physical, emotional, social, and educational needs.
2. Children with emotional disturbances should receive services in accordance with the unique needs and potential of each child and guided by an individualised service plan.
3. Children with emotional disturbances should receive services within the least restrictive, most normative environment that is clinically appropriate.
4. The families and surrogate families of children with emotional disturbances should be full participants in all aspects of the planning and delivery of services.
5. Children with emotional disturbances should receive services that are integrated, with linkages between child-serving agencies and programs and mechanisms for planning, developing and coordinating services.
6. Children with emotional disturbances should be provided with case management or similar mechanisms to ensure multiple services in a coordinated and therapeutic manner and that they move through the system of services in accordance with their changing needs.
7. Early identification and intervention for children with emotional disturbances should be promoted by the system of care to enhance the likelihood of positive outcomes.
8. Children with emotional disturbances should be ensured smooth transitions to the adult service system as they reach maturity.
9. The rights of children with emotional disturbances should be protected, and effective advocacy efforts for children and adolescents with emotional disturbances should be promoted.
10. Children with emotional disturbances should receive services without regard to race, religion, national origin, sex, physical disability, or other characteristics, and services should be sensitive and responsive to cultural differences and special needs.

Fig. 7.1 System of care philosophy.

The system of care as conceptualised by these guiding principles provides the basis for the development, implementation, operation and evaluation of systems of care at various levels from the local community to state or province levels. The role of nursing, as with any other professional discipline within this system of care, has not been specifically identified and nurses function at all levels from case management to state or province level system administration. The values and principles underlying the system serve to guide practice and to encourage collaborative efforts to achieve optimal outcomes for children and their families.

Research and the system of care

Nurses are increasingly taking a role in research on the outcomes of systems of care. While this type of research is in its infancy, there is a sense that the best available research should guide the development of systems of care. The most comprehensive evaluation of the outcomes of a system of care has been done by Bickman and his colleagues (Bickman, *et al.*, 1995), who studied a continuum of mental health services at Fort Bragg in North Carolina. Their evaluation compared case management at Fort Bragg to a more traditional system of care at Fort Campbell in Kentucky and Fort Stewart in Georgia. The continuum of services at the demonstration site was based on the principles and values of the system of care as articulated by Stroul and Friedman (1986). Four substudies comprised the evaluation: an implementation study, a quality study, a mental health outcomes study, and a cost/utilisation study. The evaluation showed that the demonstration site successfully implemented a continuum of care, which increased access to care. In the demonstration site, children were successfully treated in less restrictive environments and parents and adolescents were more satisfied with the services than parents and adolescents at the more traditional sites. There were, however, no clear differences in clinical outcomes across sites, while there were substantially higher costs per child at the demonstration site. This finding called into question the advisability of developing comprehensive systems of care in view of the emphasis on public fiscal accountability. There have been numerous debates, regarding the outcomes and what they mean, particularly for publicly funded mental health systems (see Friedman, 1996; Evans & Banks, 1996; Burchard, 1996; Henggeler, *et al.*, 1996; Weisz, *et al.*, 1996; Kingdon & Ichinose, 1996; Bickman, *et al.*, 1996).

Because this is only one study and because it focused on a continuum of mental health services, rather than a system of care across child-serving systems, systems development continues and additional evaluation efforts have been initiated. In the meanwhile, the focus has shifted somewhat to an examination of the outcomes associated with innovative programs based on system of care principles and the best practices information derived from these studies.

Best practices and nursing interventions

In recent years, a number of models of service delivery and specific interventions have resulted in positive outcomes for children and adolescents. Areas supported by recent research findings include prevention of and early intervention for mental health problems, case management, individualised services, intensive in-home services, treatment foster care, and psychotherapy and related interventions. In regard to the outcomes associated with child mental health interventions, there has been considerable discussion in the field regarding the importance of moving from efficacy studies to effectiveness studies (Clarke, 1995; Hoagwood, *et al.*, 1995).

Efficacy studies refer to those in which the investigator exercises considerable control over selection of the sample, delivery of the intervention and other conditions under which the intervention occurs. This approach characterises laboratory studies, clinical research studies and drug research, which often involves random assignment to treatment condition and sometimes participant blinding to the intervention. Effectiveness research, on the other hand, refers to studies in which a known efficacious intervention is examined with a more heterogeneous sample in a naturalistic setting. Such studies are often referred to as clinical trials in field settings, research demonstrations or services research. Meta-analyses suggest that psychotherapy, for example, is quite effective with children and adolescents under laboratory conditions, although significantly poorer outcomes are experienced in general outpatient settings (Weisz & Weiss, 1989; Weisz, *et al.*, 1995).

Because nursing is conducted in naturalistic settings and the nurse seldom has complete control over the environment and the client population receiving services, our practice is guided primarily by effectiveness research and the studies that are discussed in the following section represent primarily effectiveness research.

Prevention of mental health problems

Because of diagnostic and measurement issues, the effectiveness of prevention efforts related to mental disorders is more difficult to assess than for physical disorders. The Institute of Medicine report on *Reducing Risks for Mental Disorders* (Mrazek & Haggerty,1994) adapted a classification system on interventions that includes prevention, treatment and maintenance. In this model, therapeutic interventions are provided to persons who may meet or nearly meet the diagnostic level specified by a standard nosology, such as the United States National Center for Health Statistics's *International Classification of Diseases* (ICD)(1978). In other words, prevention is not confined to interventions that occur before the initial onset of a disorder, but also refers to interventions that reduce the length of the disorder, halt the progression of severity and recurrence, and reduce the likelihood of co-morbidity. With regard to the timing of prevention interventions, Kazdin (1993) argues that adolescence presents an important opportunity for such activities because of the transitional nature and disequilibrium normally experienced during this developmental stage. Interventions, including nursing interventions, should focus on improving competence and/or ameliorating dysfunction clearly specifying short-term and long-term goals. The follow-up period for assessment should be long enough to determine the enduring effects of the interventions as the young person moves into adulthood.

Currently, the lack of prospective epidemiological data on the incidence and prevalence of mental disorders and specific risk factors in childhood and young adulthood limits the ability to develop effective ways of preventing mental disorders. An additional challenge is the lack of appropriate instrumentation for accurately diagnosing mental disorders in young children. These issues may have slowed, but have not halted work in developing prevention interventions, particularly those for conditions such as conduct disorder and depression.

Risk and protective factors do not tell the whole story regarding the development or prevention of psychopathology. Grizenko and Fisher (1992) note that it is necessary to understand the developmental and situational mechanisms involved in the development of psychopathology. They advise that it is important to examine the way in which one variable, like aggressive behaviour in boys, increases the exposure to risk factors, such as parental disapproval and severe punishment. Such an examination may shed light on related developments, such as a chain reaction that prolongs the risk, with resulting oppositional defiant behaviours and association with a deviant peer group. Nursing assessment should, therefore, focus on examining relationships among risk and protective factors as well as identifying individual risk and protective factors.

Nursing has a holistic approach to individuals and strongly supports health promotion activities, thus making prevention interventions important nursing activities. This is as true of nursing for children, adolescents and families as it is in other areas of nursing practice. In the recent past, prevention and early intervention efforts with children and their families employed a clinical perspective in which child outcomes were seen as dependent on the presence or absence of parental pathology. The role of professionals, such as nurses, in the intervention was to conduct an assessment and to develop the remedial intervention, which might include parental counselling, support groups and behaviour modelling. The field is now moving more toward a social system perspective that applies a more family-focused approach (Darling & Darling, 1992). Family assessment is used by professionals to determine the family's definition of the situation. Interventions are then developed consistent with the family's definition of what is appropriate. Assessment includes the identification of family strengths as well as needs, making this perspective compatible with the nursing process approach.

Prevention interventions in early childhood and school

Many prevention and early intervention activities have been focused in preschool or school settings or have an educational focus, for example, Head Start, an early educational experience for children from socially and economically disadvantaged backgrounds. Additional work in schools has focused on prevention or reduction of aggressive behaviour, heavy drug use and depression through an intervention in first and second grades called the Good Behavior Game (Kellam, *et al.*, 1994). This intervention has been shown to have positive short-term effects in reducing aggressive behaviour, as compared to both active and passive control groups, and to show enduring, significant positive effects six years later as children enter middle school.

Partnerships between preschool educators and social workers have been used to reach out to families with preschool children enrolled in programs for disadvantaged children (Edlefsen & Baird, 1994). Such partnerships might reasonably include a nurse whose speciality in mental health could contribute knowledge about child development, parent-child communication skills, ways to foster child self-esteem, and information on child-rearing and discipline.

An interesting program of research conducted by Olds and his colleagues (1988) focused on improving the life course development of socially disadvantaged mothers. It was based on the premise that healthy mothers foster the development of healthy children. The original research randomly assigned women who had just given birth to their first child to an intensive home visitation program conducted by nurses or to a comparison condition of free transportation to health services and/or developmental screening for the child. The experimental program began during pregnancy and involved nurses establishing therapeutic relationships with the women. The focus was on a woman's personal strengths and the home visits continued through to the child's second birthday. The study found that, during the first four years following the child's birth, women in the experimental condition who had not graduated from high school returned to school more rapidly. Those who were poor and unmarried also showed a significant increase in the number of months employed and had significantly fewer subsequent pregnancies, postponing the birth of a second child an average of 12 months longer than women in the comparison group.

The results suggest that nurses may be able to produce improvements in many aspects of mother and child functioning that have generally been the province of several separate services. Cox (1993) reports on similar successful interventions in the UK using health visitors, often community child psychiatric nurses, or specialist nurse practitioners.

Prevention of specific mental disorders

An example of a program of prevention research targeted toward a particular mental disorder was conducted by Clarke and his colleagues (Clarke, *et al.*, 1995). The research was designed to determine whether unipolar depressive disorder can be prevented in both a general population of adolescents and a group of adolescents at risk of the disorder. Adolescents with elevated depressive symptomatology were assigned to either a cognitive group prevention intervention or a usual care control condition. The research showed that depressive disorder could be successfully prevented among adolescents who were at risk of this disorder.

Case management

Children and adolescents with serious emotional disturbances require a number of services to improve their functioning and maintain them in least restrictive environments. As noted earlier, case management plays an important role in assessment of need, linkage to services, coordination of services, and provision of ongoing support for the child and family. Case management can be defined as a mechanism for linking and coordinating segments of a system of care. Burns, *et al.* (1995) have identified seven case management models for children. These models are displayed in Fig. 7.2.

Generalist/ Service Broker Model

Primary Therapist Model

Interdisciplinary Team Model

Comprehensive Service Center Model

Family as Case Manager Model

Supportive Care Model

Volunteer as Case Manager Model

Fig. 7.2 Types of Case Management. (Models identified by Burns, B. J., Gwaltney, E. A. , & Bishop, G. K. (1995) Case management research: issues and directions. In: *From Case Management to Service Coordination for Children with Emotional, Behavioral, or Mental Disorders: Building on Family Strengths* (eds B.J. Friesen & J. Poertner), pp. 353–72. Paul H. Brookes Publishing Co, Baltimore.)

In the generalist/service broker model, the case manager is a human services professional responsible for services coordination who obtains services for the child and family based on identified need. In the primary therapist model, the case manager is a professional who provides a particular therapeutic intervention, such as cognitive behavioural therapy. A team approach is used in delivering services through the inter-disciplinary team model and one person, whose professional background varies from case to case, is usually designated as having the primary responsibility for assisting the client through the service system. In the comprehensive service system model, a lead agency such as mental health or child welfare provides basic services and linkage to services in other agencies and service sectors. The final three models use either the family, other citizens in the community or professionally trained volunteers as the case manager.

Despite the prevalence of case management, few studies have systematically investigated the outcomes for children with emotional and behavioural problems. Using a quasi-experimental design, Evans and her colleagues (Evans, *et al.*, 1993; Evans, *et al.*, 1994; Evans, *et al.*, 1996) have reported reduced hospitalisation, increased community tenure, and improved functioning in children enrolled in an intensive case management program across New York State, compared to a matched sample of eligible children who were not enrolled. Burns and her colleagues (Burns, *et al.*, 1996) found positive outcomes from a randomised field trial of case management in North Carolina. Young people with serious emotional disturbance were randomised to a multi-agency treatment team with a case manager or to a multi-agency team led by the young person's primary mental health clinician. Young people with case managers had longer participation in services, used a wider variety of services, had fewer inpatient days, used more community-based services, had increased parental satisfaction and had decreased use of alcohol. Additional research is needed to examine the outcomes of various models of case management and to explore whether differential outcomes are achieved when nurses, rather than social workers or other professionals, function as case managers. Currently only 3% of the intensive case managers employed by the statewide program in New York are registered nurses, but there are many opportunities for nurses in case management positions.

Case management as typically implemented in mental health settings focuses on a client, for example on an adolescent with a serious emotional disturbance such as conduct disorder and learning disabilities. Based on CASSP values, even when the system of care is child centred, it should be family focused and families should be full participants in all aspects of the planning and delivery of services. This is intuitively appealing because adult caregivers are generally responsible for seeking services and agreeing to specific treatments for their child and ensuring that the child complies with the treatment plan. Adult caregivers are often critical participants in the treatment plan, delivering reinforcements for positive behaviour, teaching skills, administering medications, and keeping records of the child's behaviour, to name a few activities. It makes sense, therefore, that case management should be family centred to support the individuals caring for the child and to make modifications in the child's physical and social environment. Support for the family unit and improvements in the home environment might also have an impact on the health and development of the siblings of the child client. This is a high priority area for research.

Based on initial research on intensive case management and principles of individualised care, Evans and colleagues modified the generic intensive case management model in New York State to be more family focused, creating Family-Centered Intensive Case Management (FCICM) (Evans, *et al.*, 1994). The features of FCICM included use of low caseloads (eight families), a parent advocate, flexible service money ($2000 per family per year), behaviour management skills training for parents, support groups and respite care. The latter service was available in the family's home or out-of-home on a planned or emergency basis. Assessment, linkage and advocacy continued to be important components of FCICM, as did 24-hour-a-day, seven-day-a-week availability of the case manager. Children aged 6 to 12 years who were referred to a multidisciplinary team for out-of-home placement in treatment foster care and whose families were willing to participate in a research demonstration were randomly assigned to

FCICM or treatment foster care. The study showed that children, even those referred for out-of-home placement, could be kept in their own homes with family support. Over the 18-month follow-up period, children remaining at home were not disadvantaged in terms of their self-esteem, functioning, symptoms and behaviour, and their families experienced the same levels of cohesion and adaptability as families who had placed their child in treatment foster care.

Individualised services

One of the CASSP principles is that children with emotional disturbances should receive individualised services in accordance with their unique needs and potential. In the field of children's mental health individualised services are sometimes referred to as 'wraparound', a process approach to service delivery whose goal is to do whatever is necessary to keep children at home or in their local communities in least restrictive settings. Innovative services and supports such as classroom companions, flexible service dollars, respite care, and paid companionship are examples of non-traditional supports that are employed in the wraparound process. There has been little research reported on the outcomes associated with the use of wraparound although some initial findings have been published recently (see Clark & Clarke, 1996), including positive findings for children in foster care (Clark, *et al.*, 1996) and schools (Eber, *et al.*, 1996).

It is of particular importance that nurses are familiar with the concept of individualising services through a wraparound process, as employing this approach to care may be effective in keeping children in least restrictive environments. Nurses are skilled in working with agencies and families to identify what it would take to keep a child in a particular environment. Nursing process is compatible with the wraparound process and wraparound may be a useful concept for nurses caring for children in many different types of settings.

Intensive in-home services

For many years the primary settings for the delivery of mental health services to children and adolescents were hospitals and outpatient clinics or health professionals' offices. There has been a movement over the last decade to provide service in more normalised environments such as schools (US Department of Education, 1995) and homes. In-home services have often been patterned after the Homebuilders model of family preservation, which was developed in Tacoma, Washington (Kenny, *et al.*, 1977), for child welfare populations. Such programs involve low caseloads and teach families problem solving, communication, and crisis management skills. Currently, there is a paucity of information regarding the modifications made in program models when they are used for child mental health populations and little is known about the child and family outcomes. Two programs of research in the United States are beginning to identify program outcomes.

Evans, Boothroyd and Armstrong (1997) conducted a randomised field study in the Bronx, New York, an area of intense urban poverty. In the study, children presenting at psychiatric emergency rooms and judged appropriate for in-home services were randomly assigned to one of three in-home programs. One program, Home-Based Crisis Intervention (HBCI), was a classic Homebuilders program with counsellors carrying caseloads of two families for a period of four to six weeks. A second program, Enhanced Home-Based Crisis Intervention (HBCI+), was a modification of Homebuilders, with added in-home and out-of-home respite care, a parent advocate, parent support group, flexible service money, and staff training in cultural competence and issues related to working and living in environments with high levels of violence. The third program, Crisis Case Management (CCM), was a short-term adaptation of intensive case management and featured respite care and flexible service money. All three were short-term (four to six weeks) interventions targeted to children and adolescents experiencing a psychiatric crisis and their families. Counsellors and case managers included nurses and social workers who had received specialised training in one of the program models. The outcomes of this research, recently completed, include short-term (at the end of the intervention) and longer-term (at six month follow-up) gains in self-esteem for all children. Preliminary analyses also show gains in family adaptability and cohesion in the HBCI and HBCI+ conditions which begin to degrade over time. Children who were at risk of hospitalisation and restrictive placement were successfully maintained in their normative environments at the six month follow-up. Further analyses of differential outcomes associated with the three interventions and a cost analysis study are pending.

Working with a slightly different population, Henggeler and his colleagues (Scherer, *et al.*, 1994) have shown Multisystemic Family Therapy (MST) to be effective in reducing delinquent behaviour in adolescents and cost-effective because less time is spent in restrictive service settings (jail). MST is based on a family-ecological system approach to delinquency and psychopathology, viewing the adolescent as embedded within multiple systems. The therapeutic efforts of the therapists are focused on changing transactions within and between these systems (Henggeler, *et al.*, 1986). The intervention is typically short-term, about three months, and therapists are supervised intensively. Having shown MST to be effective with juvenile offenders in both rural and urban areas, Henggeler (1994) is now conducting a randomised study in which young people aged 12 to 18 years presenting to an urban psychiatric emergency service and identified as needing immediate hospitalisation are randomly assigned to either inpatient care or MST.

The opportunities for psychiatric mental health nurses to engage in these types of intensive in-home interventions are likely to increase over the next several years as health care systems shift to managed care approaches. With an emphasis on cost containment, fewer children will be admitted to hospitals and admissions will be shorter as a greater variety of community-based services are developed. There is likely to be greater emphasis on strengthening social supports to permit children to remain in normative environments rather than placing them in more costly, restrictive residential settings.

Treatment foster care

There are some children with serious emotional disturbances who are not able to live with their natural families for some period of time. An option for these children is placement in treatment foster care homes where professional parents, who have received special training needed to care for children with mental disorders, provide care for them until they can be reuinited with their families or until another appropriate living arrangement can be found. A popular model of treatment foster care is based on a cluster model developed at People Places (Bryant, 1983). To achieve the program's goals, treatment parents are grouped in clusters of five treatments and one respite home. Only one child is placed in each treatment home and an intensive matching process is used before placement occurs. Members of the clusters meet with a family specialist, usually a master's level mental health professional, regularly for training and support. The family specialist works with the child's natural family to prepare them for reunification, when that is the goal, or for other placements.

New York State's version of treatment foster care, Family-Based Treatment (FBT), is based on this cluster model. An evaluation of FBT showed that placement tends to be relatively long (Huz, *et al.*, 1994). Children who were discharged had been in foster placement for an average of 17 months. Enrolment in the program was associated with a decrease in admissions to state psychiatric inpatient care during and following discharge from FBT. Follow-up research (Evans, *et al.*, 1994) shows that children aged 6 to 12 years enrolled in this program made gains in functioning and showed a significant reduction in symptoms at 6, 12, and 18 month follow-up periods.

Nurses are actively involved in providing therapy to children who are enrolled in FBT and could easily function as treatment parents or family specialists. In addition to the team building done by family specialists, they teach parenting skills (Snodgrass, 1986) and work intensively with natural families and community agencies. These tasks and roles are comfortable for nurses and the community setting provides the additional advantages of autonomy and the opportunity for creativity within the professional role.

Psychotherapy and related approaches

Taken in its broadest sense, psychotherapy encompasses a wide range of interventions whose purpose is to decrease or eliminate problem behaviour and to improve prosocial functioning. What these approaches share in common is the reliance on interpersonal interaction, counselling or activities that follow a specific treatment plan, and a focus on how people feel, think and act (Kazdin, 1994). Psychotherapy and related approaches can vary widely in the settings where they are offered, who is seen in treatment, the training of the therapists, and the mediums of treatment, for example, talking or play therapies. In his review, Kazdin (1988) identified over 230 different treatment techniques in use for children and adolescents, most of which have not been studied empirically. A number of meta-analyses have been conducted and they indicate that psychotherapy is better than no treatment (Kazdin, 1994) although its effects appear to be of greater magnitude under controlled rather than less controlled conditions (Weisz & Weiss, 1989).

Treating aggressive behaviour disorders

Aggressive, antisocial and conduct disorders are the problems most frequently seen in clinical practice with children and adolescents (Kazdin, et al., 1990). Currently, four promising approaches to the treatment of children and adolescents with aggressive behaviour exist. The first approach, problem-solving skills training, focuses on how children approach situations, teaches them to engage in a stepwise approach to solve interpersonal problems, and uses structured tasks such as games to teach skills. The therapist role models the stepwise process, provides cues to prompt the child to apply the process and provides the child with feedback regarding behaviour. When this approach is used in structured settings such as group homes, it may be important that all caregivers are consistent in working with the children to reinforce a child's skill in using the stepwise process.

A second approach showing positive outcomes is parent management training in which parents are taught to modify their child's behaviour at home. The focus is on altering the interaction patterns between parent and child to promote prosocial behaviour. The behaviour that will be the target of the change effort must be identified (*assessment*). Parents then learn positive and negative reinforcement procedures, negotiation skills and contracting procedures (*interventions*). These interventions are practised and their outcomes as experienced in the home are reviewed with the therapist (*evaluation*). Because this type of intervention takes place in the home, it may be embedded within program models such as FCICM and treatment foster care.

The third approach is family therapy with its focus on the family as a system. Therapeutic approaches vary widely but often include an emphasis on improving communication among family members and teaching negotiation and problem solving skills. Henggeler's MST, described above as an in-home intervention, extends these approaches beyond the family to extrafamilial systems such as the school and com-munity.

The final approach is treatment based in school or community settings. In general, these interventions involve the same techniques used in other approaches. The setting, however, often changes the focus from a single child with aggressive behaviour to larger numbers of children who can benefit from acquiring prosocial behaviours. Particularly in adolescence, school and community-based interventions can make use of peer pressure to reinforce newly acquired positive behaviours.

Nurses in a number of settings are actively involved in all of these interventions. Their roles vary from being a primary therapist to providing consultation to teachers and others working directly with children engaged in aggressive and antisocial behaviour. As with other behaviour problems, use of the nursing process, use of a variety of nursing roles, and knowledge of a system of care perspective are important in working successfully with children with aggressive and antisocial behaviour, and their families.

Future directions

The challenges for psychiatric mental health nursing in the future are related to three major trends (Pothier, *et al.*, 1990). These are the increasing number of persons diagnosed with mental illness, the shift from a psychological to a biological and neurochemical model of mental illness, and changes in the organisation and delivery of mental health care. Future directions in nursing children and adolescents with mental health problems must be responsive to these challenges. Possible future directions will be examined for the areas of education, practice and research.

Education

At the present time, few undergraduate curricula in nursing have significant psychiatric theory and clinical laboratory experiences for students. This may be the result of past curricular decisions that integrated psychiatric content into the curriculum and provided experience in applying principles of psychiatric nursing in non-psychiatric clinical settings. To attract students to this speciality area, the undergraduate content may need to be increased and additional graduate programs may be required. Most graduate programs offering specialisation in psychiatric mental health nursing provide content and practice in adult mental health. Although the core principles may be the same, specialisation in child mental health would require additional coursework and specialised clinical experience. Finke (1994) suggests that tracks or options for child mental health could be developed within graduate programs that are currently orientated towards adult mental health. As a foundation, students specialising in child mental health would need a background in normal growth and development and abnormal psychology focused on childhood. Coursework in sociology related to social problems, deviance and family would be helpful. Also of importance would be information on substance abuse. Graduate coursework might include courses on child psychopharmacology and neurophysiology as well as physical and behavioural assessment skills related to children and adolescents.

Supervised practice in clinical settings where children are found is essential, and a broad range of settings should be available. Because children with mental disorders receive services from a number of child-serving agencies at varying levels of restrictiveness, students should be exposed to these agencies and settings to develop the knowledge and skills necessary to work collaboratively as team members. In particular, experience might be gained in the following settings:

- Juvenile court and group homes
- Foster care or treatment foster care homes
- Custody hearings
- Parent support groups and parent organisations
- Day treatment, in-home and special education programs
- Supervised outpatient experience in psychotherapy and play therapy
- Head Start and early childhood settings
- Acute and longer-term in-patient experience

Case management experience is valuable in following children and families across multiple services and agencies. Work with homeless families, migrant families, or immigrant families may also be a useful experience in promoting an understanding of the relationships between social and economic factors and mental health. In all settings, the cultural diversity of the families with whom students work should be maximised in order to prepare them to work effectively with the increasingly diverse population in many practice settings.

Practice

It seems likely that the next few years will see an expansion of nursing responsibilities across a variety of settings. With managed care's focus on cost containment, as mentioned earlier, an expansion in the numbers and types of intensive community-based alternatives to hospital care is likely to occur. Nurses may assume additional responsibilities for conducting initial assessments of children referred for evaluation and treatment of emotional and behavioural problems and for screening children and adolescents in general practice settings for the presence of significant psychiatric disabilities and developmental delays. This will require enhanced assessment skills and flexibility regarding work setting.

In managed care environments, children who are admitted to inpatient settings are likely to be more acutely ill and have shorter hospital stays than in the past. Nursing's challenge will be to design and implement short-term interventions for the child and to establish relationships with family and other service providers to ensure a safe, therapeutic environment for the child at discharge. Pharmacological interventions will probably grow increasingly more targeted and nurses will be engaged in teaching caregivers about these drugs and related monitoring. More nurses will be employed in community settings providing in-home and school-based services. This will present a number of challenges to nurses including gaining relevant skills and maintaining an identification with the nursing profession. These challenges are balanced by the promise of greater autonomy and opportunities for advanced practice.

Research

The nature and scope of nursing research studies may change as psychiatry moves more toward biochemical and neurological research and the health care system is altered in its organisation, delivery and financing of services. Efficacy studies on treatment and prevention interventions are likely to remain popular.

Multidisciplinary, large-scale evaluations of system change efforts are likely to become more common. The challenge to move efficacious interventions from the laboratory into communities and systems of care will continue and nursing, hopefully, will be engaged in effectiveness studies. Studies that include cost-effectiveness and other cost analyses will become increasingly common. Because of the complex nature of systems and natural environments, nursing may need to change its approach to teaching research skills to graduate students and to fostering research activities of faculty. Specifically, nurses may be engaged in multidisciplinary research projects with a larger number of investigators from various disciplines than they have in the past. Collaborative research experiences, rather than solo experiences, may prove useful in socialising students for their eventual research role.

It is wise for nurses to remain up to date about gaps in research and priorities of funding agencies. A number of organisations have prepared lists of priority areas for research (for example, United States National Institute for Mental Health, 1990; National Institute on Nursing Research, 1996) and gaps in knowledge have been identified. Hoagwood and Hohmann (1993), for example, list several areas of high priority as identified in the *National Plan for Research on Child and Adolescent Mental Disorders* (National Institute of Mental Health, 1990). Examples of these areas include hospitalisation and residential treatment of children and adolescents, school/mental health interface, and cost containment and reimbursement mechanisms. The National Institute for Nursing Research (1996) has identified current areas of special interest including community-based nursing models, approaches to remedy or prevent cognitive impairment, and biobehavioural factors and interventions that promote immuno-competence.

Because of the relationship between the economic health of countries, the political climate and the funds available for research, it is difficult to foresee what resources will be available to support nursing research. The concerns about future funding come at an important time for nursing, which has recently acquired a critical mass of doctorally prepared nurses who engage in research and theory development. Nurses will need to increase the diversity of agencies from which they seek funding to support scholarly work and will likely need to request larger amounts of money to conduct increasingly complex projects.

Summary

Although the incidence and prevalence of childhood mental disorders have not been determined definitively, it is apparent that these disorders are relatively common and that too few of the children who could benefit from services actually receive them. Prevention interventions and interventions targeted toward remediation of specific disorders or behaviours, such as aggressive behaviours, have been shown to be efficacious, and some have been shown to be effective. Nurses have important roles to play in improving the lives of children and adolescents with emotional and behavioural problems and their families. These roles include case finding, prevention, intervention, case coordination, role modelling and advocacy. To be most effective nurses must use the nursing process and assume various roles in providing care while maintaining a system of care perspective.

It is always difficult to predict the future and is especially difficult now with the accelerated rate of change in health care delivery systems. It would seem to be reasonable, however, to prepare additional child mental health nurses. Children are being underserved and a number of prevention interventions and other interventions will continue to be developed to improve children's functioning and the quality of life for them and their families. Because of the growing emphasis on cost containment in the health care system, additional emphasis may be placed on prevention, early intervention and provision of services within homes and communities, rather than in hospitals and residential settings. Nurses have a long history of providing care in many settings including homes and schools and are, therefore, well-suited to providing services in these settings in the future. To be most effective, nurses working with children and their families will require additional knowledge, especially knowledge gained through research, regarding children and enhanced skills in physical and developmental assessment. Continuing education will become critical to keeping up with new behavioural and pharmacological interventions. Research conducted by nurses is expected to become increasingly complex and to involve multidisciplinary teams. As with other disciplines, nursing will continue to develop as a profession through the demonstration of effective approaches informed by the nursing process and confirmed by research.

Acknowledgements

The author acknowledges the generous and critical assistance of Paul G. Hillengas, Elizabeth A. Pease, and Paula Plew in the preparation of this manuscript.

References

Achenbach, T.M. (1991) *Manual for the Child Behavior Checklist 4–12 and 1991 Profile.* University of Vermont, Department of Psychiatry, Burlington, VT.

Alfaro-LeFevre, R. (1994) *Applying Nursing Process*, 3rd edn. J.B. Lippincott, Philadelphia.

Bickman, L., Guthrie, P., Foster, E.M., Lanbert, E.W., Summerfelt, W.T., Breda, C. & Heflinger, C.A. (1995) *Managed Care in Mental Health: The Fort Bragg Experiment*. Plenum Publishing, New York.

Bickman, L., Lambert, E.W., Summerfelt, W.T. & Heflinger, C.A. (1996) Rejoinder to questions about the Fort Bragg evaluation. *Journal of Child and Family Studies*, **5**, 197–206.

Brandenburg, N.A., Friedman, R.M. & Silver, S.E. (1990) The epidemiology of childhood psychiatric disorders: Prevalence findings from recent studies. *Journal of the American Academy of Child and Adolescent Psychiatry*, **29**, 76–83.

Bryant, B. (1983) *Special Foster Care: A History and Rationale*. People Places, Verona, VA, unpublished.

Burchard, J.D. (1996) The Fort Bragg managed care experiment. *Journal of Child and Family Studies*, **5**, 173–6.

Burns, B.J., Farmer, E.M.Z., Angold, A., Costello, E.J. & Behar, L. (1996) A randomized trial of case management for youths with serious emotional disturbance. *Journal of Clinical Child Psychology*, **25**, 476–86.

Burns, B.J., Gwaltney, E.A. & Bishop, G.K. (1995) Case management research: Issues and directions. In: *From Case Management to Service Coordination for Children with Emotional, Behavioral or Mental Disorders: Building on Family Strengths* (eds B.J. Friesen & Poertner), pp, 353–72. Paul H. Brookes Publishing Co, Baltimore.

Carpenito, L.J. (1995) *Handbook of Nursing Diagnosis*. 6th edn. J.B. Lippincott, Philadelphia.

Clark, H.B. & Clarke, R.T. (1996) Special issue on wraparound services. *Journal of Child and Family Studies*, **5**, 1–116.

Clark, H.B., Lee, B., Prange, M.E. & McDonald, B.A. (1996) Children lost within the foster care system: Can wraparound service strategies improve placement outcomes? *Journal of Child and Family Studies*, **5**, 39–54.

Clarke, G.N. (1995) Improving the transition from basic efficacy research to effectiveness studies: Methodological issues and procedures. *Journal of Consulting and Clinical Psychology*, **63**, 718–25.

Clarke, G.N., Hawkins, W., Murphy, M., Sheeber, L.B., Lewinsohn, P.M. & Seeley, J.R. (1995) Targeted prevention of unipolar depressive disorder in an at-risk sample of high school adolescents: A randomized trial of a group cognitive intervention. *Journal of the American Academy of Child and Adolescent Psychiatry*, **34**, 312–21.

Cox, A.D. (1993) Preventive aspects of child psychiatry. *Archives of Disease in Childhood*, **68**, 691–701.

Darling, R.B., & Darling, J. (1992) Early intervention: A field moving toward a sociological perspective. In: *Sociological Studies of Child Development* (eds P.A. Adler & P. Adler), **5**, 9–22, JAI Press, Greenwich, CT.

Dollard, N., Evans, M.E., Lubrecht, J. & Schaeffer, D. (1994) The use of flexible service dollars in rural community-based programs for children with serious emotional disturbance and their families. *Journal of Emotional and Behavioral Disorders*, **2**, 117–25.

Eber, L., Osuch, R., & Redditt, C.A. (1996) School-based applications of wraparound process: Early results on service provision and student outcomes. *Journal of Child and Family Studies*, **5**, 83–99.

Edlefsen, M. & Baird, M. (1994) Making it work: Preventive mental health care for disadvantaged preschoolers. *Social Work*, **39**, 566–73.

Evans, M.E., Armstrong, M.I., Dollard, N., Huz, S., Kuppinger, A. & Wood, V. (1994) The development and evaluation of treatment foster care and family-centered intensive case management in New York state. *Journal of Emotional and Behavioral Disorders,* **2,** 153–87.

Evans, M.E. & Banks, S.M. (1996) The Fort Bragg managed care experiment. *Journal of Child and Family Studies,* **5,** 169–72.

Evans, M.E., Banks, S.M., Huz, S. & McNulty, T.L. (1994) Initial hospitalization and community tenure outcomes of intensive case management for children and youth with serious emotional disturbance. *Journal of Child and Family Studies,* **3,** 225–34.

Evans, M.E., Boothroyd, R.A. & Armstrong, M. I. (1997) The development and evaluation of an experimental study of the effectiveness of intensive in-home crisis services for children and their families. *Journal of Emotional and Behavioral Disorders,* **5,** 93–105.

Evans, M.E., Huz, S. & McNulty, T.L. (1993) Intensive case management for children and youth with serious emotional disturbance: An emergent role for nursing? *Journal of the New York State Nurses Association,* **24,** 4–8.

Evans, M.E., Huz, S., McNulty, T.L. & Banks, S.M. (1996) Child, family, and system outcomes of intensive case management in New York State. *Psychiatric Quarterly,* **67,** 273–86.

Finke, L.M. (1994) Child psychiatric nursing: Moving into the 21st century. *Nursing Clinics of North America,* **29,** 43–8.

Friedman, R.M. (1996) The Fort Bragg study: What can we conclude? *Journal of Child and Family Studies,* **5,** 161–8.

Friedman, R.M., Kutash, K. & Duchnowski, A.J. (1996) The population of concern: Defining the Issues. In: *Children's mental health: Creating systems of care in a changing society* (ed. B.A. Stroul), pp. 69–96. Paul H. Brookes Publishing Co, Baltimore.

Gettrust, K.V. & Brabec, P.D . (1992) *Nursing Diagnosis in Clinical Practice: Guides for Care Planning.* Delmar, Albany, NY.

Grizenko, N. & Fisher, C. (1992) Review of studies of risk and protective factors for psychopathology in children. *Canadian Journal of Psychiatry,* **37,** 711–21.

Hallfors, D., McQuide, P., Brach, C. & Hutcheson, C. (1996) *First Steps: A Guide to Integrating Information for Systems Evaluation of Children's Mental Health Services.* The Technical Assistance Center for the Evaluation of Children's Mental Health Systems, Judge Baker Children's Center, Boston.

Henggeler, S.W. (1994) *Family Preservation vs. Hospitalization of SED Youths.* Grant proposal submitted to the National Institute of Mental Health.

Henggeler, S.W., Rodick, J.D., Bourdin, C.M., Hanson, C.L., Watson, S.M. & Urey, J.R. (1986) Multisystemic treatment of juvenile offenders: Effects on adolescent behavior and family interaction. *Developmental Psychology,* **22,** 132–41.

Henggeler, S.W., Schoenwald, S.K. & Munger, R.L. (1996) Families and therapist achieve clinical outcomes, systems of care mediate the process. *Journal of Child and Family Studies,* **5,** 177–84.

Hoagwood, K. (1995, Spring). *A New Study of Child and Adolescent Mental Health Services: The NIMH Multi-site Study of Service Use, Need, Outcomes and Costs in Child and Adolescent Populations (UNOCCAP).* American Public Health Association, Mental Health Section Newsletter, Washington, DC.

Hoagwood, K., Hibbs, E., Brent, D. & Jensen, P. (1995) Introduction to the special section: Efficacy and effectiveness in studies of child and adolescent psychotherapy. *Journal of Consulting and Clinical Psychology,* **63,** 683–7.

Hoagwood, K. & Hohmann, A.A. (1993) Child and adolescent services research at the National Institute of Mental Health: Research opportunities in an emerging field. *Journal of Child and Family Studies*, **2**, 259–68.

Hodges, K. (1994) *The Child and Adolescent Functional Scale*. Eastern Michigan University, Ann Arbor, MI.

Huz, S., McNulty, T.L. & Evans, M.E. (1994) *Family-based Treatment in New York State: Evaluation Report*. New York State Office of Mental Health, Bureau of Evaluation and Services Research, Albany, NY.

Kazdin, A.E. (1988) *Child Psychotherapy: Developing and Identifying Effective Treatments*. Pergamon Press, Elmsford, NY.

Kazdin, A.E. (1993) Adolescent mental health: Prevention and treatment programs. *American Psychologist*, **48**, 127–41.

Kazdin, A.E. (1994) Interventions for aggressive and antisocial children. In: *Reason to Hope: A Psychosocial Perspective on Violence and Youth* (eds L.D. Eron, J.H. Gentry & P. Schlegel), pp. 341–82, American Psychological Association, Washington, DC.

Kazdin, A.E., Siegel, T. & Bass, D. (1990) Drawing upon clinical practice to inform research on child and adolescent psychotherapy: A survey of practitioners. *Professional Psychology: Research and Practice*, **21**, 189–98.

Kellam, S.G., Rebok, G.W., Ialongo, N. & Mayer, L.S. (1994) The course and malleability of aggressive behavior from early first grade into middle school: Results of a developmental epidemiologically-based prevention trial. *Journal of Child Psychology and Psychiatry and Allied Disciplines*, **35**, 259–81.

Kenny, J.M., Madsen, B., Flemming, T. & Haapala, D.A. (1977) Homebuilders: Keeping families together. *Journal of Consulting and Clinical Psychology*, **45**, 667–73.

Kingdon, D.W. & Ichinose, C.K. (1996) The Fort Bragg managed care experiment: What do the results mean for publicly funded systems of care? *Journal of Child and Family Studies*, **5**, 191–6.

Knitzer, J. (1982) *Unclaimed Children: The Failure of Public Responsibility to Children and Adolescents in Need of Mental Health Services*. The Children's Defense Fund, Washington, DC.

Kuppinger, A.D. (1995) *ICM Crisis Home: Comfort Sheet*. New York State Office of Mental Health, Albany: NY, unpublished.

Mrazek, P.J. & Haggerty, R.J. (eds) (1994) *Reducing Risks for Mental Disorders: Frontiers for Preventive Intervention Research*. National Academy Press, Washington DC.

McBride, A.B. (1986) Theory and research: Present issues and future perspectives of psychosocial nursing. *Journal of Psychosocial Nursing*, **24**, 27–32.

Mereness, D.A. (1982) Forward: 1940–1982, The evolution of a textbook. In: *Mereness' essentials of psychiatric nursing*, 11th ed. (ed. C.M. Taylor), pp. vii–x, C.V. Mosby, St. Louis.

Morrissey, J.P., & Goldman, H.H. (1984) Cycles of reform in the care of the chronically mentally ill. *Hospital and Community Psychiatry*, **35**, 785–93.

National Institute of Nursing Research (1996) *Extramural Research and Research Training Programs*. World Wide Web (http://www.hih.gov.minr. factsht. html).

Nicholson, J. & Robinson, G. (1996) *A Guide for Evaluating Consumer Satisfaction with Child and Adolescent Mental Health Services*. Judge Baker Children's Center, Boston.

OTA (1986) *Children's Mental Health: Problems and Services*. Office of Technology Assessment, Washington, DC.

Olds, D.L., Henderson, C.R., Tatelbaum, R. & Chamberlin, R. (1988) Improving the life-course development of socially disadvantaged mothers: A randomized trial of nurse home visitation. *American Journal of Public Health*, **78**, 1438–45.

Pothier, P.C., Stuart, G.W., Puskar, K. & Babich, K. (1990) Dilemmas and directions for psychiatric nursing in the 1990s. *Archives of Psychiatric Nursing*, **4**(5), 284–91.

Reiss, B.S., & Evans, M.E. (1996). *Pharmacological Aspects of Nursing Care*. 5th Edn. Delmar Publishers, Albany, NY.

Robins, L.N. & Regier, D. (eds) (1991) *Psychiatric disorders in America: The epidemiologic catchment area study*. The Free Press, New York.

Rog, D.J. (1995) The status of children's mental health services: An overview. In: *Children's Mental Health Services: Research, Policy and Evaluation* (eds L. Bickman & D.J. Rog), pp. 3 -18, Sage, Thousand Oaks, CA.

Scherer, D.G., Brondino, M.J., Henggeler, S.W., Melton, G.B. & Hanley, J. H. (1994) Multisystemic family preservation therapy: Preliminary findings from a study of rural and minority serious adolescent offenders. *Journal of Emotional and Behavioral Disorders*, **2**, 198–206.

Snodgrass, R. (1986) *Parent Skills Training*. People Places, Inc, Staunton, VA.

Stroul, B. & Friedman, R.M. (1986) *A System of Care for Children and Youth with Severe Emotional Disturbances*. Georgetown University Child Development Center, National Technical Assistance Center for Children's Mental Health, Washington, DC.

Taylor, C.M. (1982) *Mereness' Essentials of Psychiatric Nursing*, 11th edn. C.V. Mosby, St Louis.

United States National Center for Health Statistics. (1978) *International classification of diseases, 9th revision, clinical modification*. Commission on Professional and Hospital Activities, Ann Arbor, MI.

United States National Institute of Mental Health (1990) *National Plan for Research on Child and Adolescent Mental Disorders*. (DHHS Publication No. ADM 90-1683). U.S. Government Printing Office, Washington DC.

USDE (1995) *School-linked Comprehensive Services for Children and Families: What We Know and What We Need to Know*. US Department of Education, Washington, DC.

Weissman, J., & Appleton, C. (1995) The therapeutic aspects of acceptance. *Perspectives in Psychiatric Care*, **31**, 19–23.

Weisz, J.R., Donenberg, G.R., Han, S.S. & Weiss, B. (1995) Bridging the gap between laboratory and clinic in child and adolescent psychotherapy. *Journal of Consulting and Clinical Psychology*, **63**, 688–701.

Weisz, J.R. & Weiss, B. (1989) Assessing the effects of clinic-based psychotherapy with children and adolescents. *Journal of Consulting and Clinical Psychology*, **57**, 1–6.

Weisz, J.R., Han, S.S. & Valeri, S.M. (1996) What we can learn from Fort Bragg. *Journal of Child and Family Studies*, **5**, 185–90.

Yorker, B.C. (1994) Populations at risk: Children and adolescents. In: *Essentials of psychiatric nursing* (ed. C.M. Taylor), 14th edn. 388, C.V. Mosby, St. Louis.

Zelizer, V.A. (1994) *Pricing the Priceless Child: The Changing Social Value of Children*. Princeton University Press, Princeton, NJ.

8 Therapeutic Nursing of the Person in Depression

Phil Barker

Introduction

Depression, however it is defined, is the 'common cold of psychiatry', one of the biggest human problems of the late twentieth century (WHO, 1996; Jonsson & Rosenbaum, 1993). Although 'sufferers' are most apparent among the adult (working age) populations, virtual epidemics of depressive problems are evident among older and younger age groups (Barker & Jackson 1996, 1997). The escalation of depression among older people may be a function of loss – of past role or identity – within a rapidly changing postmodern society. For younger people, the crisis may also involve loss – of future: what have young people to live for? Although critical, such speculations have no place in the discussion here, the reader [you][1] may care to consider the importance of such hypotheses for practice by consulting the original sources (Brayne & Ames, 1988; Health Advisory Service, 1995).

The characteristics of depression have changed little since Hippocrates first described *melancholia* 2500 years ago. Having developed almost twenty distinct diagnostic categories for mood disorders (APA, 1994), we are witnessing a return of the use of the term 'melancholy' (Barker, 1992). Indeed, even the most casual of reflections on the plight of humanity in the postmodern world, confirms the hypothesis that we are now living in another Age of Melancholy (Jablensky, 1987). Given the substantial literature describing the phenomena of depression (*cf* Barker, 1992; Beeber, 1989, 1996) I shall not address the issue of recognition here. Instead, I shall focus on the nurse's response to the person's *human response*[2] to depression.

The experience of depression: nursing the breakpoint

The person in depression has reached, passed or returned to a personal 'breakpoint'. 'Break' implies that something in the person has reached a limit; 'point' suggests that this limit can be defined (Harris, 1979). Descriptions of this breakpoint invariably involve complex metaphors. The person often appears like a one-legged individual who collapses when her crutch gives way. She may have a 'constitutional' weakness that predisposes her to depression. However, we can no more 'fix' the constitutional weakness than we can replace the missing limb. We can, however, look at ways of providing new supports, or try out alternative ways of coping with the loss, disability or restrictions imposed by the experience. This suggests the possibility of 'psychic healing' – growing out of distress. Such human growth represents the philosophical focus of this chapter.

I shall discuss how nurses might approach the person in depression. I shall emphasise the nurse's use of the interpersonal relationship, in particular the importance of collaboration and Socratic dialogue, that has been described in detail in the nursing literature for over 40 years (*cf* Peplau, 1952; O'Toole & Welt, 1994; Travelbee, 1969; 1971). By sharing descriptions of the 'breakpoint' experience nurses may explore the alternatives that may lend support, may help the person 'stand up' again to the rigours of everyday life.

Nursing practice has for generations emphasised medical expressive roles and functions (Cormack, 1976). In the case of people in depression, the nursing role has emphasised the administration of medication, support in the administration of ECT, observation and monitoring – especially of the suicidal patient – and highly general and non-specific forms of support. Although all such roles and functions are important, they may fail to address the core elements of the experiences of people in depression. Nursing may, in effect, be failing to address the breakpoint experience that is the common denominator of many forms of depression. This may well be one example of the 'proper focus' of nursing the person in depression (*cf* Barker, *et al.*, 1997). As a developmental activity, nursing needs to emphasise the contribution it may make to helping people use their natural resources to get back on their feet (metaphorically) and circumnavigate the breakpoint.

This chapter will emphasise the structure of the helping relationship. I shall discuss one approach which nurses might adopt toward working constructively in a one-to-one relationship. This might be termed the 'therapeutic relationship' that focuses on a formal, regular meeting to address specific problems of living. This relationship is, of course, an adjunct to the nurse's roles and responsibilities in facilitating or delivering other forms of assessment, support, observation or treatment. The approach described here is based on the author's lengthy clinical practice (20 years) in working with people in major depression.

The construction of depression

Depression takes many forms and may be a function of social circumstances, gender, ageing, organicity or loss (*cf* Beeber, 1989). In this chapter I shall focus on the form of depression that appears to be *constructed* from the person's past and present life experience. The view of depression I map here may be read as dystheoretical, drawing on a range of models and theories of the human condition, and the amelioration of human distress. The discrete influences and theoretical underpinnings may be found in Barker (1992).

Some, though not all, forms of depression arise from the person's specific views of the world and the meaningful experiences existing within it. Many people have good reasons to be depressed. Having said that, one route to the resolution of their depression is through a change of perspective, on themselves and the world that may have treated them harshly. Such a change of perspective involves addressing their view of themselves and their world and the stories they weave to provide partial descriptions and explanations of the mythic experience of being 'me'. Viewed from this perspective it is appropriate to describe people as being 'in' depression, rather than suffering from depression.

On a biological level, people are complex machines and when they break down, depression may be one outcome. People are also the stories, accounts and dreams (waking and unconscious) which are the product of this amazing machine (Leiber, 1991). In considering how we care for people in depression, we need to acknowledge the curious role played by one set of ideas in constructing another: how one '1' (the self) may construct and respond to another '1' (the experience of depression). Ironically, we may only be able to grasp the complexity of the depressed mind through use of an artificial model of the mental processes that might generate depressed thoughts and beliefs.

Stepping out on the road to freedom

Although the experience is very personal, indeed private, the 'what' of depression is quite public. The depressed person reflects on her life, her actions, her failings; on the past, the present and the future. In all these musings she reflects upon what she did or did not do: action – the very stuff of life. The emotional experience of depression *is* an expression of that stuff. All the wrongs that were committed, all the chances that were missed, all the losses and all the things that were neglected. All this: the good and the bad. Some of this is accepted by everyone as real (*consensus reality*); and some may be real only to the sufferer (*personal reality*). All these things belong in the world. We can talk about them. We can share – through language – our construction of these events. What is beyond reach is the person's interpretation of these events and the significance she gives to them. When we 'take care' of the person, we help her to share with us her personal reality and our consensus reality.

Paradoxically, some people who are depressed possess a more realistic view of the world. We should not assume, glibly, that we are reasonable and the depressive is 'irrational' – the reverse may be the case. Sharing experience within the helping relationship may encourage the person to adopt our view of the world; not because it is more rational but because it eases the business of living.

By focusing on the here-and-now experience both of you will recognise the need to grasp the nettle of choice *and* action. Although it may not feel like it, we all stand on the road to freedom: we could hardly stand any-where else. I may be afflicted by an optimistic view of the human condition, believing that people can (and do) leave the past behind them, can begin to live in the present and for the future. This does not mean that distressing experiences can be erased. However, neither does this mean that the past restrains people, like some traumatising anchor.

Helping: some possible characteristics

Eight needs are identified in Fig. 8.1 which appear to be the key stimuli for the construction of the helping relationship. These derive from the 'spiral paradigm' of depression (Barker, 1992), the theoretical ramifications of which need not be discussed here. These eight hypothetical needs serve as the basis for determining both 'what' the nurse needs to address and something of 'how' she might do it.

> The need for:
>
> 1. *Structure:* taking the lead
> 2. *Focus:* attending to details
> 3. *Nowness:* re-authoring life
> 4. *Development:* growing out of distress
> 5. *Experience:* taking the direct route
> 6. *Collaboration:* standing united
> 7. *Holism:* fumbling with the infinite
> 8. *Flexibility:* horses for courses

Fig. 8.1   The core needs of the helping relationship.

Taking the lead: the need for structure

People in depression often appear passive, if not resistive, to the nurse's attempts to help. Concentration is but one problem that can block your efforts. The person's progressive withdrawal often accompanies increased rumination and reflection (*internal*) and reduced attention to changes in her world (*external*). Your efforts to communicate may be limited by her difficulty in attending to what you are saying.

Gentle, but direct, interaction may be indicated. If the person is 'hiding' or 'retiring' from the world, she may perceive a threat which, at least, you need to acknowledge. One way to do this is to take the initiative in shaping the development of the relationship, which is akin to 'leading off' in dancing.

If you intend to develop your partnership, an understanding of what is involved must be communicated (Ley, 1988). You might consider listing what *might* be discussed:

- 'Where shall we begin?' [Pause-silence] 'Well, we might talk about...'
- 'How you feel?'
- 'How we might work together?'
- 'What kind of help I might offer you?'
- 'What you might do to help yourself?' and
- 'What you expect to happen?'

Use direct and simple language, short sentences punctuated by brief pauses. Repetition of important points throughout the discussion will help her to pick up the key messages. Finally, if you want the person to do something, ask her directly:

'I would like you to tell me how you feel right now'.

This implies that she can tell you, but is framed as a straightforward invitation. In the early stages, you may need to take direct charge of the proceedings, encouraging her to respond to your initiatives. This structure will allow her time to gain confidence in you and in her own ability to participate in this new venture. As the relationship develops she can begin to take a more proactive role. The structure provides a secure base upon which to build her confidence, gain some new experiences gradually extending herself.

Attending to details: the need for focus

The person may have a wealth of problems. Focus upon addressing these specifically, rather than in the abstract. In the early stages the focus is upon the person's present understanding of these problems. Exploration of any underlying philosophies or belief systems is best left for later. Help the person tease out the various threads of her complex life problems. You are involved in a sensitive form of human education, helping her draw out from within herself the linking threads of a generalised problem, and attaching useful descriptive labels.

'Depression' per se cannot be manipulated. It is an idea that represents a range of interacting problems of living. I caution against using this concept with the person at this stage. Many people take comfort from the diagnosis of depression: in some way it explains their experience. If appropriate, acknowledge that the person (and/or other members of the team) believes she is 'suffering from depression'. Having made this acknowledgement, encourage her to identify what life problems represent the tentacles of depression. Draw up discrete lists of her problems:

- Emotional
- Behavioural
- Motivational
- Relationship
- Physical
- Cognitive

By encouraging her to focus, you help her to identify some of the 'facts' of depression, which she can share. As long as she uses only the soft focus of depressive metaphor, it will not be clear to you exactly what her problems mean. As the relationship develops, she may find it easier to label and describe the function of problems in her everyday life; how they work for or against her interests. As she experiments with her 'rules' she may become more aware of whether or not these problems need to exist. Having focused her attention upon the everyday 'manipulation' of her problems, you can help her shift the focus to the beliefs which might have helped create them.

Re-authoring life: the need for 'nowness'

Emphasis needs to be given to the person's experience of her problems as they occur in the here-and-now. Past events are addressed only in terms of what they mean now and the problems they caused are dealt with in a problem-solving manner. Suffering, like all other experiences is constructed, and its product is here-and-now. As Keefe (1975) commented:

> 'Guilt and anxiety are children of the past and the future. To the extent that a person dwells upon the should-have-been or might-have been at the expense of living life in the reality of the present, he *suffers*' [italics added].

We are all condemned to freedom, condemned to take responsibility for shaping our lives as best we can. In so doing we must use what nature and nurture have given us. Biology, child-rearing practices, cultural mores, education and socialisation (among others), all influence the direction of our lives and conspire to bring us to this point at this time. The reasoning that we use to make choices and decisions may not always be helpful, as in depression. To that extent we are free to blame those who shaped our reasoning, our values and thinking style. We can, however, choose to follow the difficult path toward new values, new ways of thinking, a more useful form of reasoning. We are the authors of our own lives (Nelson-Jones, 1990).

Emphasis should be given to identifying what needs to be done to deal with one problem or another. Lead the person, sensitively, towards the point of existential awareness. What she did and what happened to her in the past was important; what she might do or what might befall her in the years ahead will be important. What she is doing right now *is* most important of all.

Now is the only time you will ever be given to begin changes that will result *in* your being at the place where you want to be when you die. What needs to be done? Do it (Reynolds, 1985).

Help the person become aware that as long as she is alive she is alive to the possibilities of action. We deceive ourselves by claiming that we 'can't' do this or that, or that we can only 'try'. Action is always possible, although what it might produce is, obviously, variable. It isn't necessary to want or to decide or to get it together or to motivate oneself, or to make the effort, or otherwise insert some step before the doing. It is the doing that counts (Reynolds, 1985, p. 39).

Many therapeutic approaches employ a variant of religious confession: catharsis will somehow bring emotional relief, getting in touch with feelings will somehow bring emotional enlightenment, Barker's 'spiral paradigm' (Barker, 1992) focuses upon a more radical hypothesis. The person has constructed her emotional distress; therefore, she can de-construct it, or build an alternative, more satisfying reality.

Much Western psychology operates on the notion that the 'real person' lies in the subconscious, masked by a false self which can crack under stress allowing the real 'self' to show itself. 'Person' derives from the Latin *persona*: literally, 'an actor's mask'. Although we often assume that masks express a false image, they can be inherently revealing:

> 'Why do actors wear masks in the first place? Because it is the mask that makes the actor's role clear at a single glance.'

> (Doi, 1986, p. 25)

In Japanese *omote* and *ura* mean 'face' and 'mind'. *Omote* always expresses *ura*. Changes in a person's face are assumed to reflect different expressions of her mind. *Ura* (mind) always performs *omote* (face): when people look at our 'masks', they see not only the mask but the 'mind' through the mask. William James (1890) expressed a similar view: the idea of multiple selves, expressed through different masks. A person might, however, try to keep some of these selves secret:

> 'afraid to let one set of his acquaintances know him as he "Is elsewhere" … or [the multiple selves] may be a perfectly harmonious division of labor, as where one tender to his children is stern to the soldiers or prisoners under his control.'

> (James, 1890)

All these 'selves' are true, and the process of presenting one and withholding another involves choice. In Oriental thought, the idea that people might comprise only one or two 'selves' is unrealistically limiting, perhaps even laughable. We are apparently a unity, a stream of innumerable selves following one another like a series of cinematographic pictures, so quickly that they seem one continuous whole (Blyth, 1960, p. 101).

This is not philosophy, nor even psychology. This is the very stuff of life. Encourage the person to consider that, from moment to moment, she writes the story of her life. She frames her experience in much the same way as an author plots a novel. Through its fixations with history and forward planning, our culture has lost sight of the importance of the moment. Help her recognise that the past *was*, and the future always will be, *momentary*. This is that moment within which she makes and remakes herself – she must seize it *now*.

Growing out of distress: the need for development

The therapeutic relationship provides the conditions under which the person might learn from her experience: recognising how she constructs her emotional reality, and how she might develop ways of dealing constructively with her problems. Although becoming takes place within the sessions, it needs to be supplemented by notes, recommended reading and 'real-world' assignments. Emphasise how she deals with life in general. Experimentation with specific life problems can, however, be useful in clarifying common themes and how they might be resolved. Help her develop personalised methods of coping with these problems, through repeated, systematic practice. These 'experiments' can be used later to frame broader, more flexible rules for living.

Acceptance also occupies an important place within the approach. Help her distinguish between what can and cannot be changed. Many people in depression have suffered significant losses, abusive relationships, rejection or failure. The 'trick' of living in an incomplete or hostile world involves a similar kind of acceptance. Her list of 'therapeutic desirables' – what needs to be done – may be reduced to two main categories: *need for acceptance* or *need for change*. 'My partner shows no sign of wanting to improve our relationship. I need to accept that this relationship has come to an end' (*acceptance*) or 'I need to improve my relationship with my partner' (*change*).

The threads of her personal construction need to be teased out carefully. She cannot change others. Whether acceptance or change is appropriate will be known only through direct experience. Exploring the exact nature of her thoughts about change and acceptance, and the evidence that supports them, prepares the way for experimentation. She may find it threatening or 'depressing' to accept that some of her perceived 'needs' might never be achieved. Ask her to clarify her thinking on these subjects:

- 'What *exactly* are your reasons for thinking that you cannot (accept or change) this or that?'

Ask what are her reasons, rather than why she thinks she cannot do something, The former assumes she has her reasons: the latter invites an examination of personal philosophy which may be premature. Many people in depression believe that they are 'sick', 'helpless' or 'useless'. They may need to be guided towards recognising that as long as they think they *cannot*, they *will not*. Encourage the unreasonable view: 'Believe it and you'll see it!' (Dyer, 1990) 'Believe you can and you will – believe you can't and you won't'.

Maslow (1976) took the radical view that all people with mental illness were 'cognitively wrong' rather than 'sick':

> 'Neurosis, psychosis, stunting of growth – all are, from this point of view, cognitive diseases as well, contaminating perception, learning, remembering, attending and thinking.'
>
> (Maslow 1976)

Although Maslow's consideration of cognitive processes is not as well known as those of other theorists, his hypotheses provide valuable distinctions between 'adaptive' and 'maladaptive' thinking. They bridge Oriental and Occidental models of (wo)man, which have been lost in the headlong rush toward reductionist explanations of depression. 'Healthy' people, in Maslow's (1962) view, get lost in 'doing' – they do things for their own sake, not as part of some interminable competition involving the judgement of oneself. The 'healthy' person is an end in itself, not a means to an end, something that is relative to the rest of the world, a partial success or failure. Maslow described 'unhealthy' people as owning 'deficiency cognitions'. They measure themselves primarily in negative terms – qualities they do not possess, stages they have not yet reached, etc. Psychotherapies which address 'cognitive problems' by adjusting the person's thinking style to enhance conformity to the world simply exchange one set of restrictions for another. The person who becomes depressed is distressed more by what she or her world is not than by its positive reality.

Help the person to experience her-self and her world *as it is,* accepting and changing *as she* considers appropriate or possible.

Taking the direct route: the need for experience

I have emphasised the person's experience of herself, her reflections upon her life and actions, and experience of alternative courses of action. Reflection alone, however, will accomplish little. If the person owns 'self-defeating' rules she needs to generate evidence that will help her dispute their supremacy. Changes in thinking are usually bound up with changes in action. Both must be experienced repeatedly if change is to occur. Repetition, however, means disciplined practice.

Encourage the person to examine her feelings, thoughts and actions. What relationships exist between these three facets of the individual? Keeping a diary is the simplest way she can record the thoughts and feelings that occur through the action of her day. This may appear daunting but if she is encouraged to build up this reflective record gradually, she will be able to amass considerable descriptive evidence of *how* she constructs her day-to-day experience. The authorship of her life will become more readily apparent.

Your working relationship with the person should be focused, unequivocally, upon her experience here and how. Invite her to re-play memories of events, whether recent or distant. Help her re-experience those events, encouraging her to:

Become more and more aware of where you are...
What is happening around you...
Perhaps you can hear certain sounds ... or are aware of a special smell or
    taste?
As you become more and more aware of that whole experience you
    become aware of feelings within yourself ... and you know what those
    feelings are.
As you begin to feel them again...
What is your 'private voice' saying...?
What did that whole experience mean to you?

Encourage her to recall the various sensory experiences she had at that time. Your instructions should be intentionally vague, allowing her to 'fill in the details' privately. You need not know exactly what is going on. Such vagueness can also reduce any embarrassment or shame she might feel. It may also demonstrate that you have no interest in probing her emotional recesses, or otherwise 'threatening' her. This will cement your relationship (*cf* Bandler & Grinder, 1979; Barker, 1997, pp. 246–9).

These replays sensitise her to her personal construction of reality. They are used to illustrate how she might become more aware of the experiences which lie ahead of her. An important long-term objective is that the person should spend more time in the immediate experience of her world and less time ruminating, perhaps negatively, about the world. Reynolds (1985) described how he encourages his clients to keep a daily diary, on which he comments at each session. He encourages the client to attend more and more to the actions described and to describe these in greater detail. As the client's awareness of her actions *in the world* increase, her awareness of internal feelings decreases.

The difficulty which she might experience in undertaking this transfer should not be underestimated. Providing that short periods of awareness, recorded briefly in the daily diary, are used as the starting point, the authorship of her life will grow in size and significance.

United we stand: the need for collaboration

Medicine has often emphasised the 'manipulation' of the person who is the patient, analogous to the scientist's manipulation of the laboratory conditions. Doctors often speak of the medical regimen – derived from the Latin for 'rule'. Many patients assume that this is *the* rule. Also we talk of the patient's treatment compliance – which implies that the patient needs to 'yield' to our wishes, rather than understand, agree with or sanction the proposed intervention. These suggest that the patient is literally 'under the doctor'; submitting to his expert manipulation, subjugated by his rule. Increasingly, nurses are tempted to employ similar concepts.

The person in depression needs help since she may feel helpless. This does not mean, however, that she is helpless. Take the view that the person has resources, capabilities and other non-specific strengths upon which she can draw. In seeking the solutions necessary to resolve her life problems and establish the route back to meaningfulness, the person needs guidance and support. She does not need to surrender or be taken over. She needs a partner who will help her to tread the scary path towards recovery.

The working alliance (Bordin, 1976) discourages the traditional passivity of the 'patient' and rejects the assumption that the practitioner is in any way 'all-knowing'. Instead, the 'patient' and the 'therapist' work together; learning from each other, interacting like any partnership. The kind of partnership required depends greatly upon the person's needs and what the practitioner has to offer. Initially, the relationship may be akin to that of athlete and sports coach. The person needs to develop herself in some way and agrees to try out the 'methods' favoured by the practitioner. As the person develops (changes) the relationship develops. Gradually balance is established, and the person begins to teach the nurse about 'what needs to be done'. Eventually, the person may assume a 'majority control' of the content of any session; this does not diminish the collaborative nature of the relationship, but merely shows how it has matured, like the two parties involved.

All professional efforts to 'treat' people with psychological disorders are probably, ultimately, manipulative and coercive (Masson, 1989). The person in depression should always be helped to feel in control of therapeutic services: deciding what is or is not desirable. If you are aiming to empower someone who is temporarily 'powerless', your help should be offered within an open, sharing relationship. However, although you should not pretend to be 'all-knowing', nothing is gained by pretending that you know nothing. Helping has much in common with education, you help the person learn about herself and the possible processes of change. (Although nurses are not doctors we might remember that the Latin root of 'doctor' means 'to teach'.)

It seems self-evident that people in depression need to connect with those helping them, perhaps in a more human – even spiritual – sense. In the future all mental health professions might come to:

'regard themselves as servants of larger spiritual reality conceived of as God or nature, a higher power or life energy – of which they and their patients are a part. As such, they will see themselves more modestly, as vehicles for healing rather than *its* agents, as co-participants in a process that is awesome rather than as its controlling force.'

(Gordon, 1990)

This provides an even wider, perhaps more realistic view of the therapeutic (healing) process. The therapist's task is double-edged: needing to restore both the person's and their own harmony – with nature (the world) and the inner nature (self). Those who seek help need to establish what changes they need to make and how they might make them. Those who offer help need to become aware of their capacity to enable such a process of exploration and discovery. Both are involved in defining the 'art of the possible'.

Fumbling with the infinite: the need for holism

Throughout, I have taken the view that the person does not *suffer* from depression; rather, she expresses such disturbance of mind (*ura*) through her actions or masks (*omote*) (*cf* Barker, 1992). This is a whole lived-experience (Parse, 1981). Although she may not be aware of what exactly she is expressing, to presume that what she is expressing does not belong to her (or is meaningless) is dehumanising. This applies equally to all forms of mental disturbance. As Podvoll (1990) observed, such an attitude has major implications for the kind of help offered:

'Believing that psychosis, for example, begins and ends with idiosyncrasies of the brain nullifies it as a human tragedy, and contributes to the steadily deteriorating conditions of care that today face almost all of the chronically mentally ill'.

Others have emphasised the centrality of actions in the complex functioning of the individual. The idea of 'splitting' people up into emotional, intellectual and behavioural 'selves' is questioned: 'Doing, thinking, and feeling are inseparable aspects of behaviour and are generated from within. Most of them are choices' (Wubbolding, 1988).

Rather than talk about 'suffering from a disorder', you might acknowledge the distress the person is expressing:

'Thus an angry person is said to be "angering" rather than to "be angry". Clients are encouraged to say, "Today I am guilty", or, "Last night I was depressing". Phrases like "fit of depression", "anxiety attack" or "stressful job" are meaningless.

(Wubbolding, 1988, p. 5)

Some models of mental disorder appear to 'explain away' the person's experience; taking the meaning out of the person's actions. A 'depressing' person is expressing what it means to 'be' at the moment: thoughts and feelings expressed naturally through actions – *ura* performing *omote*. She expresses the whole of her experience. You need to attend to that whole; therein lies the person.

If you embrace the person whole this will reduce the likelihood that you will rely on single reductionist methods of helping. Everything from adjustments to the diet to meditations and prayer might conceivably be of value. That depression can be nothing but a human tragedy seems so obvious that it hardly requires repeating. That people who are depressed need to consider the role of diet, prayer or contemplation as part of their 'recovery' needs to be repeated forcefully. The critic may argue that there is no evidence for the value of this 'shotgun' form of helping. The American psychiatrist James Gordon (1990) counselled against such cynicism:

'Whatever the efficacy of these approaches (exercise, dietary modification, relaxation, guided imagery and meditation) they reinforce the patient's sense of control and empowerment and the concept of health care as partnership in which both physician and patient have responsibilities.'

This is the crux of the matter. Many therapeutic systems can be used as a professional shield against the distress of the person. If you desire to be involved with the *whole person* who is in depression, you need to be ready to use the whole of your self. You cannot afford to shelter behind any of the 'screens' employed by traditional psychotherapists. Gordon (1985) acknowledged that:

'Medication (for example), particularly in an institutional setting, was often used as a tool for foreclosing, under the aegis of therapy, ideas and behaviour which were unconventional and disturbing to the staff.'

It should be apparent that more limited forms of intervention will be less taxing for the practitioner; all forms of 'processing' reduce the need to think, feel and act along with the object of the process. In all forms of psychological distress, but especially depression, there is a need for creative engagement. The helping relationship needs to be played for real.

Horses for courses: the need for flexibility

A wealth of explanations has been used down the ages to explain depression, from radical behaviourism (Ferster, 1973), through ethology (Eibl-Eibesfeldt, 1972) to psychodynamics (Gilbert, 1984). Even within these 'schools', dispute and conflict abound. In this chapter, I have given some consideration to how we might go about helping the sufferer. I remain sceptical about the emergence of any one clear indication of what, exactly, should be done. I favour the alternative view that many things might be done, indeed, the greater the range of options, the greater the likelihood of a satisfactory outcome.

We need to avoid narrow ideology, associated with any school of thought. Therein, we run the risk of developing a secular religion as a means of addressing human distress (*cf* Masson, 1989). As you engage the person you will encourage her to think, construct images, recall events, frame and re-frame the meaning of experiences, make herself up, moment by moment. Cognition is undoubtedly at the core of everyday experience, and is the medium for the messages of our everyday lives. In my own work, I include metaphors, riddles and quotes from writers as diverse as Zen masters or modern humanistic therapists as part of my helping package. I assume that many, but not all, therapeutic systems may be of benefit to the person who is depressed. There may be value in being eclectic:

> '...the dilemma is whether a therapist should practice as an ideological partisan or as an eclectic. The partisan (e.g. the psychoanalyst, the radical behaviourist, the reflective Rogerian) stays with the principles and techniques of a particular mode of therapy, whereas the eclectic uses techniques as they fit, regardless of theoretical purity.'

> (Lueger & Sheikh, 1989)

Although the scientific purist may be upset, much is to be gained from employing an eclectic, transtheoretical approach. People make changes in their lives for many reasons. Ask the person to consider the part any of the following have played in shaping the conditions that led her to choose a specific course of action:

- A chance encounter with a friend or stranger
- A traumatic accident
- A serious illness
- Reading a book, poem, newspaper or magazine article
- Viewing great works of art
- Hearing familiar or new pieces of music

- Recalling the past
- Contemplating the present
- Imagining the future
- Looking in a mirror

This list is endless. Any or all of these everyday events shape the conditions of all our personal choices, providing us with the materials which stimulate the idea of choosing, or help us to weigh up options. There is no reason why the helping process cannot accommodate such 'shapers'. There is no reason why helping needs to be focused entirely on talk and the expression of warm, empathic, genuine understanding. Effective helping cannot be based within any one rigid ideology: the person and her world are too complex for such reductionism.

Humble beginnings

Dreams and possibilities

Practical steps need to be taken to introduce the helping process:

- How does the person feel about entering into this relationship?
- What does she think the practitioner might be able to do for her?

These should be clarified at the outset, setting aside time to air these freely. If she has unrealistic expectations, clarify what is possible, given your skills and knowledge.

Laying out the relationship

Practical arrangements should also be discussed.

- How often you should meet, where, at what time, and for how long?

This allows the person to express preferences while allowing you to continue to clarify the 'possibilities'. This addition to the scene-setting is another aspect of collaboration. By discussing these in an adult, egalitarian fashion, you validate her. She is a full person who needs to be consulted, but whose every wish it may not be possible to meet. Hopefully, she will gain the impression that this will be an equal and dignified relationship.

Introducing the method

Helping will make demands on both parties. These should be re-stated, without being overly dramatic. Emphasise your belief that she can be helped, but this is most likely to happen through her active collaboration. The vital nature of the partnership may be illustrated by reference to notable partners: Sherlock Holmes and Dr Watson solving a mystery (the nurse taking, of course, Watson's dogged supporting role!), Fred Astaire and Ginger Rogers personifying rhythm. Within these relationships, *partnership reigns supreme.*

Acknowledgment should also be paid to the importance of *real-world* assignments: keeping diaries (*reflection*), and using oneself as an experiment (*self-study*)[3]. You might agree to audio-tape each session, each taking away a copy for further reflection.

The individual session

Irrespective of the care location – inpatient or out-patient unit, or the person's own home – aim to create an atmosphere conducive to continuous learning. Reinforce her status as an active, equal collaborator. The key feature of each session is the sharing of knowledge of 'what' will be done: the helping agenda. You are aiming to help the person become more aware of how she 'constructs her own reality', helping her make meaningful connections between her thoughts, feelings and events in her everyday life. Emphasis needs to be given repeatedly to her experience within the session.

- What does she think of what is being done?
- What does this mean to her?
- What can she do with this new-found perception of herself and her world?

It is common practice to allocate one hour to a session. Where the person is in severe depression, this may prove too taxing for her concentration and shorter, more frequent sessions may be more appropriate. Adjust the length of the session as she becomes better able to cope with the demands. Relate everything which happens within the session to the rest of the person's life, whether within the ward or in the 'wider world':

> 'There is a myth in our culture that something magical occurs during an hour of psychotherapy... Many people seem to believe that what happens during the golden hour is sufficiently powerful to colour the rest of the week. They seem to believe that the other 167 hours of the week have less effect than that one hour. Even some therapists agree. To succumb to this myth is to relegate $\frac{167}{168}$ of life to meaninglessness. Life must be lived moment by moment. Each moment brings possibilities for purposeful activity. Each moment carries a message, a lesson for us. There are no golden hours, only ready people.'

> (Reynolds, 1985, p. 56)

Processing the past

Let the person review, briefly, what has happened since the last session; in her everyday life, or within her personal musings or reflections. Are these problems or signs of progress? A brief review of the outcome of her real-world assignment is also desirable. What did she do and what did she think of that? Given this addition to her self-knowledge, what can she do now? Finally, allow her to recall and comment upon the events of the previous session. What does she remember addressing? What does she think of that now, with hindsight?

You aim to promote a sense of continuity between the sessions. Encourage her to recall the past sessions so that she can reinforce the 'significance' of what has been learned. She may refer to notes or diary jottings to refresh her memory. The main aim, however, is that what has happened in the recent past is recalled, interpreted from her new 'viewpoint' and added to her growing body of self-knowledge.

The art of negotiation

Negotiate the content of each session. The question 'What have you brought along today?' (Robinson, 1983) represents an ideal starter. Negotiate a realistic agenda that will address the issues you both believe are important. This may be left to the person's initiative in later stages. In the early stages, it may be valuable briefly to 'brainstorm' a list of possible contenders for the agenda. These should be ranked, collaboratively, in terms of their relative importance at this stage. Initially, the agenda will focus on developing awareness and enacting limited real-world experiments. Progressively, the focus will turn to the personal rationales that underpin her thoughts, and in turn her feelings. The uncovering and 'reality-testing' of specific beliefs about herself and the world are better left until later. By that time she will have built a solid base of self-knowledge.

The heart of the session

The major part of each session is devoted to a careful examination of the agenda item(s). Encourage her to discuss what is 'problematic'. She may describe problems with her feelings (sad, guilty, ashamed or fearful), her will or motivation (apathy, avoidance, inertia), her actions and interactions (slowness, coping, withdrawal, relationships) or her physical self (sleeping, eating and sex). Specific problems may be encountered with thinking (indecisiveness, impaired concentration and memory). She may ruminate, obsessively, about a range of other problems; worrying about where these may lead or trying to account for their origin. Encourage her to bring a personal focus to the discussion.

- 'In what way, *exactly*, is this a problem for you?'

At the heart of the session you are helping her address the personal rules which govern her perception of events, the actions of others, but more importantly of herself. You are inviting her to explore the extent to which some of the 'awfulness' of her world derives from her constructions. Having identified how she views these problems at present, you will help her to identify and consider other viewpoints: how might others perceive these events? Finally, you will help her to assess whether these 'alternative' viewpoints offer any help in reducing her distress. Where these alternatives are a radical departure from her typical mode of thought, how might she go about using or developing these viewpoints?

Where the 'problem' is not one of her construction, she needs help to explore alternative courses of action. If she has not dealt successfully with this problem to date, she may have failed to acknowledge and use possible alternative courses of action. You need to help her identify such alternative solutions, and to 'rehearse' how she might implement such problem-solving strategies.

Real-world assignments

A realistic task should be negotiated which will allow the person to explore the issues she has so far only examined intellectually and emotionally. What can she do between now and the next session which may allow her to come face-to-face with the problem which has been addressed? This assignment needs to be outlined in some detail. Translate vague ambitions to 'speak to my mother' or 'sort things out at home' into discrete actions: what will she do, with whom, where and when, *exactly*.

If necessary, discuss her reasons for saying this is desirable, facilitating her belief in the value of doing this or that now. Such assignments may prove daunting. Ask her:

- How do you feel about this?
- Do you have any lingering doubts?
- What do you think might happen?
- What might stand in the way of carrying out this assignment?
- How will you notice what takes place?

Resume

In winding up the session, summarise what she has learned.

- What seems to be most important?
- What does this mean to you?
- How did you feel about my handling of the session?

Finally, a few minutes should be left for any other comments, winding down from what may have been an emotionally-demanding period.

The therapeutic stance: gaining through losing

Here I have merely sketched the outline of the therapeutic structure. This relationship cannot be achieved without a human, honest, collaborative, egalitarian approach. These qualities, however, are unlikely to be enough, in themselves. Even love itself, where it is possible, is rarely enough. Helping the person in depression requires a kind of human caring which is often difficult to describe. There is no room here for an epistle on the art of being human and I could add little of any consequence to the available literature (*cf* Fromm, 1993). I do, however, make two suggestions for your further reflection.

The first concerns the idea of caring for the person. Here, I am thinking of a different form of caring, rendered most clearly by Robert Pirsig (1974):

> '... just sitting [is] a meditative practice in which the idea of a duality of self and object does not dominate one's consciousness... When one isn't dominated by feelings of separateness from what he's working on, then one can be said to "care" about what he's doing. This is what caring really is, a feeling of identification with what one's doing. When one has this feeling then he also sees the inverse side of caring. Quality itself.'

(Pirsig, 1974, p. 290)

Perhaps we can be most helpful (caring) by 'losing ourselves' in rapt attention. This recalls W.B. Yeats' riddle, how to tell the dancer from the dance?

Secondly, it may be worth reflecting on the awesome nature of 'coming out of depression'. The person is being coaxed out of her shell, to which she has retired to avoid the ravages of an unkind or disappointing world. You attempt to draw her out to experience the warmth of the sun, along with the occasional shower. Without her shell she is vulnerable. Despite this, you attempt to undress her 'in the cold light of day'; disrobing layer after layer of unhelpful construction. Even allowing for the melodrama of the metaphor, this is not an exercise to be undertaken lightly. Especially when we become frustrated by the apparent 'resistance' to change or 'slowness' of progress, we might all care to reflect on this metaphor.

Strengths, weaknesses and future directions

The approach to the one-to-one relationship described here derives from a clinically based research project (Barker, 1988), focused on women with major disorder. It is described by Reynolds and Cormack (1990, p. 17) as 'the first experimental examination of the role of the nurse in caring for (clients suffering from major affective disorders) mounted anywhere in the world'. The author's series of studies suggested that the person's perceived powerlessness and locus of control (Barker, 1994) were critical foci for the one-to-one relationship. Interventions which merely provided emotional support, or failed to recognise the person's need for structure and guidance, had poorer outcomes, overall.

The key strength, therefore, of the approach outlined here is its recognition of the person's sense of powerlessness. The structure inherent in the approach provides a necessary sense of security, which can gradually be withdrawn as the person gains confidence. The philosophical emphasis on human growth, rather than simply symptom reduction, also appears to validate the person and her distress as inherently meaningful. The major weakness is that the approach requires a nurse who is confident in her ability to work collaboratively, creatively and resourcefully – especially when therapeutic roadblocks are encountered. Despite the many prescriptions for practice, this approach expects the nurse to assess continuously the person's stage of development and, creatively, to introduce or develop collaboratively, appropriate interventions.

Further justification for this approach is emerging from the broadly-based *The Newcastle Need for Nursing Studies* (Barker, 1996). Preliminary findings from this series of phenomenological studies appears to suggest that when they are in the patient role, people value most the relationship with the nurse, even when it is used as a means of directing the person toward some therapeutic goal. Conversely, there have been few reports of discrete therapeutic methods, suggesting that the co-creative nature of the one-to-one relationship is valued most highly by the person *in* care.

That said, little is known about the discrete processes used within the one-to-one relationship, especially 'how' nurses acquire the confidence to *be fully* or otherwise *lose themselves* in the kind of rapt attention described in this chapter. The exploration of those discrete intra- and interpersonal processes represents a challenge for future research.

References

APA (1994) *Diagnostic and statistical manual of mental disorders prepared by the task force on DSM-IV*, 4th edn. American Psychiatric Association, Washington DC.

Bandler, R. & Grinder, J. (1979) *Frogs into Princes: Neuro-Linguistic Programing*. Real People Press, Moab, Utah.

Barker, P. (1988) *An Evaluation of Specific Nursing Interventions in Patients Suffering from Manic Depressive Psychosis*. Unpublished PhD thesis. Dundee Institute of Technology.

Barker, P. (1992) *Severe Depression: A Practitioner's Guide*. Chapman and Hall, London.

Barker, P. (1993) *A Self Help Guide to Managing Depression*. Chapman and Hall, London.

Barker, P. (1994) Locus of control in women with a diagnosis of manic-depressive psychosis. *Journal of Psychiatric and Mental Health Nursing*, 1(1) 9–14.

Barker, P. (1996) *The Newcastle Need for Nursing Studies*. University of Newcastle Upon Tyne.

Barker, P. (1997) *Assessment in Psychiatric and Mental Health Nursing. In search of the whole person*. Stanley Thornes, Cheltenham.

Barker, P. & Jackson, S. (1996) Seriously misguided. *Nursing Times*, **92**(34) 56–9.

Barker, P & Jackson, S. (1997) Mental health nursing. Making it a primary concern. *Nursing Standard*, **11**(17) 39–41.

Barker, P., Reynolds, B. & Stevenson, C. (1997) The human science basis of psychiatric nursing: Theory and practice. *Journal of Advanced Nursing*, **25**, 660–67.

Beeber, L. (Ed) (1989) *Depression: Old Problems, New Perspectives in Nursing Care*. Slack Inc, Thorofare, NJ.

Beeber, L. (1996) The client who is depressed. In: *Psychiatric Nursing: A comprehensive reference* (ed. S. Lego), 2nd edn. Lippincott, NY.

Blyth, R.H. (1960) *Zen in English Literature and Oriental Classics*. Dutton, London.

Bordin, E.S. (1976) The Working Alliance. Basis for a General Theory of Psychotherapy. Paper presented at the meeting of the *American Psychological Association*, Washington DC, September.

Brayne, C. & Ames, D. (1988) The epidemiology of mental disorder in old age. In:

Mental Health problems in Old Age. A reader (eds B. Gearing, M.L. Johnson & T. Heller). Open University Press, Bucks.

Cormack, D.F.S. (1976) *Psychiatric Nursing Observed*. Royal College of Nursing, London.

Doi, T. (1986) *The Anatomy of Self The Individual Versus Society*, p. 25. Kodansha International, New York.

Dyer, W. (1990) *Believe It and You'll See It*! Arrow Books, London.

Eibl-Eibesfeldt, I. (1972) *On Love and Hate: The Natural History of Behaviour Patterns* (trans. G. Strachan). Holt, Rinehart and Winston, New York.

Ferster, C.B. (1973) A functional analysis of depression. *American Psychologist*, **28**, 857–70.

Frankl, V. (1963) *Man's Search for Meaning* (p. 173). Washington Square Press, New York.

Fromm, E (1993) *The Art of Being*. Constable and Co, London.

Gilbert, P. (1984) *Depression: From Psychology to Brain State*, Ch 2. Lawrence Erlbaum Assoc, Hillsdale, New Jersey.

Gordon, J.S. (1985) Holistic medicine, fringe or frontier? In: *The New Holistic Health Handbook: Living Well in a New Age* (ed. S. Bliss). Stephen Greene Press, Lexington, Mass.

Gordon, J.S. (1990) Holistic medicine and mental health practice: toward a new synthesis. *American Journal of Orthopsychiatry*, **60**(3), 357–70.

Harris, A.B. (1979) *Breakpoint. Stress – The Crisis of Modern Living*. Turnstone Books, London.

Health Advisory Service (1995) *Together We Stand: Thematic Review of Child and Adolescent Mental Health*. HMSO, London.

Jablensky, A. (1987) Prediction of the course and outcome of depression. *Psychological Medicine*, **17**, 11–19.

James, W. (1890) *The Principles of Psychology*. Holt, New York.

Jonsson, B. & Rosenbaum, J. (eds) (1993) *Health Economics of Depression*. Wiley, Chichester.

Keefe, T. (1975) A Zen perspective on social casework. *Social Casework*, March, 18–22.

Leiber, I. (1991) *An Invitation to Cognitive Science*. Basil Blackwell, Oxford.

Ley, P. (1988) *Communicating with Patients. Improving Communication, Satisfaction and Compliance*, Ch 6. Croom Helm, London.

Lueger, R.J. & Sheikh, A.A. (1989) The four faces of psychotherapy. In: *Eastern and Western Approaches to Healing: Ancient Wisdom and Modern Knowledge* (eds A.A. Sheikh & K.S. Sheikh), Ch 8. John Wiley, New York.

Maslow, A. (1962) *Towards a Psychology of Being*, p. 189. Van Nostrand, Princeton, New Jersey.

Maslow, A. (1976) *The Further Reaches Of Human Nature*, Ch 20. Penguin, Harmondsworth.

Masson, J.M. (1989) *Against Therapy: Warning – Psychotherapy May Be Hazardous to Your Mental Health*. Collins, London.

Nelson-Jones, R. (1990) *Thinking Skills. Managing and Preventing Personal Problems*, Ch 3. Brooks/Cole, Pacific Grove, California.

O'Toole, A.W. & Welt, S.R. (1994) *Hildegard E. Peplau. Selected works*. Macmlllan, London.

Parse, R.R. (1981) *Man-Living-Health: A theory of nursing*. Wiley, NY.

Peplau, H.E. (1952) *Interpersonal relations in nursing*. Putnam, NY.

Pirsig, R. (1974) *Zen and The Art of Motorcycle Maintenance*, p. 290. Corgi, London.

Podvoll, E. (1990) *The Seduction of Madness. A Compassionate Approach To Recovery at Home*, p. 2. Century, London.

Reynolds, D. (1985) *Playing Ball on Running Water*, p. 27. Sheldon Press, London.

Reynolds, W. & Cormack, D. (1990) *Psychiatric and Mental Health Nursing: Theory and Practice*. Chapman and Hall, London.

Robinson, L. (1983) *Psychiatric Nursing as a Human Experience*, 3rd edn. W.B. Saunders, London.

Smail, D. (1987) *Taking Care: An Alternative to Therapy*. J.M. Dent, London.

Travelbee, J. (1969) *Intervention in Psychiatric Nursing. Process in the one-to-one relationship*. FA Davis Co, Philadelphia.

Travelbee, J. (1971) *Interpersonal Aspects of Nursing*, 2nd edn. S Saunders, Philadelphia.

WHO (1996) *Investing in Health Research and Development*, World Health Organization, Geneva.

Wubbolding, R.E. (1988) *Using Reality Therapy*. Perennial Library, Harper and Row, New York.

Notes

1. I shall refer to the reader as 'you', to expedite a simple dialogue, and the person in depression as 'her', to acknowledge that in most instances, women represent the majority of the clinical population.
2. The American Nurses Association (1980) Nursing: A social policy statement. Kansas City, MO: Author.
3. A self-help guide to managing her experience in depression may help the person learn at her own pace, and in her own time. One example is Barker (1993).

9 Communication with People Suffering from Severe Dementia

Astrid Norberg

Introduction

Communication is essential in nursing care. In caring for people suffering from severe dementia communication presents great difficulties. Yet some carers are able to transcend these problems, successfully communicate and even establish a warm rapport with people with severe dementia. In order to improve the care of this difficult and disadavantaged client group it is essential that we develop an understanding of how successful communication with a person with dementia can be established. In this chapter, research findings based on interviews with care providers about their interaction with people with severe dementia and observations/video-recording of these interactions will be presented and reflected upon.

Dementia

The symptoms of Alzheimer's disease (referred to in this chapter as dementia) make verbal communication difficult. Being able to communicate presupposes various abilities that are impaired in people with dementia. There are problems of memory, especially short-term episodic memory, problems of language, perception, attention and comprehension (APA 1994). Non-verbal communication is also problematic (Apell *et al.*, 1982; Athlin & Norberg, 1987b; Bayles & Tomoeda, 1991; Obler & Albert, 1984). Facial expressions are reduced (APA, 1994, p. 134; Asplund, *et al.*, 1991a, 1995) and gestures are less expressive (Critcley, 1964). There are reports that people with severe dementia of the Alzheimer type express a range of affective signals (e.g. Magai, *et al.*, 1996). A progressive loss of insight into one's own situation during the course of the disease has been reported (McDaniel, *et al.*, 1995) and in the final stage, the patient is often mute (Bayles, *et al.*, 1992). The fact that people with severe dementia are usually quite old (APA 1994, p. 134) must be taken into consideration when caring for them. Being old can be seen as struggling to achieve an experience of integrity, i.e. wholeness and meaning (Erikson, 1982) and cosmic transcendence (Thornstam, 1994; see Chapter 20).

There is research which shows that the competence of people with severe dementia varies in relation to environmental pressure (Svensson, 1984, based on Lawton, 1982). Overt competence, which is only a part of covert competence, is influenced by the physical and psychological care environment (e.g. Athlin & Norberg, 1987b; Sandman, *et al.*, 1988). Of course, a care provider's caring performance has consequences for the environment (Sabat, 1994; Woods, 1995). It is a well-known fact that people with dementia are very sensitive to environmental influences (e.g. Corcoran & Gitlin, 1991) and, moreover, they may be deprived of opportunities to utilise their covert competence in a poor environment.

Communication in severe dementia

People with severe dementia are described as context-bound and find abstract thinking a problem (APA, 1994). This means, among other things, that they may not understand talk about subjects that they would otherwise comprehend if they were assisted by visual cues. For example, observations of morning care sessions with patients with moderate and severe dementia have shown that the patient's understanding of instructions to perform a certain task improves in a situation where all items carry an unambiguous message (Sandman, *et al.*, 1986). The specific factors in any situation that help people with severe dementia to understand are, of course, related to types of impairments, such as agnosia and apraxia.

Thus it is true to say that various aspects of communication are affected in people with severe dementia (Athlin & Norberg, 1987b). Dementia causes people to send weak and unclear communicative clues that are difficult for care providers to interpret. Even if the care providers send cues that are adapted to the abilities of people with severe dementia, these people will still have problems interpreting them. They may also have difficulty in taking the initiative to respond. The time needed for reaction is prolonged and people with severe dementia are easily disturbed by other stimuli in the environment. Despite all these difficulties there are care providers who often or occasionally seem to understand such people and also are able to make themselves understood.

Video-recordings (Ekman, *et al.*, 1993; Ekman & Norberg, 1993; Jansson, *et al.*, 1993; Kihlgren, *et al.*, 1994, 1996; Sandman, *et al.*, 1988; Åkerlund & Norberg, 1986), observations (Hallberg, *et al.*, 1995; Lindgren, *et al.*, 1992; Sandman, *et al.*, 1986; Zingmark, *et al.*, 1993), and audio-recorded interactions (Edberg, *et al.*, 1995; Ehrenberger Hamilton, 1994; Hallberg, *et al.*, 1993; Frank, 1995) have shown that communicative cues from people with severe dementia can be understood.

Lucidity

Episodes of lucidity may suddenly and unexpectedly occur. Research has claimed that patients may function by being aware of their situations on two levels: on one level they are aware of the situation but on the other level they are not (Miesen, 1993). This makes communication a sensitive issue. During one study on sensory stimulation of people with severe dementia a patient for example suddenly and unexpectedly became lucid for a few minutes (Norberg, *et al.*, 1986). This patient, a woman with severe dementia, had been lying curled up in a foetal position and had no verbal communication for two years. When she was stimulated by music and firm touching two types of response were elicited: a change in the rate of eye blinking and mouth movements. No other reactions could be identified on video-recordings. However, at one meal when she was being spoon-fed she swallowed badly and coughed. When she could breathe again the care provider said with delight: 'Now it is OK!'. 'Yes', the women answered, 'I think so too'. The nurse lifted the glass and showed it to the woman saying: 'You have some milk left'. 'Yes, I can see that', the patient answered, 'but I wish to save it'. After that the woman remained silent for another year before she died.

Similar experiences have been described by Åkerlund and Norberg (1986) during conversations in groups; by Bleathman and Morton (1992) from validation therapy; by Bright (1992) in connection to listening to music; by Kitwood and Bredin (1992) when intersubjectivity was established with the care provider; by Sabat and Harre (1992, p. 452) in a 'heightened emotional state'; by Kitwood (1993) in settings where care was centred on the person, and by Gibson (1994) in connection with reminiscence work. Swane's (1996) research found that these moments of lucidity were frightening for families.

Episodes of lucidity have been captured on videotape (Ekman, *et al.*, 1993; Kihlgren, *et al.*, 1994, 1996; Sandman, *et al.*, 1988; Åkerlund & Norberg, 1986). Spontaneous episodes of lucidity have been reported to occur mostly when the patients are acting closely together with a care provider who makes no demands of them, and regards them as valuable human beings whose behaviour is a meaningful expression of their experiences (Norberg, 1996). Further research is necessary to question the assumption that the self or personhood of people with severe dementia is destroyed. Episodes of lucidity in people with severe dementia challenge care providers to create an undemanding atmosphere that fosters close contact.

What do episodes of lucidity tell about what it means to suffer from dementia? The philosopher Karl Popper and the neuroscientist John Eccles, in their book *The self and its brain* (1977), proposed a model of a human being based upon a neuro-scientific perspective. They reflected on the literature concerning the functions of the brain and suggested that there is an integrating instance, which they called the self, that uses the brain like a musician uses his or her instrument. The musician can only demonstrate his or her skills when the instrument functions. This model seems to fit in with observations of episodes of lucidity as well as with the possibility that one can be in close contact with people with severe dementia, who can be seen as existing 'fenced in within their tattered brain' (Norberg, *et al.*, 1994).

Perceptions

Communication relies upon perception of the person with whom one is communicating. It has been suggested that the care provider's outlook on life affects the way in which they regard and communicate with the person with severe dementia (Asplund, 1991). Several studies have shown that there are care providers who see the patient with severe dementia as an object (Athlin, *et al.*, 1990), and leading, of course, to serious consequences for both communication with the person and for the care given. Other care providers perceive the patient as a subject (Athlin, *et al.*, 1990). This can be done in various ways, for example, by seeing the patient as the person he or she used to be, as a child or as a suffering old person. Asplund and Norberg (1993) reported that professional care providers responded differently to a picture of a person with severe dementia and to a picture of an infant. A person with severe dementia was seen as painful, apathetic, suffering, weak, afraid, sad, cold, dark, rough, and ugly, whereas the infant evoked positive responses.

Barnett (1995) stated that it is important for care providers to uphold the personhood of dementia sufferers by seeing the divine essence of the person that remains unchanged by the condition. This view will be mirrored as love in the eyes of the care providers and positively affects the dementia sufferers. This, Barnett stated, can only come from 'that place deep within us which is only reached through our own brokenness, fear and confusion' (p. 42). Barnett was probably trying to express the phenomenon that Johnston (1978) wrote about as looking with the eye of love.

Care providers have difficulty expressing why and how they can regard the person with severe dementia as a valuable human being. One way of expressing this regard is to use metaphors. The choice of metaphor is certainly connected to the care provider's outlook on life (*cf* Norberg, 1996). They may use the Jewish metaphor that you see God's face behind the patient's face or the Christian metaphor that when you care for the patient you care for Christ – hungry, naked and sick.

In order to understand how some care providers are able to communicate with people with severe dementia despite all the communication difficulties we will now turn to research that has investigated the interaction between care providers and people with severe dementia. For the remainder of the chapter we will discuss and reflect upon the data generated by interviews with care providers and observations and video-recordings of their interactions with people with severe dementia.

Integrity promoting care

Video-recordings of interactions between patients and skilled and trained care providers revealed positive interactions (Kihlgren, *et al.*, 1994, 1996). An approach to care known as 'integrity promoting care' promotes the patient's experience of trust, autonomy, initiative, industry, identity, intimacy, generativity and integrity (wholeness and meaning) during all care activities. This approach to care is inspired by Erikson's (1982) theory of the 'eight stages of man'. In response to integrity-promoting care, patients who communicated in a fragmented way changed and appeared more integrated in the integrity-promoting climate, they even disclosed competence and strengths that had previously been hidden. Kihlgren (1992) interpreted these findings as related to motherly support, preservative love and confirmation of the person with severe dementia as a valuable human being. It is evident that the care providers in this study were focusing on the experiences of the patients with severe dementia.

Covert competence

Ekman's (1993) study of dementia in immigrant populations revealed video-recordings that disclosed patient competence that had hitherto been hidden. In interaction that promoted an experience of wholeness and meaning, mainly in interactions with bilingual care providers, (Ekman, *et al.*, 1993) patients appeared to react to the melody of speech rather than to words (Ekman, 1993). This observation is reminiscent of observations that infants react to the tone of their mothers' voices (*cf* Fernald, *et al.*, 1989). Good interactions were characterised by the care providers' virtues such as patience, honesty, generosity, forgiveness, consideration, softness, trust, harmony, joy; humility, and a positive attitude to life; respect for the patient; communion, i.e. a deep contact; will, i.e. the care provider showing interest, concern and a desire to understand and help.

Observations in group-dwellings for people with moderate and severe dementia showed that, in calm situations where no demands were made on the patients, the patients and their care providers seemed to understand each other without words (Zingmark, *et al.*, 1993, Norberg, *et al.*, 1994). In this kind of situation the patients were seen as exhibiting an experience that was labelled 'being at home'. The connection between the patient and his or her care provider was labelled 'communion', which describes a deep contact without demands. The quality of this contact seems to be 'love'. Care providers were also observed to move very flexibly in 'time' and 'space'. In fact, carers interpreted the communications of people with severe dementia about past time and places as revealing messages about emotions related to the *present* (Norberg, 1994; Norberg, *et al.*, 1994; Zingmark, 1994).

Interpretation was undertaken of video-recorded interactions at a psychogeriatric clinic between care providers and patients with severe dementia who were regarded as being unable to communicate their feelings and desires (Jansson, *et al.*, 1993). Data about the patients (facial expressions, vocalisations, single words) and the care providers (verbal utterances, care activities and awareness of the care context) were incorporated into a narrative for each patient. The process was based upon Sundén's (1959) theory about the communication of Christians with God in prayer. Sundén argued that Christians' knowledge of Bible stories allows them to identify with biblical characters when they find themselves in difficult situations. By identifying with that person they anticipate the voice of God and therefore interpret things that happen as God's voice. Analogously, care providers can be seen as starting with the preunderstanding that there is meaning in the patient's communicative cues and that this meaning is implicit in the situation. They then create a narrative that discloses the meaning. However, only a fragmented picture emerges from an assessment of the meaning of selected facial expressions by means of a registration of patterns of motor movements linked to emotions (Asplund, *et al.*, 1995). It appears, therefore, that care providers participate in the narrative by actively filling in missing pieces in the puzzle of communication of severe dementia sufferers. This narrative, moreover, is also dependent upon the care provider's intuitive grasp of the whole (*cf* Hellner & Norberg, 1994).

Narratives

In order to be able to complete the puzzle of such fragmented communication it is necessary to know the patient's story. This knowledge can be used to fill in gaps between the fragments that the patient presents. Thus the care provider can help the patient to create nice episodes that fit the patient's overall life story. For example, a woman with severe dementia who had been a Christian believer suffered attacks of severe anxiety. A nurse tried to calm the patient by talking about God. 'Who is God?' the woman asked. 'I remember the name but I do not remember who he is'. Then the nurse put herself in front of the woman, clasped her hands and started to pray. 'Dear Lord', she said and the patient continued. In her prayer she showed that she was aware of the situation, she exhibited an episode of lucidity. 'Dear God', she said, 'please, take care of the nurses and help them with their difficult work'. When she had finished her prayer she opened her eyes and asked: 'Where am I? Where am I?' She appeared as confused as before her prayer (Norberg, *et al.*, 1994).

This story shows that in order to help the patient, awareness of her life story must be coupled with knowledge of the effect of the damage to her brain. After this episode the nurse was able to calm the patient by helping her into her bed, sitting at her side reading prayers. The situation can be interpreted as follows. This woman had positive memories from similar situations in her childhood. The situation evoked expectations of love. She also had positive experiences of approaching God. Thus the situation evoked double positive expectations of love. If the patient had experienced a different life history, the situation might have frightened instead of calmed her.

There have been suggestions that people with severe dementia regress to a state that resembles infancy (e.g. Asplund, *et al.*, 1991b; Hurley, *et al.*, 1992; Sandman, *et al.*, 1990; Sclan, *et al.*, 1990). For example, people with severe dementia often exhibit clinging and demanding behaviour that can be interpreted as attachment-seeking behaviour (Wright, *et al.*, 1995). The person may be seen as a Russian doll with a nucleus of early developed abilities encased in layers of abilities later developed (Norberg, *et al.*, 1994). Such a view implies that theories about infants and children may be used to understand the experiences that are expressed by the behaviour of people with severe dementia. It should however be emphasised that when the environmental influences are optimal the person with dementia may suddenly react as an adult or even as a wise old person (Kihlgren, *et al.,* 1996). Berg-Brodén (1992) suggested that the term 'ingression' would be a more proper term than 'regression' to describe adult use of early behaviour.

'Maternal thinking'

The fact that there are care providers who seem to understand their patients with severe dementia although they cannot give any rational reasons for this understanding (Athlin, *et al.,* 1990; Åkerlund & Norberg, 1990), can be interpreted in analogy with Pawlby's (1977) discussions of interaction between infants and their mothers. Pawlby argued that mothers impute meaning to the infant's incomprehensible cues and the infant gradually makes the imputations his or her own meaning. It could, by analogy, be regarded as also good for people with severe dementia to feel that they are regarded as a person with feelings, thoughts and desires, even if care providers would impute different meanings. For example refusal behaviour during meals may be regarded by the care provider as an expression of a wish to be left alone or as an expression of a need for contact. The problem with Pawley's model is that only the care provider determines the meaning, and the person with severe dementia then becomes the care provider's creation, i.e. an object (Norberg, 1996). Care providers have to strike a balance between imputing too much meaning to the patient's cues and ignoring the possibility that there might be some meaning to be interpreted (Asplund, *et al.,* 1995).

In interview, care providers, at a group dwelling for people with moderate and severe dementia, often referred to their personal experiences of mothering of children or relating to their own mothers when they tried to explain how they could understand the residents (Häggström & Norberg 1996). Callery (1997) considered that a mother interprets her child's behaviour within the context of the child's normal pattern of behaviour. The mother can make intuitive judgements about the child's feelings and well-being as maternal knowledge is acquired in close contact with the child, whom the mother knows intimately.

The term 'maternal thinking' denotes a familiar phenomenon and is intended to be understood as a metaphor used to express a kind of close mainly non-verbal care that could be performed by men as well as by women (*cf* Pringle, 1995). Häggström (1997) emphasised that a less emotionally loaded word is needed to avoid the risk of degrading people with severe dementia, a word that expresses attentive love and closeness (*cf* Ruddick, 1990, pp. 10–12) and also emphasises respect for the person's previous life (*cf* Thomasma, 1984).

Ekman and Norberg (1993) described the relationship between the carer and the person with dementia as a deep human contact beyond words – a communion, sharing in another's experience with no attempt to change what that person does or believes. This is the same kind of relationship, described by Stern (1985), that obtains between an infant and its mother. By 'being with', 'sharing', or 'joining in', the care provider helped the patient to express ideas of which he or she was only dimly aware and was unable to express unaided. Communion implies that the care provider takes for granted that there is meaning in the patient's verbal and non-verbal expressions. The care provider is thus sensitised to the patient's speech and actions and seems to understand them.

Communion

Communion can be understood as moments of a unique togetherness, a shared understanding and acceptance between the care provider and the person with severe dementia (*cf* van Kaam, 1959). Communion seems to occur even where the parties relate to a different time and space. People with severe dementia may experience that they are in their childhood home with their parents, while the care provider's experience is that they are in a nursing home in the present. The important prerequisite for communion seems to be a shared affective state, rather than a shared cognitive interpretation of that state (*cf* Norberg, 1994; Norberg, *et al.*, 1994). The sharing does not imply any symbiosis; Zizioulas (1993) emphasised that communion does not mean suppressing the person but on the contrary it includes freedom for the person.

Affect attunement

Stern (1985) described affect attunement between mothers and their infants as a process where the mother starts imitating the infant's actions until she tunes into his or her affective state. From that shared affective state she can slowly affect him or her and for example change his or her mood. Thus, when comforting an infant the mother starts by sharing the infant's agitated rhythm and then she slowly reduces it by gradually reducing the speed and intensity of her movements, tone of voice and the like. Affect attunement might be one explanation for the quite common observations that people with severe dementia exhibit most integrity when acting slowly in calm situations (Ekman, *et al.*, 1993; Hallberg, *et al.*, 1995; Kihlgren, *et al.*, 1994). According to Häggström (1997) 'three concepts together: "maternal thinking", "communion" and "affect attunement" form a pattern of understanding that can be achieved beyond words'.

There are several researchers who have reported similar observations. For example, Kitwood (1993), Kitwood and Bredin (1992), Harrisson (1993) as well as Gibson (1994) think that care providers can help people with severe dementia to keep mental fragments together, which will promote their experience of well-being. People with severe dementia may communicate about the present via the past. The care provider should listen with an open mind and try to grasp the emotional content of the message. By listening again and again to the patient the message may become more and more fully expressed and the care provider can gradually build up an understanding of its content. This presupposes that the care provider does not feel threatened by the message and dares to accommodate it. The care provider helps the patient to fill in missing parts in his/her message, to create a whole. The care provider thus fulfils the patient's initiated actions.

Sovereign utterances

The perspective of the Danish philosopher K. Lögstrup (Bexell, *et al.*, 1985, Lögstrup, 1971) offers a means to understand communion and communication with people with severe dementia. He described a human ethic based on a phenomenological analysis of life. Lögstrup thought that when we encounter other people we may be captured by spontaneous or sovereign utterances of life such as trust, sympathy, open speech, mercy and joy. But if we try to produce, use or control these positive phenomena they will be destroyed. What we must do is create situations that allow for and nurture the spontaneous utterances of life and we must avoid destroying them.

Lögstrup emphasised that it is basic to human life that we meet each other with trust. The occurrence of trust cannot be explained. In fact, what must be explained are situations where trust does not occur. When another human being is hurt our basic reaction is to become seized by sympathy and mercy. This does not have to be explained – it is the situation where this does not occur that has to be explained. Relating to other human beings means that we have power over them. In fact, we can hurt or even kill each other. We are responsible for each others' lives – in a literary or metaphorical sense. We are interdependent as parts of the same situation and of each other's lives.

Sometimes the spontaneous utterances of life are not grasped, a conscious effort has to be made to interpret the situation. Lögstrup emphasised that when we encounter another person we meet with an ethical demand to take good care of the other's life. When interpreting the ethical demand we sense the situation of which we and the others are part. In order to sense we must be open to receiving and sharing experiences with other people. Interpretation of our intuition is made against the background of our preunderstanding. When interpreting the ethical demand we are for example guided by norms and values, for example, the norm about love to our neighbour. The norms and values are parts of our outlook on life. Another important part of the preunderstanding is our idea of what it means to suffer from dementia.

It seems that affect attunement and being in communion are phenomena that might be described as spontaneous utterances of life. This acting in communion appears spontaneous, when we go deep enough into a situation, we no longer have any choice of action, we just know what ought to be done. Lögstrup's writings of course are concerned with ethics. However, in my view ethical reasoning must be connected with communication theory. Ethical problems arising in care as narrated by care providers are often related to problems of communication. Care providers, for example, related that they faced an ethical problem when deciding how to treat patients with severe dementia who exhibit refusal-like eating behaviour. This predicament was clearly related to their communication problems, as they could not feel certain about the patients' wishes and feelings (Jansson & Norberg, 1992).

A problem connected with affect attunement and communion is that care providers must be able to cope with sharing negative and sometimes horrifying affective states in order to help the patient towards a more positive affective state. Nurses were interviewed concerning their thoughts about experiences with patients with severe dementia who were vocally disruptive in their behaviour. The nurses articulated anxieties about dissolution, and about being abandoned (Hallberg & Norberg, 1990). It seems logical that those care providers who have these thoughts would interact closely with their patients. However, it was evident from observation that nurses spent no more time with noisy patients than with the patients who did not scream (Hallberg, *et al.*, 1990). Furthermore, they interacted with the screaming patients mainly when they performed tasks, they talked very little to the patients and then in a task-orientated way. They said things like: 'Open your mouth! Swallow!' (Hallberg, *et al.*, 1993). This lack of congruence between what the nurses thought they ought to do and what they did do can be understood from their reported experiences. The noisy patients evoked in the nurses feelings of being insufficient and powerless and, in order to avoid these feelings, nurses avoided the patients who evoked them.

Negative affective states

Care providers need help to contain negative affective states. To this end Hallberg started systematic clinical supervision for nurses to help them gain power over their negative feelings. Positive results of systematic clinical supervision for nurses were noted both for patients and for nurses (Hallberg & Norberg, 1993). Lögstrup emphasised our interdependence. This interdependence is very apparent in the care of people with severe dementia (e.g. Norberg & Asplund, 1990). In interviews with care providers we find those who say that caring for a patient with severe dementia is meaningless work in that they get nothing back from the patient. These care providers talk about the patient as an object or as socially dead. They express the feeling that they only work in dementia care, they do not care for those with dementia.

Other care providers tell us they find care work with the patient with severe dementia such meaningful work and they get so much from the patient. They talk about patients with respect as valuable human beings and they seem proud of their work. It appears that the perception of the patient is of the utmost importance. If the patient is seen as a valuable person, then the work caring for the patient appears important and the care provider who performs such important work is also a valuable person (*cf* Hegel, 1967; Norberg, 1996).

The question remains, as to how is it possible to learn to communicate and be in communion with people with severe dementia. In interviews good care providers often relate experiences that could be labelled border experiences: 'Before I thought and felt so and so, but when my mother died, I understood. Since that event I see and feel and think in another way'. It could also be a child who died. The care providers relate experiences that made them touch the holy and that made them change their outlook on life. We cannot give students and care providers these kinds of experiences but when they do occur we can help them reflect on them and gain from them because these situations can lead to fear and result in negative effects (*cf* Jansson & Norberg, 1992).

Conclusion

In order to be open enough to be grasped by spontaneous or sovereign utterances of life and to share the patient's experiences care providers need the ability to look with the eye of love. In order to be able to interpret what we sense we need to combine knowledge of the patient's life story with knowledge about the brain damage and open ourselves to the holy in the person. Writings about looking at a person with severe dementia with the 'eye of love' are based on a religious outlook on life. Yet there must be ways to do research into achieving a better understanding of the phenomenon. Likewise the observations that concepts arising from the care of infants can be used to understand some observed phenomena in the care of people with severe dementia also ought to be further investigated in relation to how the effects of various types of brain damage affect behaviour.

References

Åkerlund, B.M. & Norberg, A. (1986) Group psychotherapy with demented patients. *Geriatric Nursing*, **7**, 83–4.

Åkerlund, B.M. & Norberg, A. (1990) Powerless in terminal care of demented patients: An exploratory study. *Omega*, **21**, 15–19.

APA (1994) *Diagnostic and statistical manual of mental disorders prepared by the task force on DSM-IV*. 4th edn. American Psychiatric Association, Washington DC.

Apell, J., Kertesz, A. & Fisman, M. (1982) A study of language functioning in Alzheimer's patients. *Brain and Language*, **17**, 73–91.

Asplund, K. (1991) *The experience of meaning in the care of patients in the terminal stage of dementia of the type. Interpretation of non-verbal communication and ethical demands.* Umeå University, Medical Dissertation New Series No 310, Umeå.

Asplund, K. & Norberg, A. (1993) Caregivers' reactions to the physical appearance of a person in the final stage of dementia as measured by semantic differentials. *International Journal of Aging and Human Development*, **37**, 205–15.

Asplund, K., Norberg, A., Adolfsson, R. & Waxman, H.M. (1991a) Facial expressions in severely demented patients – a stimulus-response study of four patients with dementia of the Alzheimer type. *International Journal of Geriatric Psychiatry*, **6**, 599–606.

Asplund, K., Norberg, A. & Adolfsson, R. (1991b) The sucking behaviour of two patients in the final stage of dementia of the Alzheimer type. *Scandinavian Journal of Caring Sciences*, **5**, 141–7.

Asplund, K., Jansson, L. & Norberg, A. (1995) Expressive facial behaviour in patients with severe dementia of the Alzheimer type (DAT). A comparison between unstructured naturalistic judgements and analytic assessment by means of the Facial Action Coding System (FACS). *International Psychogeriatrics*, **7**, 527–34.

Athlin, E. & Norberg, A. (1987a) Caregivers' attitudes to and interpretations of the behaviour of severely demented patients during feeding in a patient assignment system. *International Journal of Nursing Studies*, **24**, 145–53.

Athlin, E. & Norberg, A. (1987b) Interaction between the severely demented patient and his caregiver during feeding. A theoretical model. *Scandinavian Journal of Caring Sciences*, **1**, 117–23.

Athlin, E., Norberg, A. & Asplund, K. (1990) Caregivers' perceptions and interpretations of severely demented patients during feeding in a task assignment care system. *Scandinavian Journal of Caring Sciences*, **4**, 147–56.

Barnett, E. (1995) Broadening our approach to spirituality. In: *The new culture of dementia care* (eds T. Kitwood & S. Benson), pp. 40–43. Hawker Publications in Association with the Bradford Dementia Group, London.

Bayles, K.A. & Tomoeda, C.K. (1991) Caregiver report of prevalence and appearance order of linguistic symptoms in Alzheimer's patients. *The Gerontologist*, **31**, 210–16.

Bayles, KL., Tomoeda, C.K. & Trosset, M.W. (1992) Relation of linguistic communication abilities of Alzheimer's patients to stage of disease. *Brain and Language*, **42**, 454–72.

Berg-Brodén, M. (1992) *Psykoterapeutiska interventioner under spädbarnsperioden* [in Swedish: Psychotherapeutic interventions during the period of infancy]. Förlagshuset Swedala, Trelleborg.

Bexell, G., Norberg, A. & Norberg, B. (1985) Ethical conflicts in long-term care of aged patients. An ontological model of the care situation. *Ethics & Medicine*, **1**, 44–6.

Bleathman, C. & I. Morton I. (1992) Validation therapy: Extracts from 20 groups with dementia sufferers. *Journal of Advanced Nursing*, **17**, 658–66.

Bright, R. (1992) Music therapy in the management of dementia. In: *Caregiving in dementia. Research and applications* (eds G. Jones & B.M.L. Miesen), Ch 10, pp. 162–80. Routledge, London.

Callery, P. (1997) Maternal knowledge and professional knowledge: co-operation and conflict in the care of sick children. *International Journal of Nursing Studies*, **34**, 27–34.

Corcoran, M. & Gitlin, L.N. (1991) Environmental influences on behaviour of the elderly with dementia: principles for intervention in the home. *Occupational Therapy in Geriatrics*, **9**, 5–20.

Critcley, M. (1964) The neurology of psychotic speech. *British Journal of Psychiatry*, **110**, 353–64.

Edberg, A.K., Nordmark, Sandgren, Å. & Hallberg, I.R. (1995) Initiating and terminating verbal interaction between nurses and severely demented patients regarded as vocally disruptive. *Journal of Psychiatric Nursing*, **2**, 159–67.

Ehrenberg Hamilton, H. (1994) *Conversations with an Alzheimer's patient. An interactional sociolinguistic study*. Cambridge University Press, Cambridge.

Ekman, S.L. (1993) *Monolingual and bilingual communication between patients with dementia diseases and their caregivers*. Umeå University, Medical dissertation. New series No 370, Umeå.

Ekman, S.L. & Norberg, A. (1993) Characteristics of the good relationship in the care of bilingual demented immigrants. In: *Monolingual and bilingual communication between patients with dementia diseases and their caregivers* (ed. S.L. Ekman), pp. 139–58. Umeå University, Medical dissertation. New series No 370, Umeå.

Ekman, S.L., Robins Wallin, T.B., Norberg, A. & Winblad, B. (1993) Relationship between bilingual demented immigrants and bilingual/monolingual caregivers. *International Journal of Aging and Human Development*, **37**, 37–54.

Erikson, E.H. (1982) *The life cycle completed. A review.* WW Norton & Company Inc., New York.

Fernald, A., Taeschner, T., Dunn, J. & Papousek, M. (1989) A cross language study of prosodic modifications in mothers' and fathers' speech to preverbal infants. *Journal of Child Language*, **16**, 477–501.

Frank, B. (1995) People with dementia can communicate – if we are able to hear. In: *The new culture of dementia care* (eds T. Kitwood, S. Benson), pp. 24–9. Hawker Publications in Association with the Bradford Dementia Group, London.

Gibson, F. (1994) What can reminiscence contribute to people with dementia? In: *Reminiscence reviewed, perspectives, evaluations, achievements* (ed. J. Bornat), pp. 46–60. Open University Press, Buckingham.

Hallberg, I.R., Norberg, A. (1990) Staff's interpretation of the experience behind vocally disruptive behaviour in severely demented patients and their feelings about it, an explorative study. *International Journal of Aging and Human Development*, **31**, 295–305.

Hallberg, I.R., Luker, K., Norberg, A., Johnsson, K. & Eriksson, S. (1990) Staff interaction with vocally disruptive demented patients compared with demented controls. *Aging*, **2**, 163–71.

Hallberg, I.R. & Norberg, A. (1993) Strain among nurses and their emotional reactions during 1 year of systematic clinical supervision combined with the implementation of individualized care in dementia nursing. *Journal of Advanced Nursing*, **18**, 1860–75.

Hallberg, I.R., Norberg, A. & Johnsson, K. (1993) Verbal interaction during the lunch-meal between caregivers and vocally disruptive demented patients. *American Journal of Alzheimer's Care and Related Disorders & Research*, **8**, 26–32.

Hallberg, I.R., Holst, G., Nordmark, Å. & Edberg, A.K. (1995) Cooperation during morning care between nurses and severely demented institutionalized patients. *Clinical Nursing Research*, **4**, 78–104.

Harrisson, C. (1993) Personhood, dementia and the integrity of a life. *Canadian Journal on Aging*, **12**, 428–40.

Hegel, G.W.F. (1967) *The phenomenology of the mind.* [German original 1807], pp. 228–9. Harper and Row, New York.

Hellner, B.M. & Norberg, A. (1994) Intuition: Two caregivers' description of how they provide severely demented patients with loving care. *The International Journal of Aging and Human Development*, **38**, 327–38.

Hurley, A.C., Volicer, B.J., Hanrahan, P.A., Houde, S. & Volicer, L. (1992) Assessment of discomfort in advanced Alzheimer patients. *Research in Nursing & Health*, **15**, 369–77.

Häggström, T. (1997) *Formal carers' understanding of residents with severe dementia in a group dwelling.* Licentiate Thesis. Department of Advanced Nursing, Umeå University, Umeå, Sweden.

Häggström, T. & Norberg, A. (1996) Maternal thinking in dementia care. *Journal of Advanced Nursing*, **24**, 431–8.

Jansson, L. & Norberg, A. (1992) Ethical reasoning among registered nurses experienced in dementia care. Interviews concerning the feeding of severely demented patients. *Scandinavian Journal of Caring Sciences*, **6**, 219–27.

Jansson, L., Norberg, A., Sandman, P.O., Athlin, E. & Asplund, K. (1993) Interpreting facial expressions in patients in the terminal stage of the Alzheimers Disease. *Omega,* **26,** 319–34.

Johnston, W. (1978) *The inner eye of love.* Harper & Row, New York.

Kihlgren, M. (1992) *Integrity promoting care of demented patients.* Umeå University, Medical Dissertation New Series No 351, Umeå.

Kihlgren, M., Hallgren, A., Norberg, A. & Karlsson, I. (1994) Integrity promoting care of demented patients. Patterns of interaction during morning care. *International Journal of Aging and Human Development,* **39,** 303–19.

Kihlgren, M., Hallgren, A., Norberg, A. & Karlsson, I. (1996) Disclosure of basic strengths and basic weakness in demented patients during morning care, before and after staff training. Analysis of video-recordings by means of the Erikson theory of 'eight stages of man'. *International Journal of Aging and Human Development,* **43,** 219–33.

Kitwood, T. (1993) Towards a theory of dementia care: The interpersonal process. *Ageing and Society,* **13,** 51–67.

Kitwood, T. & Bredin, K. (1992) Towards a theory of dementia care: Personhood and well-being. *Aging and Society,* **12,** 269–87.

Lawton, M.P. (1982) Competence, environmental press and the adaptation of older people. In: *Aging and the environment. Theoretical approaches* (eds M.P. Lawton, P.G. Windley & T.O. Byerts). Springer Publishing House, New York.

Lindgren, C., Hallberg, I.R. & Norberg, A. (1992) Diagnostic reasoning in the care of a vocally disruptive severely demented patient. A case report. *Scandinavian Journal of Caring Sciences,* **6,** 97–103.

Lögstrup, K.E. (1971) *The ethical demand* [Original Danish, 1956]. Fortress Press, Philadelphia.

Magai, C., Cohen, C., Gomberg, D., Malatesta, C. & Culver, C. (1996) Emotional expressions during mid- to late-stage dementia. *International Psychogeriatrics,* **8,** 383–95.

McDaniel, K.D., Edland, S.D. & Heyman, A. (1995) The CERAD Clinical Investigators. Relationship between level of insight and severity of dementia in Alzheimer disease. *Alzheimer Disease and Associated Disorders,* **9,** 101–104.

Miesen, B.M.L. (1993) Alzheimer's disease, the phenomenon of parent fixation and Bowlby's attachment theory. *International Journal of Geriatric Psychiatry,* **8,** 147–53.

Norberg, A. (1994) Ethics in the care of elderly with dementia. In: *Principles of health care ethics* (ed. R. Gillon), pp. 721–32. John Wiley & Sons Ltd., Chichester

Norberg, A. (1996) Caring for demented people. *Acta Neurologica Scandinavica,* **165,** 105–108.

Norberg, A., Melin, E. & Asplund, K. (1986) Reactions to music, touch and object presentation in the final stage of dementia. An exploratory study. *International Journal of Nursing Studies,* **23,** 315–23.

Norberg, A. & Asplund, K. (1990) Caregivers' experience of caring for severely demented patients. *Western Journal of Nursing Research,* **12,** 75–84.

Norberg, A., Zingmark, K. & Nilsson, L. (1994) *To be demented. Human being fenced into a tattered brain* [in Swedish]. Bonniers, Stockholm.

Obler, L.K. & Albert, M. (1984) Language in aging. In: *Clinical neurology of aging* (ed. M. Albert). Oxford University Press, New York.

Pawlby, S.J. (1977) Imitative interaction. In Scaffer HR. *Studies in mother-infant interaction* (ed. H.R. Scaffer), pp. 203–24. Academic Press, London.

Popper, K.R. & Eccles, J.C. (1977) *The self and its brain. An argument for interactionism.* Routledge, London.

Pringle, K. (1995) *Men, masculine and social welfare.* UCL Press, London.

Ruddick, S. (1990) *Maternal thinking. Towards a politics of peace.* The Women's Press Ltd, London.

Sabat, R.S. (1994) Recognizing and working with remaining abilities: Toward improving the care of Alzheimer's disease suffers. *American Journal of Alzheimer's Care and Related Disorders and Research,* **9,** 7–16.

Sabat, S.R. & Harré, T. (1992) The construction and deconstruction of self in Alzheimer's disease. *Ageing and Society,* **12,** 443–61.

Sandman P.O., Norberg, A., Adolfsson, R., Axelsson, K. & Hedly, V. (1986) Morning care of patients with dementia of Alzheimer's type. A theoretical model based on observations. *Journal of Advanced Nursing,* **11,** 369–78.

Sandman, P.O., Norberg, A. & Adolfsson, R. (1988) Verbal communication and behaviour during meals in five institutionalized patients with Alzheimer-type dementia. *Journal of Advanced Nursing,* **13,** 571–8.

Sandman, P.O., Norberg, A., Adolfsson, R., Eriksson, S. & Nyström, L. (1990) Prevalence and characteristics of persons with dependency on feeding at institutions for elderly. *Scandinavian Journal of Caring Sciences,* **4,** 121–7.

Sclan, S.G., Foster, J.R., Reisberg, B., Franssen, E. & Welkowitz, J. (1990) Application of Piagetian measures of cognition in severe Alzheimer's disease. *Psychiatric Journal of the University of Ottawa,* **15,** 223–8.

Stern, D.N. (1985) *The Interpersonal World of the Infant.* Basic Books, New York.

Sundén, H. (1959) *The Religion and the Roles. A psychological study of piety.* Diakonistyrelsens bokförlag, Stockholm.

Swane, C.E. (1996) *Hverdagen i demens. Billeddannelser og hverdagserfaring i kulturgerontologisk perspektiv* [in Danish: Everyday life with dementia. Images and experience in a cultural gerontological perspective]. Munksgaard, Köpenhavn.

Svensson, T. (1984) *Aging and Environment. Institutional Aspects.* Studies in Education. Dissertations No. 21. Linköping University, Department of Education and Psychology, Linköping.

Thornstam, L. (1994) Gero-Transcendence: A theoretical and empirical exploration. In: *Aging and the religious dimension* (eds L.E. Thomas & S.A. Eisenhandler). Auburn House, London.

Thomasma, D.C. (1984) Medical Ethics and Humanities. Freedom, Dependency, and the freedom of the very old. *Journal of the American Geriatric Society,* **32,** 906–14.

van Kaam, A.L. (1959) The nurse in the patient's world. *American Journal of Nursing,* **12,** 1708–10.

Woods, B. (1995) The beginning of a new culture in care. In: *The new culture of dementia care* (eds T. Kitwood & S. Benson). Hawker Publications in Association with the Bradford Dementia Group, London.

Wright, L.K., Hickey, J.V., Buckwalter, K.C. & Clipp, E.C. (1995) Human development in the context of aging and chronic illness: The role of attachment in Alzheimer's disease and stroke. *International Journal of Aging and Human Development,* **41,** 133–50.

Zingmark, K., Norberg, A. & Sandman, P.O. (1993) Experience of at-homeness and homesickness in patients with Alzheimer's disease. *American Journal of Alzheimer's Care and Related Disorders and Research,* **8,** 10–16.

Zingmark, K. (1994) *Promoting an experience of at-homeness in people with Alzheimer's disease.* Licentiate Thesis, Umeå University, Umeå.

Zizioulas, J.D. (1993) *Being as communion. Studies in personhood and the church.* St Vladimir's Seminary Press, Crestwood, NY.

10 Older People with Mental Health Problems: Maintaining a Dialogue

Jan Reed and *Charlotte Clarke*

Introduction

We have chosen to focus this chapter around the theme of 'maintaining a dialogue with older people'. There are multiple reasons for this: in the literature on mental health care (and indeed, all other forms of health care) for older people, talking *about* older people and their problems seems to be quite common. Talking *with* their families is less common, but it still seems to be advocated more frequently than talking *with* older people themselves. As practitioners and researchers with experience of talking about and with older people, we feel that nurses dismiss the voice of older people too easily, and run the risk of delivering care which is inappropriate and ineffective as a result.

The idea of talking *with* older people seems deceptively simple, but exploring the reasons why it does not happen leads us into the murky area of ageism, where assumptions are made that older people display uniform characteristics of decay and decrepitude as an automatic consequence of their age. We begin this chapter with an exploration of ageism – we feel that it is only when we start to address this that we get closer to any form of dialogue with older people. We also explore the inherent paradoxes in moves towards the inclusion of family and carers in the therapeutic activity of nurses and therapists. While this move makes sense, and can be seen to represent a more holistic view of the individual as a member of society and of a social network, it also carries some risks. If we focus on carers because we think that those for whom they care, older people, are irremediable or unable to respond to our efforts, then we come very close to pushing the older person out of the picture – of talking *about* them rather than *with* them.

We are, of course, aware that in the very act of writing a chapter about mental health care for older people we run the risk of being ageist. To say that there are certain mental health problems that only affect older people seems to separate them off from everyone else, and of course, it is inaccurate. Older people experience the same range of mental health problems as every other group in society, the difference being that the care and support that they receive is shaped by ideas about the inevitable decline of age. This affects the way in which therapy is tinged by therapeutic pessimism, and the way that assessment of need is coloured by over-simplistic views of the mental health problems of older people.

This chapter is not a detailed discussion of the incidence and manifestation of mental health problems in older people, nor does it provide detailed guidelines on how to use specific therapeutic techniques or strategies. To do this would take a book, not just a chapter, and so we have decided to concentrate on the most important issues, the principles on which interventions should be based. We firmly believe that without an awareness of these principles, practitioners cannot deliver the care that older people deserve.

Ageism and therapeutic pessimism

The most important issue for practitioners working with older people to be aware of is the issue of ageism: the discrimination against people on the grounds of their age. The stereotypes that are promulgated about older people, by society at large and by practitioners themselves, colour and shape all approaches to practice in an invidious way. From assessment, through planning and in evaluation, the expectations and goals of practitioners are developed against a background of therapeutic pessimism – the low expectations we have of the capacity of older people to respond to therapy, to exercise self-awareness and insight, and to participate in any reflective processes.

One of the puzzling things about ageism, as Hughes (1995) points out, is that while other 'isms' apply to characteristics such as gender or race which people are born with, and which cannot be acquired in any other way, old age is something that people grow into, and it is something which potentially faces all of us. Viewing older people as separate and different from the rest of us, therefore, is an impressive feat of mental gymnastics. As Thompson (1992) has commented 'Old people are always *other* people, never oneself however old one may be'. Perhaps an additional element of ageism, however, is that we do not quite succeed in this feat, and we retain some degree of awareness that we ourselves may become old one day, while we will not become a different race or gender. Our negative images of older people then, are to some degree, negative images of ourselves in the future, and the discomfort we feel with this future is manifested in the discomfort we feel about older people.

This discomfort translates into a range of different policies and practices in health care for older people. The history of service provision for older people in Western society demonstrates this vividly. Macintyre (1977), in her discussion of old age as a 'social problem', has suggested that at one point in the social history of the UK at least, older people were not distinguished as a specific group of people needing support – they were just regarded as poor or infirm and their age was not used as an identifier. Minois (1989) makes similar comments in his history of old age, that at certain periods of Western history older people do not seem to be identified as a particular group. This state of affairs has, however, changed, as Minois chronicles, perhaps as a reaction to increased longevity that has made older people, initially a rare phenomenon regarded with admiration and wonder, a commonplace feature of the social world.

Macintyre (1977) identifies the beginning of the British recognition of the 'special case' of older people as occuring about the end of the nineteenth century. With industrialisation and the consequent demand for labour, older people were left without the means to secure their livelihood, and without their families to support to care for them. Poor relief criteria emphasised a demonstrated willingness and ability to work. However, it became apparent that for older people unemployment was due to frailty rather than idleness, and, furthermore, this frailty was likely to increase with a consequent diminishing of their future employment prospects. It made no sense therefore, on humanitarian grounds, to treat older people in the harsh way that other poor people were treated.

The 'problem' of old age, however, is subject to differing definitions. Macintyre outlines two. Firstly, the problem can be seen as a problem of how to provide the best care for older people, commensurate with their needs and with the rewards that society feels are due to them. Alternatively, the problem of old age may be formulated as the need to meet basic needs as cheaply as possible, with minimum demand on the public purse. This second formulation, of course, carries with it a notion of older people as presenting a drain on the resources of society, rather than making a contribution to it. The negative views of old age inherent in the 'cheap as possible' approach to provision for older people, therefore, constitutes a form of ageism that is built into services. This view pushes us to think of expenditure on older people as unlikely to provide any returns.

The contributions that older people make to society are not easy to assess, particularly if we only think of financial contributions, such as those arising from paid employment. Those in paid employment contribute taxes, they buy products and services which in turn guarantee employment for others. Older people, however, are excluded from this type of participation by employment policies both at a company and society level, which enforce retirement at specific ages, and replace salaries with much lower pensions. As Phillipson (1972) argues, this enforced economic redundancy contributes to the idea that older people are socially and economically redundant too. Ageist policies breed ageist attitudes, and ageist attitudes breed ageist policies.

By regarding older people as making little current or future contribution to society, services for older people are reliant on recognition of past contributions for their justification and rationale. In other words, we provide care and support for older people, not because we think that they are contributing to society (as younger adults might, or as we ourselves do). Nor do we think older people will contribute to society in the future (as children might as they grow up). Our obligations derive from the view that at some distant point they 'had' a life, and were involved in events that we think were probably important (for example, raised a family or fought in a war).

The way in which we think of our work, in terms of contributing to the general good, then, is developed in a context where the people for whom we care are seen as making limited contributions to the general good. While it is not necessarily the case that care is only valued if it is given to people who are valued, practitioners are part of the society in which they work, and are aware of the views that predominate, even if they don't agree with them. For practitioners working in the mental health field, social prejudices and stereotypes about the people that they care for remain a common feature of conversations that they have with others about what they do for a living. Justifying this work by appealing to the future contributions to society that people with mental health problems may make if they are helped now is one strategy that can be used. Work with older people with mental health problems, however, is difficult to justify on these grounds. This is because of the assumption that older people are unlikely to make current or future contributions to society. Nurses are then reduced to lame arguments for 'warehousing', as Evers (1981) described it, as an act of sympathy or charity for older people who are simply waiting to die.

The notion of warehousing, of course, stems from more than assumptions of a limited future for older people. It also stems from therapeutic pessimism – the assumption that older people are unlikely to respond to any therapeutic interventions. This pessimism is partly derived from general views and ideas about the cognitive and psychological abilities of older people, in that they are seen as rigid in their ideas and limited in their capacity for insight and change. As Banks and Blair (1997) have commented, these assumptions are also evident in some of the professional literature on mental health problems in older people, with certain forms of therapy regarded as unsuitable because of the limited abilities of older people.

Freud, for example, dismissed the idea of psychotherapy for older people, because he believed them to be 'no longer educable' (Hildebrand 1982). This view has led to a widespread exclusion of older people from such facilities, as Butler, *et al.* (1991) have described: 'Individual psychotherapy is *least* available to older people compared to other age groups.' They also go on to comment about the irony of Freud's pronouncement – 'we would barely know of him had he died before the age of 40, since his finest work was done in the postmeridian period of his life' (p. 405).

Freud's pessimism is echoed in a number of developmental theories that either ignore older age by finishing at 'adulthood' or describe it as a period of withdrawal from the world. Perhaps the most notorious of these theories is that postulated by Cummings and Henry (1961) in their 'disengagement theory'. This theory proposed that the process of growing old was a process of reducing activity and contact with others, and increasing concern with personal experiences in a narrower social sphere. Disengagement theory, not unexpectedly, has been the subject of fierce criticism, primarily from those who argue that the withdrawal of older people from wider social activity is not a matter of choice, but it arises from the exclusion of older people by financial constraints and negative attitudes. In other words disengagement is not a personal developmental stage, but an artefact of the culture and society in which older people live.

Reaction to disengagement theory, then, is often concerned with challenging the stereotypes that this theory appears to be reinforcing. There is certainly plenty of empirical evidence to support this reaction, ranging from investigations of 'structured dependency' (Townsend, 1981), such as the ways in which older people are excluded from the workplace and financial self-sufficiency, to case histories and evaluations of therapy initiatives with older people which have indicated that they can be as responsive as other age groups (see Butler, *et al.* 1991, for a discussion of these). These rejections of disengagement theories and their like, however, can sometimes run the risk of enforcing equally rigid views of older people, which perhaps, again, owe much to our own experiences and views. By emphasising the potential for activity in older people, we may be applying ideas derived from our own experiences and values, and in effect be arguing that older people should behave in the same way as younger people do, if they want to age 'successfully'.

One theory of 'successful' ageing, was in fact, named 'activity theory' (Havighurst 1963), and suggested that those who remain active and socially integrated are happier and experience more satisfaction with life. As Victor (1988, p. 44) puts it, however, 'Ageing is conceptualised as a continuous struggle to remain middle-aged'. Again, as with disengagement theory, attempts to sum up the experience of ageing, and particularly to capture 'successful' ageing seem simplistic, and carry with them their own problems of stereotyping, and the imposition of younger peoples' ideas and interpretations on the experiences of older people.

Interestingly, perhaps one of the most insightful comments about this dilemma comes from Jung, who does not seem to have shared the dismissive attitude of Freud:

> 'We cannot live in the afternoon of life according to the program of life's morning, for what was great in the morning will be little at evening, and what in the morning was true, will at evening have become a lie. I have given psychological treatment to too many people of advancing years, and have looked too often onto the secret chambers of their soul, not to be moved by this fundamental truth.'

> (Jung C.G. (1933) *Modern man in search of a soul*, quoted in Butler, *et al.*, 1991)

The ageist attitudes that persist in the care of older people with mental health problems compound the pessimism that surrounds the future for very many people. Since a degree of cognitive decline has been considered 'normal' in advancing years there has been apathy about seeking diagnosis and a trajectory of continual decline, particularly in dementia, has been regarded as inevitable. Indeed, it is largely the recognition of dementia in younger people that has triggered the current drive for early diagnosis and intervention in dementia (Keady & Nolan, 1994). Were dementia confined to people beyond the age of retirement, perhaps the level of activity in the field would be considerably less. Similarly, depression in older people has been relatively unstated and the estimated prevalence of depression in older people as ranging from 10% to 65% (Gurland & Cross, 1982) has made little impact on health promotion strategies and health care policies.

These views, however, are not solely advanced by health and social care professionals. Such is the stigma of being seen to be mentally incapacitated, individuals themselves seek to hide their cognitive losses (Keady, 1997; Robinson, *et al.*, 1997). Managing their cognitive loss becomes an increasingly dominant part of their life and is a very private experience. Only at some later stage is the difficulty revealed to family members and later again to others such as health care professionals.

The stigma would not exist of course did we not have such difficulty distinguishing between the ill-health problems of an individual and their sense of self and being. This issue is not exclusive to people with mental health problems. Indeed people who use a wheelchair are familiar with being ignored since their weak legs supposedly result in a weak brain – an interesting linkage given the reductionist approach to ill-health which pervades Western health care systems and which usually fails to recognise any association between differing aspects of the body. To be identified then as having a mental health problem is to bring the very essence of self into question. In particular for older people with dementia, Sabat and Harre (1992) argue that the norm is for people to be considered as ceasing to exist as a person once they are believed to have dementia, a stance they and others argue powerfully against. Kitwood and Bredin's (1992) influential work has pushed for a recognition of the 'personhood', or that essence which remains, of people with dementia.

However, the biomedical dominance of health care renders it hard to see beyond the continual decline of mental illness in older people. But to link the decline of cognitive functioning with the decline of self perhaps may be as errant as to equate weak legs with a weak brain. Just as older people become 'disconnected' with the rest of society if society sees fit to cast them off (as disengagement theory and economic theories of older age portray it), then so do the boundaries between cause and consequence in the experience of mental illness become fuzzy. Does mental illness cause a loss of self, or does society's assumption that it does (and therefore denial of opportunities to demonstrate otherwise) result in an apparent link between cognitive loss and self?

Biomedically, in dementia care, and to a lesser extent for people with depression, there is an overwhelming portrayal of someone with little ability to communicate and with very little chance of recovery. It is only when we look beyond the biomedical model that any hope emerges. Psycho-social models of health and ageing emphasise the role of social engagement (Havighurst, 1963) and of reconciliation with the past (Banks & Blair, 1997). However, often the ways of operationalising such models lead to an emphasis on a normative view of the world which further perpetuates the distinctions between 'them' as potentially and actually out of touch with 'reality', and 'us' who's reality is supposedly correct. Such sentiments are underpinned by ageist views that hold the middle-aged adults' world as true and correct. Hence, childhood is spent being exhorted to attain this adult perspective of the world, and people in later life are seen to be becoming increasingly out of touch with it (see Chapter 9).

One consequence of becoming out of touch with the dominant middle-aged world view is that older people with mental illness are seen as shedding layers of function: they may be no longer economically functional or even very good at being physically functional. Emotional functioning, however, has been recognised as persisting and hence modes of management have been established to respect this, most notably validation therapy. However, one disadvantage of this perceived preservation of emotional functioning is that older people have been equated to a childhood state of emotiveness in which rationality and objectivity play no part. Similarly, and unlike children, such an emotional level of cognitive functioning has resulted in older people being understood as incapable of learning other than by rudimentary behaviour modification programs.

One remarkable shift, however, has been a displacement of the older person as the centre of care activity. The combination of ageist attitudes and overwhelming pessimism about improvement in health status has rendered the person with mental illness as something to be simply attended to – they are no longer truly a person to be cared about. For example, respite care offers families opportunity to 'forget about' their relative, families are urged to get on with their own lives, the implication being that the older person with mental illness no longer has a life worth being involved with. The warehouses of older people (and this can be someone's own home as well as a larger institution) attempt to meet their physical needs, and at the best, their emotional needs, but few attempt to meet the needs of a whole person.

The primary focus of care has become the family carer. The visibility of carers has multiplied over the last few decades, thanks in part to pressure groups – in Britain for instance the Carers National Association. Services either sought to relieve them of the 'burden' of caring (through day and respite care or even long-term admission) or provided them with 'support' (for example, through carer support groups). The charitable organisation, the Alzheimer's Disease Society, has always held the family carer to be their focus for support, and care offered to people with Alzheimer's Disease has sought to be of primary benefit to carers. The view of caring as undesirable and even harmful to family carers has of course been promulgated over the last two decades by a succession of research studies (for example, Zarit, *et al.*, 1985; Chenoweth & Spencer, 1986). The ageism attached to the older people themselves has transferred to carers such that they are seen to need to be freed from their dependent so that they can get on with their lives (whatever that may be).

With family carers as a focus of care, professional carers free themselves of the hopeless task of restoring health to the older person with mental illness. Family carers provide a more fruitful avenue for care, with the possibility of an optimistic outcome in the future through psycho-educational intervention (Richardson, *et al.*, 1994). But for many years family carers have been seen variously as a social problem to be ignored (Pitkeathley, 1989) or exploited (Nolan & Grant, 1989). Only now are we beginning to emerge from the quagmire of legitimacy of caring for family carers. In Britain, legislation now requires the needs of family carers to be assessed (Carers (Recognition and Services) Act 1995), thus arguably rendering them themselves a form of patient to be cared for (Clarke, 1997).

The threat to us all now is that family carers may follow a similar history in policy and practice as did older people with the resultant discrimination and straddling of health and social care boundaries. Just as Macintyre (1977) identifies the end of the nineteenth century as the beginning of the UK recognition of the 'special case' of older people, so may the end of the twentieth century come to be recognised as the beginning of the 'special case' of family carers. If this does indeed prove to be the case, then we need learn from the example of older people and ensure that identification and visibility does not lead to discrimination. In the rush to care for the carers it must not be forgotten that family carers are, like older people, vulnerable to economic inactivity and have limits placed on their opportunities for social interaction as a result of their caring activities. Indeed, many are also older themselves.

In practice though, full legitimacy of caring for the carer results in inextricable dilemmas. Not only must the professional carer recognise the care needs of both the older person and their carers independently, but they must also balance these needs when they are in conflict. So often that which most effectively meets the needs of one will compromise the care of the other. Carers of younger adults and children have long complained that it is the dependant's voice that is privileged. For older people with mental health problems this is certainly not always the case. Respite care, for example, for someone with dementia may well result in a deterioration of cognitive functioning (Twigg, 1989) yet is a common intervention to allow the carer a break. Similarly, the use of medication to 'restrain' a confused person, so that they cease to wander around at night-time, is tolerated because of the benefit it brings to the carer (Clarke & Heyman, 1997).

Positive approaches to mental health care for older people

Butler, *et al.* (1991, p. 406) argue that

'any evidence pointing towards older people as untreatable is usually to be found in the minds of therapists rather than in empirical studies. Powerful forces of counter transference and cultural prejudice are at work, including personal fear and despair over ageing and death. Therapeutic pessimism and nihilism are inappropriate, invalid and inhumane.'

We would fully support this statement, but we are well aware that changing practice and attitudes is something that it is very easy to advocate but much more difficult to implement.

Frameworks for practice

There are, however, a number of frameworks and strategies that can be harnessed in this effort, which provide clear principles for therapy or guidelines for practice. They range from 'grand theories' of human development and ageing, to specific techniques developed for work with older people. There are also, of course, a range of theories and therapies that have not focused on older people, and are used with all age groups. We feel it important to focus on these more specific approaches. We turn now to discuss some of the general theories of human development that have a positive analysis of older age, before moving on to the mental health problems that older people most commonly experience, and the strategies which have been used to address these problems.

Perhaps the most obvious theoretical frameworks which can be harnessed in understanding older people in positive ways are those which are generally termed 'humanistic psychology', not least because they are positive about humankind in general, and have an emphasis on life-long growth and development, rather than deficits and difficulties.

Carl Rogers (1970), for example, developed a form of 'client-centred therapy' which emphasised human capacity for growth and development throughout life. In addition to this emphasis, Rogers also asserted that the relationship between the therapist and client should be one where the client was afforded 'unconditional positive regard'. Furthermore he emphasised that the therapeutic effort should be focused on the future rather than, as in other forms of psychotherapy, concentrating on the analysis of past experiences.

Similarly, Maslow (1970) proposed a developmental, humanistic model of personal growth which suggested a hierarchy of needs that people attempt to satisfy in order to facilitate personal development. Built in to this model is the notion that personal development is life-long, indeed it can require a life time to progress. First in this hierarchy are physiological needs, for example food, which are basic requirements for life. Once these needs are met, then individuals can progress on to meeting socio-psychological needs such as intimacy and security. Maslow's final set of needs, at the top of the hierarchy, is about 'self-actualisation', the need to achieve personal fulfilment and acceptance of the self.

Another model of life-long development, which is often referred to in discussions of older people, is Erikson's (1963) description of life stages. These stages do not end, as many such theories do, with 'adulthood', but describe stages of older age. Erikson's stages were described in relation to what he postulated as the key tasks of each stage – for example the infant needs to develop a sense of trust. Another way of thinking about Erikson's stages is in terms of the tensions he describes – for the baby this would be a tension between trust and mistrust. The later stages of development, middle age and old age, are characterised by firstly the task of developing 'generativity', the concern in supporting and guiding the next generation, and in old age the task of attaining 'ego integrity'. Ego integrity is only sketchily described, but involves developing a sense of meaning and order in one's life – the alternative that Erikson proposes is disgust and despair (Erikson, 1986).

Positive practice models

The models and theories in psychology and psychotherapy, such as those outlined above, offer frameworks that emphasise potential rather than deficits in older people. These ideas are echoed in a range of other theories and models in caring professions such as social work and nursing. Perkins and Tice (1995) for example, have described a 'Strengths Perspective' in social work which builds on strengths by 'focusing on the common thread of survivorship, and examining how people live, and sometimes thrive, in oppressive environments' (p. 83). They describe how many older people become permanent patients, receiving only custodial care rather than active therapy. These people, they argue, are diverse in terms of social group and personal experiences, but their common thread is that they have survived. They argue, therefore, that practice can draw on these 'untapped reservoirs of client accomplishment and resources', and in so doing, the relationship between older people and those who provide services for them will be enhanced.

Perkins and Tice refer to Saleebey's (1992) model of a strengths perspective, which was developed for general social work practice. The principles of this model are, however, particularly relevant to practise with an undervalued group of clients such as older people. Saleebey's model is contrasted with predominant problem orientated models which are centred on the professional's definitions of problems and demonstrate a linear rather than holistic approach to problem solving. In a problem-orientated model the client is expected to be cooperative and passive and compliant with whatever services are offered to them. In contrast, the strengths perspective emphasises the collaborative nature of the client–professional relationship and sees the client as an active decision maker within a community which affords resources and opportunities.

In nursing, too, a number of nursing models provide positive frameworks for practice with older people with mental health problems. This provision, however, is often through the general support they give to notions of individualised non-stereotypical care for all clients, rather than any specific consideration of the issues in the care of older people with mental health problems. One theoretical notion that is specific, however, is the idea of 'self-transcendence' as a resource for mental health in later life. Reed defines self-transcendence as 'an expansion of self-boundaries and an orientation toward broadened life perspectives'. She argues that self-transcendence is not only a natural resource for older people, but is also a significant correlate and predictor of mental health in older adults. The notion of changing self-boundaries links into many developmental theories of ageing – self-boundaries being conceptual divisions between the self and the external world which provide a sense of identity, connectedness and wholeness (Young & Reed, 1995). In infancy the boundaries are undifferentiated, in adolescence they may be self-centred, and in later life they may be transcended, and the focus moves towards the interdependence of oneself with others. This interdependence is achieved by 'the expansion of one's conceptual boundaries inwardly through introspective activities, outwardly through concerns about other's welfare, and temporally by integrating perceptions of one's past and future to enhance the present' (Young & Reed, 1995, p. 340). Mental health problems, argue Young and Reed, arise when 'conceptual boundaries are not clearly defined, or are too expansive or restrictive for a particular phase of life' (p. 340). They propose that therapeutic efforts to promote self-transcendence could involve meditation, life review and peer-counselling as well as group psychotherapy.

This model of self-transcendence is clearly open to some criticisms – particularly the idea that such transcendence is desirable where maintaining boundaries seems to be part and parcel of the culture. There are also some questions about the empirical evidence for the ideas underpinning this model – whether it is simply speculative or whether it is capable of being tested or grounded in empirical data. Despite these prudent caveats, however, this model is an example of a framework that extends the idea of development beyond simple 'adulthood ', and offers some direction to therapy.

An appreciation of the personhood of people, particularly those with dementia, has been vigorously advocated by a number of writers. Personhood is described as that social part of existence in which human beings relate to others. At the front of the field in Britain is Tom Kitwood, working within the Bradford Dementia Group (see, for example, Kitwood & Bredin, 1992). Kitwood has considered the uniqueness of individuals, and the role of a knowledge of that uniqueness, in seeking a care approach which values people. It is therefore a humane approach to care which urges people to focus not on the cognitive dysfunctioning but rather to focus on the essence of being a person: an essence which it is proposed persists despite mental illness. However, Kelly and Field (1996) argue that whilst a core sense of self and identity persists, the consequences of chronic illness have to be 'incorporated permanently into conceptions of self and are likely to become a basis for the imputation of identity by others'. The consequences of such an imputation are articulated by Sabat and Harre (1992) who draw on social constructivist theory to illustrate the destructive pattern of social interactions engaged in with people with mental illness which undermines any sense of 'self'. These destructive patterns of social interaction are referred to by Kitwood as a 'malignant social psychology' (Kitwood, 1990).

Kitwood and Bredin (1992) propose that people should be cared for within a framework that preserves their 'personhood'. However, the conventional mode of interaction emphasises the importance of functioning within the domains which are known to those without mental illness, and there is a failure to acknowledge any other form of reality. Shomaker (1989), Frank (1995) and Crisp (1995), however, illustrate the reality and rationality of someone with mental illness that exists without constraints of, for example, notions of the present time (temporality).

An interactional stance regards people as existing 'in relationship' (Kitwood & Bredin, 1992). As cognitive ability changes, so interrelationships must take over if 'personhood' is to be maintained, a view also supported by Sabat and Harre (1992). Kitwood and Bredin (1992), and also Kitwood (1993) argue for relative well-being in older people with mental illness and identify four 'global sentient states' which must be protected if well-being is to be maintained: a sense of personal worth, a sense of agency (control of personal life or self-determination), social confidence, and hope.

Only very recently has a perspective of care emerged that emphasises older people with mental health problems as in relationship with others. There need not be the dichotomy of inevitable decline in people with dementia and optimism for family carers. Indeed family carers do not necessarily share this optimism themselves, so much are their lives coexistent with that of the person they care for. Put aside for one moment the theories of biomedical decline, withdrawal from society, loss of personhood and the 'struggle to remain middle-aged'. Focus instead on the family unit, which continually shifts in function as it accommodates both its resources and the demands placed on it from within and outside. A professional focus on either the older person or their family carer exacerbates divisions within the family unit to the detriment of both.

Other models of care do exist and are well established in some fields of psychiatry. To date these have rarely been applied to the care of older people with mental health problems. Family nursing (Friedemann, 1993) has gained in popularity in the United States. It is described as being practised on three levels: the individual level in which the family is viewed as the context of the individual; the interpersonal level in which the family is conceived of as a number of dyadic and triadic units; and the systems level in which the family has its own structural and functional components which interact with outside environmental factors. Family therapy similarly conceives not of individuals but of the family unit which is amenable to health care intervention. The implicit inclusion of older people in these modes of intervention is reflected by Richardson, *et al.* (1994, p. 236), writing that 'the idea of family work with older adults essentially reflects the recognition that older people are family members too'.

The practice context

Whatever the therapeutic model used, however, practice must take into account not just the internal psychodynamic processes of the older person, but their relationship with the world that they live in, their social and economic status. In addition, practice must also take into account the way that social and economic factors combine with mental and physical health problems to make management of these problems very complex. We have already touched on Townsend's idea of 'structured dependency', where older people are excluded from economic activity by employment restrictions. But the impact of this dependency extends beyond the social exclusion and stigma that is the lot of the poor in Western societies. Financial problems mean that some life experiences are denied to some older people – social activities, travel, and cultural activities, all cost money and a reduced ability to participate means a reduced quality of life. Furthermore, some health problems, mental or physical, can be coped with more effectively if people can spend money on them – aids and adaptations, facilities such as telephones, help with housework, for example.

One aspect of ageing that seems to be generally accepted then, is the reduction in disposable income that ageing and retirement can bring, and this has a widespread impact on the ability of older people to cope with health problems. The increasing incidence of health problems, and in particular 'multiple pathology' where people experience more than one health problem, in line with increasing age is also something that is generally recognised (Bennet & Ebrahim, 1995). While it is by no means inevitable, this means that an older person with a mental health problem may well have some physical problems and also be in financially straightened circumstances.

To address these problems in any sensible way, a range of different professionals and agencies, with different areas of expertise and responsibility need to be brought together. This multidisciplinary working is essential, but also problematic. Trying to establish some sort of team approach is a desirable goal, to avoid duplication of effort or conflict of intervention – with so many different people with different knowledge bases and goals this is a real danger. Trying to work out how this can be achieved, however, is a much more difficult problem.

The problems of multidisciplinary teamwork are well-documented elsewhere (see, for example, Pearson & Spencer, 1997) but there seem to be at least two main issues that need to be resolved – firstly who should be in the team? and secondly, how it should be managed? The members of the team will be partly determined by client need – a housing problem will need someone with housing expertise, and a medical problem will need medical intervention, for example. Problems arise when needs for specialised input are not identified or recognised, which suggests that a 'standard' team, with consistent members needs to be set up. This is the policy of some agencies, but may result in unnecessary and expensive involvement of staff.

Such teams are also usually only logistically feasible if the members are all employed by the same agency, or where agencies have agreements with each other about working together. Where a number of different agencies need to be involved and where there is no agreement over collaboration, it can become very difficult to guarantee or monitor inputs. Agreements over collaboration also need to take into account different types of responsibility and roles – who is the lead agency, and under what circumstances? For nurses working for mental health agencies therefore, they may find themselves as the key professional coordinating a multitude of different agencies and workers, where there may be no agreement over priorities and responsibilities. Conversely the nurse may be 'called in' as an afterthought or even as a last resort, when different people have tried to address a client's needs and failed. This may give the nurse *carte blanche* to do whatever they see fit, or may result in a very precisely defined role and activity.

Whatever the problems of multidisciplinary working, it must be remembered that, for many older clients, this is the only appropriate way to work – a system of 'serial referral' where older people get passed from agency to agency with little continuity or coherence is destructive and demoralising. The challenge for nursing, therefore, is to work out some ways of managing teamwork in a range of different practice contexts, where they are required to play a range of different roles. As health care professionals we are, however, confined in our actions to those areas of life to which we have legitimate access. Consequently, it is not just a lack of appreciation of the relevance of social networks that makes it difficult to work within them. The structural divisions of health and social care, hospital and community care, and multiple professional care also make it difficult to engage with older people and their social worlds. Such a reductionalist approach to care delivery mitigates against knowing, and effectively working with, an individual's whole life.

Perhaps one response to this has been the emergence of self-help groups, possibly initiated by health care professionals, but increasingly coming under the umbrella of voluntary organisations. Such groups have multiple functions. Firstly, the use of the internal energy of the group to provide support, education and motivation to each other; and secondly, the exertion of pressure on professional and political groups to recognise and respond to the needs of group members. Effective though such groups can be, they are not equitable in their accessibility (for example, due to population dispersion, frequency of diagnostic label, and the predominantly 'middle class and white' membership) and are certainly not immune to the cloaking of the true recipient of care. For example, in Britain the Alzheimer's Disease Society directs its interventions for the benefit of the family carers and acts as a pressure group, not for people with Alzheimer's Disease but for their relatives.

Principles of practice

The following brief summary of therapeutic strategies covers a number of interventions that have been developed or adapted for use with older people. We have, for example, neglected bio-medical approaches, such as drug therapies or ECT, not because we feel these approaches to be unimportant (they are far too commonly used to be thought of in that way) but because the nurse's role is largely confined to observation and monitoring, rather than taking a leading role in initiating and directing such treatment. The summary we provide below concentrates on the principles on which the selected therapeutic strategies are based.

Let us look then at various approaches to the care of older people with mental health problems and disentangle some of the implications of each in terms of a non-discriminatory framework. It is a useful starting point to draw these together under two guiding principles of care: View older person as a unique individual; View older person as a social being connected to society rather than disengaged.

View the older person as a unique individual

Just as minute particles appear under the magnification of a microscope, so the perceived amorphous mass of older people unfolds as a number of individuals, stark in their variations, if we adjust our focus. It is the mechanism for such an adjustment that we need to examine. Thus approaches which concern themselves with the biography of the older person can be of particular value, for example life review and reminiscence therapy. For example, Hargrave (1994) reports on the process of making videos with older people to capture and create meaning of their past, and Murphy & Moyes (1997) describe the wide variety of mediums such as photographs which can be used to provide a multisensory approach. Whilst life review and reminiscence have the ostensible purpose of helping the older person come to terms with their past, they also allow others, be they family members or professional staff, a window into the past world of the older person.

One debate that can be distinguished in the literature is between past-orientated therapies, such as life review/reminiscence therapy and future-orientated strategies, which encourage clients to look forward. One view is that therapies which focus on the past run the risk of denying older people a future, in other words that they are negative in their focus (Sherman (1991) discusses this view in more detail). Another view is that approaches which include past experiences recognise the skills and insights that older people may have developed and contribute towards feelings of self-esteem, integration and a sense of self.

Basing care delivery on a respect of the individuality of each older person requires that we regard them not only as past people but also as present people. In other words, that we regard their present existence as of value. However, the pathology orientated health care system and problem led approach to care delivery implicitly view ability as irrelevant to care unless it is absent. Consequently, with little recognition of the skills and insights that remain intact, older people are gradually stripped of their abilities as their health fails.

Rather than deliver care which is problem driven, one alternative is to adopt a strengths perspective in assessment and care management, as described by Perkins and Tice (1995). Kitson (1991) sought to understand why nurses in geriatric wards are content to deliver depersonalised care, arguing that the therapeutic function of nursing (TNF) (or caring role) needed to be described as an integrated nursing theory. An integrated nursing theory is needed with the

'ability to identify patients' individual self-care needs, to organise a system of care that is patient-dominated rather than task-orientated, to identify the most appropriate nursing action to help maintain a patient at his or her optimal level of self-care, and to be able to provide a sensitive, personal and compassionate service that ensures patient dignity and self-respect' (p. 220).

Moreover, the dominant approach to care management values the norm. For people with mental health problems this is particularly problematic. Unless their conceptualisations of themselves and their world accords with that recognised by the vast majority of 'well' people then their thoughts are not valued. There has been a long tradition of interventions that seek to keep older people 'in contact' with reality (or at least that reality known of to others). Reality orientation, for example, strives to remorselessly reinforce the 'facts' of time, place and person (for an early and thorough account see Holden & Woods, 1982). There is no room for any other reality, for acknowledgement that older people with mental health problems may work within a differing framework in which time and place become irrelevant. Kitwood (1995) differentiates between the old and new cultures of dementia care. He argues that the old perspective of dementia views it as a disease in which personality and identity are progressively destroyed, whilst the new perspective accepts dementia as a disability, the quality of care being crucial to the experience of dementia.

Mental health issues that manifest themselves in problematic behaviour, such as wandering and agitation, have been subject to symptomatic management through techniques such as behaviour modification. As Kitwood (1995) emphasises, such approaches require the behaviour to be controlled. Kitwood (1995, p. 10) writes that 'managing the behaviour of another means a disregard of that person's own frame of reference, their struggle for life and meaning'. The alternative is to regard the individual as having a right to agency and a purpose in their actions. The meaning of the action is as much our responsibility to discover.

There is a further range of interventions that seek to promote the well-being of older people with mental health problems. These include, for example, dance and music activities which Palo-Bengtsson, *et al.* (1997) describe as instilling 'a sense of wholeness and meaningfulness into the whole life cycle' through attention to the resolution of previous developmental stages in Erikson's (1986) model of life-long development.

View of the older person as a social being connected to society rather than disengaged

Broaden the field of view a little and we see that older people are not in fact numerous independent individuals but exist within social constellations of kin and friendship. At times they can be seen to be the centre of such a constellation, at others they are peripheral, but vital, to the activity of the grouping. Knowing of, understanding, and working with this wider social group is the philosophy underpinning family centred modalities of care which, as discussed earlier, neither displaces the older person or their family from the attention of care but rather seeks to work within the system. Family systems therapy, for example, has much potential for therapeutic effectiveness in this field (Benbow, 1997) but remains under-researched and therefore an unknown intervention (Richardson, *et al.*, 1994).

When looking at the psychotherapeutic techniques and interventions which are used or advocated for use with older people, such as reality orientation and reminiscence therapy, one recurring debate is whether therapy should be group or individually based. As Butler, *et al.* (1991) have argued, individual psychotherapy seems to be rarely offered to older people, perhaps because those who practice individual psychotherapy may well be influenced by Freud's negative ideas about older people and therapy generally. The arguments for group approaches seem to be divided between a tacit acceptance of these negative ideas, by arguing the 'cost-effectiveness' of the approaches with growing numbers of older people, and more positive arguments derived from theoretical models of life-span development. Finkel (1990), for example, suggests that concerns about cost and the availability of trained professionals often underpin decisions to adopt group modalities to therapy. It is difficult to avoid speculation that the debate over cost-effectiveness includes, at some level, a consideration of the assumed outcomes of therapy with a group that is largely regarded as unlikely to show much improvement.

There are, however, more positive reasons for advocating group approaches to therapy. Some of the theories and models outlined above, for example, stress the importance of interaction with others as a means of personal growth, and the refutation of disengagement theories in part depends on asserting the importance of the social world in the lives of older people. Aside from this use of the group as a replication of social experiences, there is also a strong tradition that asserts that group therapy affords a particular and unique therapeutic input arising from group dynamics (see for an early example of this argument, Foulkes, 1964). There is also some evidence to suggest that older people prefer group approaches to psychotherapy (Berland & Poggi, 1979), although this may well depend on a number of contextual factors, and should not be taken as an indicator that all forms of therapy with older people should be group based.

Some care interventions actively seek to allow the older person to engage with others. Gibson (1997, p. 134), for example, describes how the use of

'knowledge of a person's past to hold them in present relationships is one of several creative means which can be used to maintain warm caring mutual relationships and stave off encroaching frightening retreat into isolation'.

Here reminiscence and life history work clearly play a part, but also of considerable importance is an understanding of communication modes with older people with mental illness. For example, Crisp (1998), who draws on experiences of her mother's illness of dementia (Crisp, 1995), sets out a number of ways of fostering interactions. In particular, the use of confabulation by the older person is argued to be a way of re-establishing sense and meaning of the past and the present, and needs to be recognised as such to allow effective communication with others. Whitworth, *et al.*

(1998) set out such an assessment and management framework implemented by speech and language therapists which promotes effective communication between older people with dementia and their family carers.

There is a need also to be attentive to the interactions which older people with mental health problems have with both each other and their families. Perhaps there has been an underestimation of the significance of the exchanges between older people. Reed and Payton (1996) found in their study that relationships with fellow residents were an important factor in the satisfaction that older people felt with nursing and residential homes. The therapeutic function of such interaction remains uncertain, although Foster (1997) suggests that there is the potential for enhancing the well-being of older people.

Conclusion

In assessing the adequacy of the various interventions that exist for older people with mental health problems we think it is useful to refer back to the four global sentient states described by Kitwood and Bredin (1992). If an intervention promotes all of these states then it will be an intervention that is non-discriminatory for those with mental illness and non-discriminatory for those who are older. Let us restate them:

- A sense of personal worth
- A sense of agency (self-determination)
- Social confidence
- Hope

We would argue, that it is through respect for their personhood, irrespective of age and mental health, and through respect for their social existence, that the shroud of discrimination can be removed and older people as individuals be seen, to not just exist, but to be valued by themselves and others.

References

Banks, E.J. & Blair, S.E.E. (1997) The contribution of occupational therapy within the context of the psychodynamic approach for older clients who have mental health problems. *Health Care in Later Life*, **2**, 85–92.

Benbow, S.M. (1997) Therapies in Old Age Psychiatry: Reflections on Recent Changes. In: *State of the Art in Dementia Care* (ed. M. Marshall). Centre for Policy on Ageing, London.

Bennet, G.C.J. & Ebrahim, F. (1995) *The Essentials of Health Care in Old Age*, 2nd edn. Edward Arnold, London.

Berland, D.I. & Poggi, R. (1979) Expressive group psychotherapy with the ageing. *International Journal of Group Psychotherapy*, **29**, 16–28.

Butler, R.N., Lewis, M. & Sunderland, T. (1991) *Ageing and Mental Health: Positive Psychological and Biomedical Approaches*, 4th edn. Macmillan, New York.

Carers (Recognition and Services) Act (1995) HMSO, London.

Chenoweth, B. & Spencer, B. (1986) Dementia: the experience of family caregivers. *The Gerontologist*, **26**, 267–72.

Clarke, C.L. (1997) In sickness and in health: remembering the relationship in family caregiving for people with dementia. In: *State of the Art in Dementia Care* (ed. M. Marshall). Centre for Policy on Ageing, London.

Clarke, C.L. & Heyman, B. (1997) How Families and Professional Carers Appraise Risks for People with Dementia In: *Risk, Health and Healthcare: A Critical Approach* (ed. B. Heyman). Chapman & Hall, London.

Crisp, J. (1995) Making sense of the stories that people with Alzheimer's tell: a journey with my mother. *Nursing Inquiry*, **2**, 133–40.

Crisp, J. (1998) Towards a Partnership in Maintaining Personhood. In: *Dementia Care: Developing Partnerships in Practice* (eds T. Adams & C.L. Clarke). Balliere Tindall, London.

Cummings, E. & Henry, W. (1961) *Growing Old: The Process of Disengagement*. Basic Books, New York.

Erikson, E. (1963) *Childhood and Society*, 2nd edn. Norton, New York.

Erikson, E. (1986) *Vital Involvement in Old Age*. Norton, New York.

Evers, H. (1981) The creation of patient careers in geriatric wards: aspects of policy and practice. *Social Science and Medicine*, **15**(A), 81–8.

Finkel, S.I. (1990) Group psychotherapy with older people. *Hospital and Community Psychiatry*, **41**, 1189–91.

Foster, K. (1997) Pragmatic Groups: Interactions and Relationships Between People with Dementia. In: *State of the Art in Dementia Care* (ed. M. Marshall). Centre for Policy on Ageing, London.

Foulkes, S.H. (1964) *Therapeutic Group Analysis*. Allen and Unwin, London.

Frank, B.A. (1995) People With Dementia Can Communicate – If We Are Able to Hear. In: *The New Culture of Dementia Care* (eds T. Kitwood & S. Benson). Hawker Publications, London.

Friedemann, M. (1993) The Concept of Family Nursing. In: *Readings in Family Nursing* (eds G.D. Wegner & R.J. Alexander). Lippincott, Philadelphia.

Gibson, F. (1997) Owning the Past in Dementia Care: Creative Engagement with Others in the Present. In: *State of the Art in Dementia Care* (ed. M. Marshall). Centre for Policy on Ageing, London.

Gurland, B. & Cross, P.S. (1982) Epidemiology of psychopathology in old age. *Psychiatric Clinics of North America*, **5**, 11–26.

Hargrave, T.D. (1994) Using video life reviews with older adults. *Journal of Family Therapy*, **16**, 259–67.

Havighurst, A. (1963) Successful ageing. In: *Process of Ageing, Vol. 1* (eds R.H. Williams, C. Tibbets, W. Donahoe). University of Chicago Press, Chicago.

Hildebrand, H.P. (1982) Psychotherapy with older people patients. *British Journal of Medical Psychology*, **55**, 19–28.

Holden, U.P. & Woods, R.T. (1982) *Reality Orientation*. Churchill Livingstone, London.

Hughes, B. (1995) *Older People and Community Care: Critical Theory and Practice*. Open University Press, Milton Keynes.

Keady, J. (1997) Maintaining Involvement: a meta concept to describe the dynamics of dementia. In: *State of the Art in Dementia Care* (ed. M. Marshall). Centre for Policy on Ageing, London.

Keady, J. & Nolan, M.R. (1994) Younger onset dementia: developing a longitudinal model as the basis for a research agenda and as a guide to interventions with sufferers and carers. *Journal of Advanced Nursing*, **19**, 659–69.

Kelly, M.P. & Field, D. (1996) Medical sociology, chronic illness and the body. *Sociology of Health and Illness*, **18**, 241–57.

Kitson, A.L. (1991) *Therapeutic Nursing and the Hospitalised Elderly*. Scutari Press, Middlesex.

Kitwood, T. (1990) The dialectics of dementia: with particular reference to Alzheimer's disease. *Ageing and Society*, **10**, 177–96.

Kitwood, T. (1993) Towards a theory of dementia care: the interpersonal process. *Ageing and Society*, **13**, 51–67.

Kitwood, T. (1995) Cultures of Care: Tradition and Change. In: *The New Culture of Dementia Care* (eds T. Kitwood & S. Benson). Hawker Publications, London.

Kitwood, T. & Bredin, K. (1992) Towards a theory of dementia care: personhood and well-being. *Ageing and Society*, **12**, 269–87.

Macintyre, S. (1977) Old Age as a Social Problem: Historical Notes on an English Experience. In: *Health Care and Health Knowledge* (eds R. Dingwall, C. Heath, M. Reid & M. Stacey). Croom Helm, London.

Maslow, A.H. (1970) *Motivation and Personality*, 2nd edn. Harper and Row, New York.

Minois, G. (1989) *History of Old Age*. University of Chicago Press, Chicago.

Murphy, C. & Moyes, M. (1997) Life Story Work. In: *State of the Art in Dementia Care* (ed. M. Marshall). Centre for Policy on Ageing, London.

Nolan, M. & Grant, G. (1989) Addressing the needs of informal carers: a neglected area of nursing practice. *Journal of Advanced Nursing*, **14**, 950–62.

Palo-Bengtsson, L., Ekman S-L. & Ericsson K. (1997) Nurses' opinions, ideas and beliefs about dancing and movement to music in Swedish and Finnish nursing home settings. *Health Care in Later Life*, **2**, 93–106.

Pearson, P. & Spencer, J. (1997) *Promoting Teamwork in Primary Care: A Research Based Approach*. Arnold, London.

Perkins, K. & Tice, C. (1995) A Strengths Perspective in Practice: Older People and Mental Health Challenges. *Journal of Gerontological Social Work*, **23**, 83–97.

Phillipson, C. (1972) *Capitalism and the Construction of Old Age*. Macmillan, London.

Pitkeathley, J. (1989) *It's My Duty, Isn't It? The Plight of Carers in Our Society*. Souvenir Press Ltd, London.

Reed, J. & Payton, V.R. (1996) *Working to Create Continuity: Older People Managing the Move to the Care Home Setting*. Centre for Health Services Research Report No. 76, Newcastle upon Tyne.

Richardson, C.A., Gilleard, C.J., Lieberman, S. & Peeler, R. (1994) Working with older adults and their families – a review. *Journal of Family Therapy*, **16**, 225–40.

Robinson, P., Ekman, S-L., Meleis, A.I., Winbald, B. & Wahlund, L-O. (1997) Suffering in silence: The experience of early memory loss. *Health Care in Later Life*, **2**, 107–20.

Rogers, C.R. (1970) *On Becoming a Person: A Therapist's View of Psychotherapy*. Houghton Mifflin – Sentry Edition, Boston.

Sabat, S.R. & Harre, R. (1992) The construction and deconstruction of self in Alzheimer's disease. *Ageing and Society*, **12**, 443–61.

Saleebey, D. (ed.) (1992) *The Strengths Perspective in Social Work Practice*. Longman, New York.

Sherman, E. (1991) *Reminiscence and the Self in Old Age*. Springer, New York.

Shomaker, D.J. (1989) Age disorientation, liminality and reality: The case of the Alzheimer's patient. *Medical Anthropology*, **12**, 91–101.

Thompson, P. (1992) 'I don't feel old': Subjective ageing and the search for meaning in later life. *Ageing and Society*, **12**, 23–47.

Townsend, P. (1981) The Structured Dependency of the Elderly: a creation of social policy in the twentieth century. *Ageing and Society*, **1**, 5–28.

Twigg, J. (1989) Not taking the strain. *Community Care*, **77**, 16–19.

Victor, C. (1988) Approaches to the Study of Ageing. In: *Mental Health Problems in Old Age: A Reader* (eds B. Gearing, M. Johnson & T. Heller). John Wiley and Sons, Chichester.

Whitworth, A., Perkins, L. & Lesser, R. (1998) Communication in Dementia Care: A Partnership Approach. In: *Dementia Care: Developing Partnerships in Practice* (eds T. Adams & C.L. Clarke). Balliére Tindall, London.

Young, C.A. & Reed, P. (1995) Elders' perceptions of the Role of Group Psychotherapy in Fostering Self-Transcendence. *Archives of Psychiatric Nursing*, Vol. IX, 338–47.

Zarit, S.H., Orr, N.K. & Zarit, J.M. (1985) *The Hidden Victims of Alzheimer's Disease: Families Under Stress*. New York University Press, New York.

11 Personality Disorder: Finding a Way

Ruth Gallop

Preliminary issues: definitions

This chapter addresses some of the challenges confronting nursing staff when caring for clients diagnosed with personality disorders (PD). The identification of personality disorders as categories of distinct and discrete psychiatric nomenclature is an area of controversy and ambiguity. Personality, as defined below, represents our very being and nature and is comprised of traits or enduring characteristics Defining personality disorder is not a straightforward task. PD is usually defined as an 'enduring pattern of inner experience and behaviour' that is inflexible and pervasive and leads to problems in social and occupational functioning. Criteria listed within the Diagnostic and Statistical Manual for Mental Disorders of the American Psychiatric Association (DSM) combine symptoms and traits so it is difficult to know if a PD is truly reflective of a stable set of maladaptive characteristics/traits. Many of our clients experience symptoms that can range from mildly egodystonic to severe and disabling symptoms. Furthermore, PDs come and go from the nomenclature of the DSM. The passive aggressive PD and the hysterical PD have disappeared. Borderline schizophrenia has become schizotypal PD. In the most recent version of the diagnostic and statistical manual (DSM-IV), the term Multiple Personality Disorder (MPD) has disappeared and been replaced by Dissociative Identity Disorder (DID). And even when the term MPD was used the diagnosis MPD was not listed with other PDs but with Dissociative Disorders.

The diagnosis Borderline PD (BPD), in particular, has been fraught with controversy. BPD has been shown to be interrelated with approximately a dozen other diagnoses. Stone (1992) suggests the diagnosis BPD be replaced with the category 'Unstable PD'. Other authors, as shall be discussed, suggest abandoning the term altogether. The existence of specific PDs may also be an expression of our current society. As Masterson suggests, concern about finding one's true self has become a North American (at least) obsession and may contribute to the identification of disorders of identity such as BPD and Narcissistic PD (1988). Consequently, the notion of PD is problematic and should be approached with some caution.

Outline of chapter contents

This chapter has been organised to guide the reader first through a brief overview of the multideterminants of personality and a review of the major categories of PD. Key nursing issues associated with working with clients with PD from the eccentric and avoidant clusters will be highlighted. The balance of the chapter is devoted to the issues central to caring for clients who display the self-harm behaviours and immature defense mechanisms that are often the source of nursing difficulties.

Frequently when nurses find themselves angry or frustrated in their work with clients, or speak of difficult clients, it is in response to the characterologically frustrating portion of the client's personality. This is not to suggest that all 'difficult' clients are personality disordered. However, the clinical treatment and management problems discussed in this chapter are typical (if indeed one can generalise about the human condition) to a lesser or greater degree to those problems described repeatedly by nurses working with clients presenting major treatment and management difficulties. The most challenging clients are usually clients with a diagnosis from the dramatic-erratic cluster of personality disorders such as borderline personality disorder (BPD); antisocial personality disorder (APD); narcissistic personality disorder (NPD). For this reason the focus of the nursing management and treatment section will be on:

(1) Understanding why these clients are so challenging
(2) Setting realistic treatment goals
(3) Identifying and applying conceptual frameworks that can be used for planning care
   - *Object*-relations theory and the understanding of Counter-transference
   - Dialectical behavioural therapy
(4) Using contracts

Theoretical models of personality development can take many forms: systems theory, psychoanalytic theory (Freudian, object-relations, self psychology, relational theory); learning theory, interpersonal theory, to name a few. For this chapter, an explanatory model grounded in object-relations theory will be the predominate model used to guide understanding.

What is personality?

Each of us has a personality. It is a unique collection of traits or styles that comes together to represent our way of being in the world and relating to others. While each personality is unique, there are sufficient commonalties in styles to allow us to speak of differing kinds of personalities and to differentiate the components of these personalities into traits (Stone, 1993). These traits or lifelong styles are present in all of us. We can all think of individuals who have particular styles: people who always make lists, people who keep their homes immaculate and organise others; people who are always apologising; people who are described as having a 'chip on their shoulder'. However, most people's personality style does not interfere with the fundamentals of living: the ability to have meaningful and stable relationships, and to live and work in the world with a reasonable degree of happiness and satisfaction. A person with a healthy personality expects to succeed in work and relationships and has a realistic sense of self and self worth. Sometimes traits or styles become so rigid and maladaptive that they interfere with these fundamentals resulting in distress and impaired functioning. In these circumstances the individual may be described as having a personality disorder. According to Merikangas and Weissman (1986) PDs can be found in approximately 10% of the American population. Only a few of these people will find their way into the mental health system. Some, particularly those with Narcissistic PD and Histrionic PD, may refer themselves for psychotherapy.

Conceptually, personality can be considered along a continuum of norms and extremes. While there are many ways to depict the variation in traits, Stone (1993) describes a schema of personality traits reflecting a set of 24 typical traits and extremes. These traits and their concomitant extremes are shown below (see Fig. 11.1). This figure illustrates the schema for an

abrasive	tactless	polite	courtly	obsequious
stingy	tight	thrifty	generous	prodigal
irresponsible	procrastinating	punctual	compulsive	punctilious
unfeeling	cold	sympathetic	oversensitive	maudlin
vampish	seductive	receptive	coy	prudish
randy	pushy	(sex-)assertive	reserved	inhibited
domineering	bossy	(work-) assertive	unassertive	submissive
paranoid	suspicious	trusting	naïve	gullible
abusive	irritable	calm	phlegmatic	spineless
ruthless	exploitative	fair	deferential	meek
chaotic	sloppy	neat	meticulous	fussbudget
vengeful	bitter	forgiving	philosophic	altruistic
brittle	rigid	flexible	yielding	flabby
aggressive	hostile	agreeable	friendly	overfriendly
defiant	uncooperative	cooperative	super-accommodating.	
bigoted	dogmatic	openminded	easily swayed	"as-if"
unscrupulous	devious	honest	scrupulous	overscrupulous
garrulous	talkative	communicative	laconic	taciturn
extraverted	outgoing	at ease	shy	reclusive
disloyal	uncommitted	faithful	fawning	clingy
pretentious	affected	modest	humble	self-effacing
reckless	impulsive	spontaneous	hesitant	fearful
obnoxious	disagreeable	likeable	charming	charismatic
boorish	philistine	cultured	mannered	precious

Fig. 11.1 Personality trait scheme for obsessional man. (From *Abnormalities of Personality: Within and Beyond the Realm of Treatment* by Michael Stone. Copyright © 1993 by Michael H. Stone. Reproduced with the permission of W.W. Norton & Co Inc, New York.)

obsessional man. Notice how the pattern moves from the central 'average' position to extremes on numerous traits.

In Fig. 11.1, the so called 'normal' person is described as adhering fairly close to 'typical' traits while the disordered individual varies according to a particular set of traits The more the traits move to the extremes, the more likely a full blown PD will be evidenced. Using this model, one can see how realistic treatment goals would not be directed at changing an individual's fundamental personality structure but be directed at bringing the extremes closer to the norm. A person crippled by compulsive behaviour that prevents him/her from leaving the home, because of the necessity to check and re-check the house, will never become a carefree, casual person. However, with appropriate therapy, that person may be able to modify behaviour such that after careful checking he or she can leave the house and be in the world.

Origins of personality

Early views that an infant was born a *tabla rasa* upon which a personality was imposed are now considered defunct. Instead the schools of 'nature versus nurture' have come to recognise that both nature and nurture have a considerable part in the development of personality. Even a cursory examination of new babies or discussion with new parents will reveal that all babies are not born alike. Babies appear to be born with specific temperaments: easy-going, cuddly, alert, dozy, fussy, doesn't like to be held, easily comforted, and so forth. No doubt temperament influences parental responses and may shape nurturing responses, but first there is temperament. Circadian rhythms seem to be genetic: a 'morning' person is hard to change, just as it is hard to be a 'morning' person if you are not born that way. In addition to temperament, researchers and clinicians describe resilience. Resilience – the notion that some individuals can withstand greater levels of psychological or physiological assault than others – helps us to understand why the same set of circumstances may affect children differently. Resilience and its concomitant vulnerability are probably acquired both by heredity and environmental factors (Kroll, 1993). For instance, all children who are sexually abused do not develop a BPD or a dissociative identity disorder. While variables of intensity of experience such as age of onset, duration, and relationship of abuser can influence outcome, so can resilience or genetic vulnerability of the child. Researchers have suggested that as much as 50% of personality can be considered to be genetically determined. Research into PDs suggests that polygenic factors rather than a specific genetic factor, such as in a disease like schizophrenia, play a role in the formation of PDs (Stone, 1993). However, it is likely that as much as 50% of personality is explained by nurture and other variables.

A number of theoretical models have been postulated to understand the development of personality. These models include the drive theory of Freud and the many psychodynamic models that have developed from the evolving and rethinking of psychoanalytic concepts. Writers such as

Winnicott, Mahler and Masterson, to name just a few, have all contributed to our expanded understanding of personality and PD. Many of these writers derive from the school of object-relations and have focused on understanding how our early experiences with others are central to the development of a sense of self (personhood or personality) and our ability to form satisfying relationships as adults. Object relations theorists (Mahler, 1972; Masterson & Klein, 1989; Winnicott, 1965a, 1965b, 1965c) speak of internal representations or objects that develop during childhood and represent the internal image of an external object. Initially a child's sense of self is based on others' responses and perceptions. If the parenting responses are primarily positive and non-critical the child will develop an internalised sense of self as a worthwhile person. According to Winnicott (1970), a child who receives 'good enough' mothering (or caretaking, since either parent or a significant other can provide the care) develops a suffi-ciently internalised sense of self to tolerate being alone in the world and have the capacity to self-soothe as an adult. 'Good enough' mothering is mothering that protects from overwhelming anxiety and attends to the individual rhythms of the child. Feeling valued and encouraged to grow and experiment, being allowed to make mistakes without being perceived as bad or a failure are all essential experiences for a positive sense of self.

The quality of early childhood experiences is clearly a significant factor in the development of personality and/or a sense of self. It is during early childhood that an individual acquires the internal 'glue' that enables him or her to deal with the frustrations, disappointments and successes of life. It is during the early years of life that a child learns about being in the world with others. As will be seen in discussion of specific PDs, childhood experiences that are predominately negative, such as always demanding obedience and being good, physical abuse, neglect, rewarding dependent behaviour and withdrawing approval for independent behaviour or pre-dominately inconsistent parenting can contribute to the development of a PD.

Finally, cultural norms and times also determine 'normal' personality. Acceptable behaviours for women in one culture may be perceived as disturbed or disordered in another. Life events that may in Western cul-tures contribute to the development of a PD, might in a different culture such as in China or a Muslim country be expressed as somatic symptoms (Stone, 1993).

The impact of childhood abuse on personality development

The high prevalence of histories of childhood abuse (physical and sexual) in both the general population and psychiatric populations has raised the question of the role of abuse in the aetiology of PDs, as well as other psychiatric disorders (Briere, 1992; Herman *et al.*, 1989; Kroll, 1993). It is worth noting that childhood abuse occurs in a dysfunctional family so that efforts to tease apart the contribution of the abuse versus the con-tribution of the general dysfunctional environment is extremely difficult.

It has been recognised for some time that a history of sexual abuse (particularly severe, and ritualistic abuse) is a causal factor in the development of a dissociative identity disorder. Parental abuse must have a negative impact on the forming personality since it represents a fundamental betrayal of the trust, predictability and positive regard so essential to the development of a positive sense of self. In a recent study, Gallop and co-researchers found that nurses who had been sexually abused as children had significantly lower levels of self-esteem than nonabused nurses, and experienced significantly more current distress. This distress manifested particularly in the areas of being in abusive relationships, overuse of medication and body image difficulties than the matched nonabused nurses (Gallop, *et al.*, 1995).

As Stone (1993) points out, not all physically abused children become adult abusers. However, there is a higher incidence of a history of physical abuse among felons with APD, suggesting that childhood abuse increases the risk for development of APD. More recently, increasing attention has been paid to the role of childhood abuse in the aetiology of the BPD (Arntz, 1994; Herman, 1992; Kroll, 1993). Studies have shown that 70 to 80% of women diagnosed with BPD have histories of childhood physical and/or sexual abuse. These numbers compare to a rate of 20 to 35% in controlled comparison groups of women with other psychiatric diagnoses (Herman, *et al.*, 1989; Ogata, *et al.*, 1990; Bryer, *et al.*, 1987). Kroll (1993) speaks of a Post Traumatic Stress Disorder/borderline person who displays 'ongoing, intrusive symptoms and maladaptive personality styles related to early traumatic experiences' (p. *xv*). However the PTSD/borderline person is different from a person experiencing PTSD after an event such as a car accident. In the case of PTSD/BPD, the personality is in the developmental stage thus the sense of self and symptoms are closely linked to the abuse experience. This not the case for the person suffering PTSD after an accident. A person who would meet Kroll's criteria for PTSD/BPD is going to require therapy that will differ in focus if not intent from traditional psychodynamic and cognitive PTSD models. Readers are referred to Kroll's text for a detailed discussion of the relevant therapeutic issues (Kroll, 1993).

Overview of personality disorders

The DSM-IV (American Psychiatric Association, 1994) describes three clusters of personality disorders: the eccentric cluster, the dramatic cluster and the avoidant cluster. It is important to reiterate that many individuals display traits that would incline them to be labelled 'narcissistic', 'compulsive', 'paranoid', 'histrionic'. For example, many highly successful people such as Hollywood 'stars' might be considered narcissistic. However, only when these traits are 'inflexible, maladaptive, and persistent and cause significant functional impairment or subjective distress do they constitute' personality disorder.

Each cluster is briefly reviewed. For the first two clusters key principles for nursing management are highlighted. The balance of the chapter focuses on a detailed discussion of working with the character-ologically difficult client: clients with diagnoses from the dramatic-erratic cluster.

The eccentric cluster

This cluster includes the paranoid, schizoid (SPD) and schizotypal PD (STPD). Clients with the schizoid and schizotypal PD share features. They tend to be loners. They do not wish for social contact and often find attempts by health professionals to establish therapeutic relationships with them intrusive and anxiety provoking. Of the three disorders in this cluster, the individual with STPD is much closer in characteristics to the schizo-phrenic person showing evidence of thought disorder. Research has shown a strong genetic link between schizophrenia and STPD (Siever, *et al.*, 1985) and a weaker link between schizophrenia, SPD and SPDT suggesting a schizophrenia spectrum (Stone, 1993). There is less research evidence linking a genetic factor to the evolution of the paranoid PD. People with paranoid disorders are rarely hospitalised. With appropriate supports many individuals with eccentric cluster disorders live reasonably inde-pendent though eccentric lives. If these supports are provided by family, the individual may never be known to the health care system and employment might be found that allows solitary work. However, many choose to live isolated eccentric existences on the streets. Hospitalisation, with its forced socialisation is stressful and may result in symptom exacerbation. Intervention is usually only required when traits or behaviours interfere with the client's ability to live safely in the community. This may happen when paranoid thinking or social anxiety inhibits the ability of the person to buy food, collect welfare benefits, or seek medical intervention for an acute medical condition. A person with a paranoid PD in a high stress work situation may develop suspicions about co-workers that interfere with his or her ability to function in the job and intervention by a health care worker may be necessary. The person with a paranoid PD is unlikely to stay engaged in any therapeutic endeavour given his or her inability to trust others.

Sustaining a therapeutic relationship with a nurse is difficult for these clients. Closeness and trust are unlikely to develop. The ideal relationship will often mimic the ideal parent: there when necessary or needed but undemanding for the balance of the time. For some clients, the telephone provides a useful cool medium to maintain contact. The lack of face-to-face contact feels less invasive and threatening. The client can initiate the con-tact although the nurse may suggest that if he or she has not heard from the client after an agreed upon period of time the nurse will call. The client can hang up the telephone when they wish, providing a sense of control. The nurse must be prepared for appointments not being kept or for the client turning up without an appointment. For many of these clients, the main goal is to help them recognise there is a place or person they can go to when help is needed.

The avoidant cluster

This cluster includes the avoidant, dependent and obsessive-compulsive PDs. Both the avoidant and dependent PDs are marked by feelings of inadequacy, hypersensitivity to criticisms and a need for reassurance. However, the avoidant PD contrasts with the dependent PD in focus. The avoidant PD is primarily concerned with avoiding embarrassment or humiliation while the dependent PD is pre-occupied with being taken care of (DSM-IV). The clinging, submissive behaviour of the person with a dependent PD often arouses negative feelings in care providers precipitating increasing anxiety in the client and an increase in clinging behaviour reinforcing the experience of rejection they fear. This self-fulfilling prophecy makes changing behaviour extremely difficult. Given the current priorities of nursing to increase the client's autonomous behaviour and increase the client's role in planning care and decision making, the behaviour of the client with a DPD can be frustrating. Efforts by nurses to promote participation in decision making or assuming increasing responsibility for health care may be experienced as rejection leading the client into greater efforts to be dependent. Nurses need to be careful that their behaviour does not become sadistic and rejecting in response to the client's increasing anxiety at the nurse's attempts at promoting autonomy and decision making. The nursing role requires the provision of a predictable environment in which the nurse keeps his or her word. The nurse needs to be proactive, seeking out the client, so that anxious, clinging behaviour is not promoted.

The dramatic-erratic cluster

These personality styles are marked by intense, often fluctuating, affect. While many of the disorders share characteristics, the PD in this cluster can be discriminated from each other. Anti-social personality disorder (ASPD), borderline personality disorder (BPD) and histrionic personality disorder (HD) share a tendency for impulsivity. Individuals with ASPD and narcissistic personality disorder tend to be exploitative and unempathic, however, ASPD show tendencies of aggression and impulsivity not present in NPD. Both ASPD and BPD use manipulation but for differing ends: the ASPD for power the BPD in order to be taken care of. It is easy for the nurse after a few negative encounters with these clients to lose sight of their pain and distress and respond to them as 'bad' people. Within the health care system, the client with a BPD is the most likely to be hospitalised.

Often the reason for hospitalisation is actual or threatened self-harm activity. Females are over represented in the diagnosis BPD (76% of all diagnosed BPDs). This observation is noteworthy given the possible role of abuse in the aetiology of BPD and the high rates of childhood abuse among female psychiatric clients in general. It is important to recognise that all personality disorders exist along a continuum. Rosenbluth and Silver (1992) talk of a borderline syndrome and state that the range of symptoms and disruption is highly variable, suggesting that PDs that require hospitalisation are closer to the high end of the continuum. Given that the diagnosis using DSM-IV criteria requires only a certain number of items to be present for the diagnosis to be applied, it is important to recognise the PDs of this cluster can be highly variable both within and across clusters. Clients with narcissistic or histrionic PD are more likely to be found in psychotherapy, few being hospitalised (Stone, 1993). Persons with APD are more likely to be found in the forensic setting or on adolescent units where they have been placed for anti-social acts such as truancy; theft; fire-setting; physical cruelty to animals or other persons. Stone has argued that several PDs may be present in any one individual person and that multiaxial or dimensional approaches to evaluating personality may provide a clearer picture of the person's style associated behaviours. Vaillant (1992) suggests that the focus of work with PD should be on the immature defensive styles so many clients exhibit.

Working with personality disorders: problems for nurses?

Working with personality disordered clients is a major challenge for nurses (if not all mental health professionals). Working with these clients, whether in the acute stage, the community or long-term therapy, is often a source of frustration and intense feelings for the nurse. By definition, the disorder represents the persona – not a set of clinical symptoms layered onto a personality. The disorder is the person – what you see is who he or she is; the characterological structure. Each individual possesses within his or her personality a set of coping mechanisms commonly known as defence mechanisms that control impulses and urges via behaviours that in 'normal' situations are socially acceptable and harmless to the individual. Unfortunately, the constellation of immature defence mechanisms frequently used by the clients with PDs, particularly in the dramatic cluster, evoke intense affect in clinicians. Defense mechanisms include splitting (with idealisation and devaluation), projection, projective identification, denial, and turning against self (including self-harm). These clients demonstrate such fluctuations in affect (for example believing a nurse is wonderful one day and awful the next) that novice nurses experience tremendous disappointment and subsequent anger. The extreme traits of the client may resonate with areas of difficulty of the nurse. For example, nurses who like to feel competent and in control may have difficulties with clients who are clingy and dependent (because of the nurse's own unresolved dependency needs). Consequently, working with clients with PDs requires the nurse to be able to be reflective and consider the meaning of his or her own behaviour and feelings. The defensive structure of some clients, particularly those diagnosed with a BPD is very effective at destabilising the treatment team, causing conflict amongst and between disciplines. All treatment settings need to think very carefully about treatment goals so that the goals are realistic otherwise both clients and staff will suffer.

Nurses who choose, or are required to, work with clients with PDs, should seek clinical supervision in order to reflect on practice and explore the many counter-transference issues that occur and re-occur regardless of the years of experience working with these clients. As Kroll (1993) points out it is hard to avoid making mistakes working with BPD – even for experienced therapists. The research suggests that the effectiveness of psychotherapy or other therapies in moderating the characterological structure is limited. Interestingly, the most effective outcome research findings utilised two very differing methods of therapy: psycho-dynamically based (Stevenson & Meares, 1992) and cognitive-behaviourally based (Linehan, *et al.*, 1991). Both studies used manual driven training techniques for the therapist and involved close supervision suggesting that close supervision of the therapist may be the best therapy for a BPD (Kroll, 1993).

'In any work with these clients, nurses must retain a fundamentally empathic stance. Life experience has not provided for these individuals a positive sense of worth or self-esteem. An attitude of acceptance and interest in the subjective experience of the client is perhaps the most therapeutic quality the nurse can provide.'

(Gallop, 1997)

Many nurses are likely to see clients with PDs only in times of crisis: acute suicidal behaviour or parasuicidal behaviour for BPD; or when traits become so maladaptive that the client cannot function: compulsion stops the person from going out, or eating, or interferes with safety and self-care. Clients with an APD are usually found in the forensic system. Nurses may see these clients for assessment before trial. Sometimes these clients use hospital if they feel they risk a term of prison. Again because this *is* the personality, most clients with an APD experience their traits as egosyntonic and do not experience distress (only concern if caught in criminal or harmful activity or if in a 'one down' position). As nurses move into the community and into an expanding health promotion and illness preven-tion scenario, they are more likely to come into contact with clients, who, while not requiring intensive psychiatric intervention, are experiencing personality difficulties that interfere with the quality of life. For example, men and women who have experienced an abusive childhood may appear to have personality traits that interfere with relationships, self-esteem and the ability to trust others (Briere, 1992). Many nurses working in commu-nity settings are providing mental health services to self-harming clients who ten years ago would have been hospitalised. Nurses working in the community face the additional challenge of working in the client's home and frequently do not have adequate clinical back-up available.

Working with clients with PDs often provides minimal professional gratification or reinforcement of the therapeutic competence of the nurse (Gallop & Wynn, 1986; May & Kelly, 1982). Because of the characterological nature of the difficulties and the lengthy therapeutic interventions required to effect change, setting any kind of goal that involves change in the short term is unrealistic. This lack of effecting change may feel antithetical to the nurse's need to 'make the patient better'. Long-term treatment should be only conducted by nurses with advanced training or education in psychotherapy who possess a solid understanding of long-term treatment processes. Long-term treatment will inevitably include the experience of the client 'feeling worse', if insight is to be acquired and the defence structure explored and this can be frightening for the therapist if under-standing is inadequate or supervision and support unavailable.

As stated earlier, our understanding of PDs is further complicated by notions that traumatic experiences during childhood may be responsible for a large number of cases currently diagnosed as PDs (particularly BPD). The interpersonal difficulties, lack of trust, and the view of the external world as a hostile place become more understandable in a world where the fundamental trust is betrayed and the child is left powerless and silenced by those upon whom he or she depends. Nurses must consider how this potential reconceptualisation of the disorder will affect their under-standing, and the treatment and management of clients.

Since BPD is the most frequent PD seen in psychiatric settings and the most problematic in the community setting, the client with BPD will be used as a focus to understand treatment and management challenges.

Characteristics of the BPD

The diagnosis BPD has become a pejorative label for the 'difficult' client. Vaillant (1992) suggests that the label 'borderline' is a reflection of countertransference difficulties and urges clinicians to focus on strategies for managing the primitive defence mechanisms. The DSM-IV (p. 654) describes BPD as

'a pervasive pattern of instability of interpersonal relationships, self-image and affects and marked impulsivity beginning by early adulthood'.

BPD is characterised by impulsivity, suicidal or self-mutilating behaviours, frantic efforts to avoid real or imagined abandonment, chronic feelings of emptiness, severe dissociative symptoms or transient stress-related para-noid ideation and affective instability. It is noteworthy that 'severe dis-sociative symptoms' is an addition to the DSM-IV criteria and was not present in DSM-III. Dissociation, a breakdown in connections among thoughts, feelings, behaviours and memories designed to reduce distress, either consciously or unconsciously, is common among abuse survivors (Briere, 1992).

Setting realistic treatment goals

Treatment goals: short stay

There is general consensus that the use of hospitalisation for the BPD client should be restricted to a short stay for the purpose of reducing acute suicidal or parasuicidal (self-harm) behaviours and returning the client to the more chronic state associated with this disorder. If this is the case then the role of nursing is one of supportive therapy, and providing a structured environment with clear limits that reinforces reality and focuses on the here and now. Exploratory models of therapy are to be avoided. By focusing on the here and now the nurse explores the changes in the present context of the client's life (social activities, work, housing) that may have precipitated the hospitalisations and what can be done to ameliorate the precipitants. For example, a client may be hospitalised following an overdose because her therapist has gone on vacation, or a boyfriend has left town, or a sister is getting married (all events which may precipitate feelings of abandonment). The here and now focus will address supports for the client, exploring the use of day hospitals and/or the use of a backup therapist on a regular rather than ad hoc basis. The client with a BPD has difficulty with the experience of sadness or loss and may not link the abandonment event to the self-harm behaviour. The client may recount feeling bored or restless before taking the overdose but will usually not describe feelings of anxiety, depression, or emptiness, all feelings that may have precipitated the overdose. This lack of linkage between affect and behaviour is suggestive of dissociative behaviour. Even where treatment goals of short stay hospital focus on the here and now, nurses still need to understand the psychodynamic or theoretical models of the BPD if they are to remain empathic and sensitive to the pain of these clients.

The very nature of hospitalisation is regressive and the pull to regression in the hothouse of the hospital often means that facilitating discharge is highly problematic. This fear of the client regressing often means that staff energies are focused on discharge or 'getting the patient out'. This message can be quickly conveyed to the client who in response to fears of abandonment, directs all her energy at 'staying in'. Consequently all energies of staff and client are focused on opposing goals and treatment goals may be lost in the process. Short-term hospital care of the BPD requires an attitudinal shift on the part of staff. Nurses and other clinicians must see brief hospitalisations (often frequent) as a part of a continuing process. The client will need hospitalisation from time to time and the hospital should convey the message to the client that they will be there when and if he or she needs care. Conveying this message helps the client to leave without a sense of real or imagined abandonment. If nurses accept the need to be available for short but perhaps frequent rehospitalisations, then nurses can convey to the client over the long term an important message about acceptance and belief in the worth of the client.

Treatment goals: long term

According to Kroll (1993), in the United States, the majority of psychotherapy for clients with BPD is conducted by Master's prepared nurses, psychologists or social workers. The reason for this is not clear. Since these clients do not respond to psychopharmacological interventions, the appeal of working with these clients for physicians may be reduced. Many nurses are connected to public clinics in which their right to choose clients may be limited. Few physicians find the client with BPD an attractive client. Therapy is stormy and often the client is disruptive, demanding access at all hours and demanding emergency contact. Nursing has increasingly identified a professional role in helping vulnerable clients. Since the majority of BPD clients are women, and many of these women have histories of abuse, they may be seen as a more appropriate client group for nurses than physicians.

Long-term treatment is directed at either *characterological restructuring* (psychodynamic models), or *reframing* the self-destructive behaviour (cognitive model). Both of these theoretical models will be discussed below. Any long-term treatment requires a theoretical model to drive the process. In addition, nurses involved in long-term treatment should seek advanced education, psychotherapy training and supervision. No clinician, regardless of years of experience is immune from the intense countertransference responses these clients can precipitate. Ideally, supervision should be provided by an objective expert who is not in a line authority position. Supervision can also be provided by peers or colleagues who work with difficult clients, as long as they are not involved in the direct care of the client.

In any work with these clients, nurses must retain a fundamentally empathic stance. Life experience has not provided for these individuals a positive sense of worth or self-esteem. An attitude of acceptance and interest in the subjective experience of the client is perhaps the most therapeutic quality the nurse can provide. To be unempathic by belittling the distress reinforces the pejorative image so frequently associated with these disorders (Gallop, *et al.*, 1989).

The need for a conceptual framework

If a nurse is to work effectively with a client he or she must have a conceptual framework or theoretical model for understanding his or her client's behaviour or way of being in the world. While this is true for all clients, it is exquisitely true for clients with PDs. Without a conceptual framework or theoretical model of understanding, the client will quickly be seen as 'bad' and the nurse will experience feelings of anger and therapeutic invalidation (Gallop, Kennedy & Stern 1994). Given the often dramatic and difficult behaviours of these clients it is too easy to be reactive rather than proactive. In research on 'difficult' clients, nurses have described patients' self harm behaviours as deliberate, and manipulative. When asked why clients behaved this way, nurses stated it was to seek attention or drive the nurse 'crazy' (Gallop & Wynn, 1986). With this kind of explanatory model client's pain and distress will be ignored, denied or misunderstood. While the client may be seeking attention by the behaviour, the nurse must consider the degree of internal distress (conscious or unconscious) that precipitates these self-harm behaviours and recognise that if the only way attention can be gained is by self-harm behaviours, then this is a harsh reflection of the client's sense of self and self-worth. With a theoretical framework, the nurse can understand, strategise and plan clinical interventions. Below two conceptual approaches for working with BPD are discussed. In one chapter, frameworks can only be outlined. Hopefully, the interested reader will seek further understanding and application of these models.

The object-relations model: problems in the separation-individuation phase

Psychodynamic models of the BPD have moved from drive theory and investigations of the oedipal phase to a focus on the caretaker-infant relationship and the developmental tasks of early childhood. Earlier in this chapter, when considering origins of the personality, the essential elements of effective early caretaking were briefly outlined. Explanations of the dynamic underpinnings of the BPD focus on problems in the separation-individuation phase of a child's development particularly in the 18–36 month phase of development. Many of these models derive from the work of Mahler (1986), who first described the tasks of separation – individuation when the child moves away from being a lap baby, dependent on the mother, towards becoming an autonomous striving person. According to Mahler, effective mothering (or caretaking) facilitates the development of a sense of autonomy and self. Effective mothers (or primary caregivers) reward and encourage independence. They take pleasure in their child's accomplishments yet still are available to provide the 'emotionally' refuelling necessary to facilitate the integration of positive and negative aspects of self and others. On the other hand, mothers who do not encourage autonomy, reward dependence and clinging. These mothers withdraw love and approval in response to independent activity, do not facilitate the integration of good and bad aspects of self and others and cause these good and bad aspects to be kept apart or split.

The reason for this, according to authors such as Masterson (1976), is that the primitive ego of the toddler cannot tolerate the risk of withdrawal of the love of mother so that movement towards autonomy becomes linked with fears of abandonment. Thus, the child can be dependent and feel good (i.e. loved) or be independent and feel bad or abandoned (plus the associated rage, emptiness and guilt). This separation (splitting) of good and bad results in the failure of internalised whole representations (necessary for object constancy) and a lack of a sense of inner security. The child and later the BPD adult cannot call up soothing positive internal representations to comfort the self. Winnicott describes how the ability to self-soothe is an essential capacity for tolerating being alone (1970). The BPD client has great difficulty being alone in the world. As suggested earlier, many women with a diagnosis of BPD have histories of abuse. Object relations theory has been used to understand the developmental crisis of the abused child. According to Herman (1992, p. 59) the child:

'must find a way to develop a sense of basic trust and safety with caretakers who are untrustworthy and unsafe. She must develop a sense of self in relation to others who are helpless, uncaring or cruel'.

Herman (1992) suggests the child resolves this dilemma by the use of splitting and the use of dissociation – shutting off the abuse from conscious memory and/or constructing an explanation of the abuse as justified by her badness.

Application of the object-relations model

The consequences of a lack of internal 'object constancy' and the need to defend against real and/or imagined abandonment are the dynamics that get re-enacted over and over again in the therapeutic relationship with the client who has a BPD. It is during the course of hospitalisation that these dynamics can be seen most clearly. Numerous authors have described the clinical problems that are an expression of these dynamics (Brown, 1980; Gallop, 1985; Colson, *et al.*, 1986). In the short hospital stay, understanding enables the nurse to avoid re-enacting with clients the disappointments and difficulties of the past. Often the course of hospitalisation is stormy and marked by the use of a primitive set of defence mechanisms which are the result of the faulty development described above.

The key defences are denial; idealisation; devaluation; projective identification and projective dissociation (splitting). Projective identification and dissociation allow external objects to be perceived as all good or all bad (affect is projected) thus enabling positive (love) and negative (hate) affects to be kept apart (split).

Projective identification differs from simple projection insofar as the client's need to control the person who receives the projected self or other representation. Adler (1992, p. 259) has described this mechanism in the context of the therapeutic alliance. The client attempts to

'remove an unacceptable or cherished part of himself by placing it into the therapist. The client then interacts with the therapist in a way that provokes the therapist to respond to him in consonance with the projected fantasy'.

The task of the therapist (nurse) is to contain the projection, understand or use this understanding to help the client gain insight into the reasons for the projection rather than react with the affect of the projection. These intense projected affects (love, hate) are often the source of the counter-transference responses so problematic in clinical management.

Idealisation and devaluation are further expressions of this lack of integrated objects. The client may idealise a nurse and claim that only he or she understands her (the client) and can save the client, thus temporarily fulfilling the client's need for the caring mother who requires dependency. Idealisation is often found coupled with devaluation: the projection of the negative affect onto another staff member who doesn't understand, is stupid or is insensitive and represents the client's own sense of inadequacy and rage.

At the beginning of treatment or hospitalisation there is often a brief honeymoon phase (idealisation) followed by regression (back to clingy dependent). The idealisation is rapidly replaced by disappointment because demands can never be met (devaluation, fears of abandonment and rage), The client continues to seeks a rescuer – such as a nurse who 'truly' understands her (idealisation), and views the others as bad and unworthy (devaluation, projective identification and splitting). Of course, the nurse is bound to fail (devaluation, further splitting, projective identification and rage). This cycle is repeated endlessly and can happen within days, and at times, within hours. Even though the acute suicidal phase may have passed, efforts to help the patient move towards discharge may be experienced as rejection (re-evoking the abandonment depression) and so the cycle continues. Throughout all this, the nurse and other staff experience the projections of the patient and experience intense feelings of like/dislike and interdisciplinary strife (Gallop, 1985). Often these intense affect storms are accompanied by acting out behaviours such as slashing; verbal abuse; suicidal gestures; and other regressive behaviours. As I have described in previous work

> Staff are left not only to pick up the pieces but also feeling in pieces. As recipients of the good and bad part-object representations of the borderline patient, the staff becomes a collective representation of the patient. Meanwhile the patient is left empty, dependent upon the responses of the staff bearing his projected part-object representations
>
> (Gallop, 1985, p. 8)

The arousal of fears of abandonment (although rarely conscious) can be based on clinical staff behaviours that are not associated in the minds of the staff with abandonment. For example, a compliment to an inpatient that she is looking well can be interpreted as 'you think I'm ready for discharge' and precipitate an overdose, or the failure of a preoccupied nurse to respond to a patient's greeting can be experienced as rejection and lead to self-mutilating behaviour.

Countertransference responses

The intense feelings aroused in nurses can be considered countertransference responses. Early views of countertransference described it as unconscious – an expression of the therapist's own internal conflicts about significant people in his or her own life, and always negative. More recent views of countertransference consider the understanding of countertransference feelings to be an important tool in the understanding of the therapeutic relationship and can be in response to the defensive style of the client as well as internal conflicts (Burke & Tansey, 1985). The primitive defences of the BPD client precipitate corresponding affects in many clinicians. Projective identification and devaluation (expressions of rage, inadequacy and fear of abandonment) often precipitate in staff feelings of retaliatory anger; expressions that the client's behaviour is bad and deliberate, and the belief that the client can't use hospitalisation or treatment to her benefit, and that she should be discharged or terminated. Projective identification and idealisation precipitate rescue fantasies and anger at other staff 'who clearly don't understand the pain and suffering of this client and only if the staff made a heroic effort this "hospitalization" or "treatment" could change the course of the client's life'. Other nurses believe the patient is simply manipulative, attention-seeking and bad, and unable to use the hospital or community care, and should be discharged from care. Neither viewpoint is accurate but put together, staff can begin to understand the dynamics of the client and see how each staff represents a part-object projection.

As previously indicated, even the most experienced staff get caught in the intense affects of the countertransference. Certainly staff with greater insight and understanding resolve the conflicts more quickly, and are able to use this understanding in the interest of the client, but counter-tranference still happens. It is essential that nurses recognise that intense feelings of like/dislike, or other conflictual feelings, are expressions of projective identification or countertransference and not expressions of the clinical reality. Nurses need to be able to recognise behavioural and affective changes in themselves that may be cues that a countertransference dilemma exists. Examples of behavioural changes include:

(1) Excusing or explaining away client behaviour you would not excuse in another client
(2) Spending too much or too little time with a client
(3) Changing your schedule unreasonably to accommodate a client
(4) Feeling that other staff don't really understand the client or care in the way that you do
(5) Feeling that the client is getting away with behaviour and should be punished
(6) Setting up an impossible contract designed to fail

Contracts

Much has been written about the utility of contracts with BPD clients. Often contracts are used too late and are used to get rid of problem clients so that staff do not have to reflect on their treatment failure. Under these circumstances the contract represents not a thoughtful proactive negotiation between patient and staff but a countertransference response. A clinical example illustrates the problem:

> Jane, a young female client, was admitted following an overdose. The goal of hospitalisation was to return her to her chronic suicidal state versus her current acute suicidal state. According to the nursing staff, once in the hospital Jane's behaviour started to regress. She began scratching her arms and burning herself with cigarette stubs. Fearing further regression, nursing staff were reluctant to place her on close observation, feeling the increased attention of close observation would reward the regression and precipitate further regressive behaviour.

Her primary nurse contracted with Jane that if she felt she would self harm she would approach the nursing staff to talk about it. During the evening shift, the nurses had little contact with Jane since this would be seen as providing attention in response to attention seeking behaviours. That night Jane inflicted serious burns on her chest spelling out the word 'PAIN'.

Jane could not meet the requirements of the contract. Her behaviour was already too regressed. She was beyond being able to seek out staff and was driven by impulse. She craved attention and used self-harming behaviours as her means to attain it. If she were capable of more appropriate and less pathological means of obtaining attention Jane would probably not have required hospitalisation. The nurses felt manipulated. Her behaviour was manipulative, i.e. designed to meet her needs and she did not know how else to do this. Jane needed to receive attention before the acute self-harm behaviour. She needed frequent short interactions. Frequency is essential. Brief interactions focus on the here and now. They are exploratory in nature. Brief interactions limit the intensity of the interaction and are more tolerable for staff. Because of her inability to retain good feelings, Jane will quickly drain of the emotional feeding provided by the interaction and quickly feel hungry or empty so that frequency is necessary. More than one nurse should be involved with Jane during this regressed time so that if one is not available another familiar nurse is present. Nurses need to keep each other fully informed of any treatment decisions. Treatment decisions that will affect Jane's privileges on the unit should be told to her with more than one staff member present so that splitting is diminished. Unfortunately, in this clinical illustration the nurses saw Jane as trouble rather than troubled and this no doubt intensified the feelings of abandonment she experienced.

Setting behavioural expectations

While the use of contracts to control difficult behaviours that have already occurred is problematic and reactive rather than proactive, setting behavioural expectations at the time of admission can be helpful. One way to do this is by providing for all clients on admission a set of behavioural expectations (see Fig. 11.2). A similar set of expectations can be used for time limited community/outpatient clinical services.

Figure 11.2 shows an example of admission documents in which the information sheet states clearly the date of admission and the anticipated date of discharge. Additional information is also provided: Clients are told that the focus of treatment will be to deal with the specific precipitants of hospitalisation and to reduce acute symptoms. They are also told what behaviours will not be tolerated and the consequence of these behaviours (discharge or transfer). All ward activities are listed and it is indicated which ones the client must attend. Clients are informed on which day team meetings are held and informed that decisions concerning unit privileges and weekend passes will only be discussed at those meetings, thus avoiding using all interaction times as bargaining sessions. Key personnel: primary nurse, therapists are identified on the sheet. The purpose for e.g. On this unit, we try to develop treatment plans that are tailored to your needs: however some basic rules apply to all patients.   The   following   actions   will   lead   to   immediate discharge, or transfer to a secure institution:

(1) fire setting
(2) substance abuse or weapons on unit
(3) physical attack on staff

You will be admitted to this unit for a maximum of   weeks.

The date today is _____

You will be discharged no later than _____

From time to time after this date you may need re-admission. This unit and its staff will be available for that purpose.

We expect all patients to:

(1) attend meals in dining-room
(2) attend group therapy
(3) meet twice weekly with therapist
(4) have daily contact with assigned nurse
(5) attend O.T.

You are exempt from the above as listed below   date

_____   _____

_____   _____

This will be re-assessed _____

Failure to attend the above may indicate to us that you feel unable to utilise the hospitalisation in which case we will discuss early discharge.

Gallop, 1997

Fig. 11.2   Example of an admission document.

providing this material is to reduce the perception of staff responses to acting out behaviour as precipitous, personalised and punitive.

Clients know these rules from the beginning. Often the client will test the rules and several admissions and discharges are required before the client realises that staff mean what they say. Re-admission is not denied but must be re-negotiated. Sometimes a client becomes acutely suicidal in response to being told they are to be discharged because of acting out behaviour. One response is not to discharge the client but place him or her on close observation and not permit the client to take part in any ward activities or leave the unit. This gets boring after a day or so and usually discharge is possible. Clients are not allowed to bargain returning to full program on the promise that the behaviour precipitating discharge will not recur. To do this would lead to escalating tests of staff limits. While it might be argued that structure and expectations such as these described are too rigid, they do provide a predictable environment in which clients feel safe. Constantly changing behavioural expectations or tolerated limits of behaviour conveys a frightening message to clients: it suggests that the client's rage is so frightening and destructive that if staff confront the rage, it might destroy the clinician. Unit expectations need not dehumanise the staff. In fact, having clear expectations allows staff to focus on affect and current distress. Similar contracts of behavioral expectations can be negotiated with clients in the community. A critical part of the contract will focus on what will be the therapist's response to self-harm threats or behaviour. The therapist must make it clear to the client that the client can talk about and express any feelings he or she wishes in sessions (including angry feelings about the therapist) but certain behaviours will have consequences (including termination of therapy).

The psychodynamic model has held great appeal to clinicians for many years. Truly understanding the psychodynamic model so that the nurse can be sensitive to the pain of the client that lies behind the angry, manipulative and self-harm behaviour is one of the greatest challenges caring for these clients. It is too easy to learn the words and miss the music. Nurses can quickly identify splitting and other angry and difficult behaviours but that is insufficient if the nurse does not then proceed to attend to the pain and distress driving that behaviour.

Dialectical behavioural therapy

The dialectical behavioural therapy model of Linehan (1987) was developed as an outpatient treatment model for chronically suicidal or self-mutilating BPD clients. According to Linehan, three bimodal behavioural patterns dominate the style of the BPD client.

Pattern 1: Emotional vulnerability versus invalidation
In this pattern the BPD client is unable to regulate emotional responses. Suicidal or other self-destructive behaviours are maladaptive responses to overwhelming and painful affect. Cognitively clients pay attention to only

vivid negative affect experiences and usually have difficulty recalling or experiencing positive affect states. Many clients come from environments where affective experiences were never validated. For example, homes in which parents or significant others trivialised or ignored the experience of painful emotions. Failure is explained as not trying hard enough or lack of discipline. Presenting a positive mental attitude and smiling in the face of adversity is valued so that failure to meet these expectations results in disapproval or criticism (withdrawal). As a result, the individual is exquisitely sensitive to emotional stimuli but experiences validation only for extreme expressions.

Pattern 2: Helplessness versus apparent competency

In most situations the client approaches problems with a passive, helpless stance eliciting problem solving from others. Although the person may appear competent, this facade may thwart the very support and encouragement needed to use what competencies he or she has. It is relevant to see the comparisons with the conflict about dependence and autonomy outlined in the psychodynamic model.

Pattern 3: Unrelenting crisis versus inhibited grieving

According to Linehan, the BPD client is in a chronic state of crisis, feeling constantly overwhelmed. The chronic state of crisis prevents the client from the grieving that must occur over the history of loss, disappointment and trauma. The chronic state of crisis further explains the apparent overreaction, given the sense of helplessness, to minor events (or psychological slights).

Treatment goals

The outpatient treatment program designed by Linehan (1987) is devised to reframe the self-destructive behaviour as habitual behaviour in response to these behavioural characteristics. Individual or group work is directed at increasing interpersonal skills in conflictual situations; increasing internal regulation of unwanted emotions; developing skills to tolerate emotional distress until change occurs and learning self-management skills. Linehan has developed specific therapeutic techniques, training programmes and manuals for interested therapists.

Nursing goals

Gallop (1992) has considered the utility of this model for the inpatient treatment. She suggests that cognitive dialectical behaviour therapy may provide a reframing for nurses of client's behaviour that will have positive benefits for both staff and client. By viewing the self-destructive response as habitual, nurses may become more tolerant. Seeing the BPD client as someone in a chronic state of crisis, exquisitely sensitive to affect yet inexperienced in receiving responses to appropriate displays of emotion makes the intense affective storms of the BPD understandable. Arntz (1994) extends this cognitive model to suggest that since most BPD clients have chronic traumatic childhood experiences, they develop cognitive schema based on assumptions of self as powerless, bad, and existing in a dangerous world. Nurses and therapists attempting cognitive work still need to focus on the development of a therapeutic relationship grounded in trust (reliability and consistency) before setting about modifying schema and dealing with trauma experiences.

Nurses using the DBT model must develop rapid assessment skills for new admissions. All BPD clients with a history of impulsive or self-destructive behaviour should be assessed for problems with impulsivity and dangerous or reckless behaviour. After identification, designed to differentiate these clients from clients who are clinically depressed and at high suicidal risk, clients move into a treatment program geared to helping them control impulsive and self-destructive behaviour. Harborview Medical Center in Seattle, Washington, has developed a program for frequent utilisers with self harm behaviours. It is a multi-step programme grounded in a combination of post-traumatic stress theory, cognitive therapy theory and dialectical behaviour theory. It includes planned admissions, individualised contracts, staged interventions and skills training. Much of the therapy (in and outpatient) is conducted by advanced practice mental health nurses. During the first stage (often over several admissions) the focus is on safety and the development of the contract. The contract focuses on planned versus emergency admissions. Clients are required to negotiate admissions and will not be admitted directly from emergency or other facilities. Self-harm behaviours are targeted. Clients enter into skills acquisition via either cognitive or DBT therapy or therapy directed at management of anxiety and panic.

In facilities that do not have a formal program and are short stay, goals must by necessity be limited. For many patients, developing the insight to recognise that impulsivity and self-harm behaviours are a response to affect is an enormous task. Helping a client consider that these responses may change over time is another important nursing task. For many of these clients the notion of change is hard to accept. Nurses can work with clients to help them recognise triggers and precipitants of self-harm behaviours. By doing this, the nurse helps the client link the behaviour to the painful affect and increases the client's self-awareness. Gallop (1992) has identified a number of areas appropriate for exploration which may help increase self-awareness. These areas include identification of cues such as a build up of tension; reconsideration of habitual responses and an exploration of whether or not the client wants help controlling impulsive behaviours. In longer stay facilities or in community settings, trained nurses can lead groups for self-harming clients. In these groups clients learn to identify patterns of behaviour that were acquired as a result of real pain and real hurts. The past is not trivialised but acknowledged as the source of patterns and assumptions about self which now influence all interactions but are inappropriate for current situations.

Conclusion

Throughout this chapter, it has been reiterated that personality change is extremely difficult. Goals when working with PD clients must be modest. The so-called symptoms of distress reflect deeply integrated beliefs about the badness or worthlessness of self. To work effectively with clients a conceptual framework is essential. Without a framework, nurses respond only to behaviour and lose sight of the distress of individuals. In addition, the nurse must have the capacity to reflect upon his or her own behaviour and responses to clients. Often this is difficult both for the novice nurse and the experienced nurse. The novice nurse is easily swept up in the wish to rescue. The experienced nurse may lose empathic abilities after multiple encounters with these challenging clients or else feels he or she knows it all and is beyond having countertransference difficulties. The successful nurse acknowledges her own limitations, recognises the complexity, and seeks supervision. Working with these clients requires a fundamental belief in the value and inherent worth of the individual. Nurses who possess and can display a fundamental acceptance of the client, and demonstrate warmth, positive regard and genuineness as espoused by Rogers (1957) will facilitate the greatest growth regardless of theoretical framework.

References

Adler, G. (1992) The myth of the therapeutic alliance with borderline patients revisited. In: *Handbook of Borderline Disorders* (eds D. Silver & M. Rosenbluth). International Universities Press, Madison, Conn.

American Psychiatric Association (1994) *The Diagnostic and Statistical Manual of Mental Disorders – Version IV*. American Psychiatric Association, Washington DC.

Arntz, A. (1994). Treatment of borderline personality disorder: A challenge for cognitive-behavioural therapy. *Behaviour Research Therapy*, **32**(4), 419–30.

Briere, J. (1992). *Child Abuse Trauma: Theory and Treatment of the Lasting Effects*. Sage Publications, Newbury Park, Calif.

Brown, L.J. (1980). Staff countertransference reactions in the hospital treatment of borderline patients. *Psychiatry*, **43**, 333–45.

Bryer, J.B., Nelson, B.A., Miller, J.M., & Krol, P.A. (Nov. 1987). Childhood sexual and physical abuse as factors in adult psychiatric illness. *American Journal Psychiatry*, **144**(11), 1426–30.

Burke, W. & Tansey, M. (1985) Projective identification and the countertransference turmoil: Disruptions in the empathic process. *Contemporary Psychoanalysis*, **21**, 372–402.

Colson, D., Allen, J. & Coyne, L. (1986) An anatomy of countertransference: Staff reactions to difficult psychiatric hospital patients. *Hospital and Community Psychiatry*, **37**, pp. 923–8.

Gallop, R. (1985) The patient is splitting: Everyone knows and nothing changes. *Journal of Psychosocial Nursing and Mental Health Services*, **23**, 6–10.

Gallop, R. (1992) Self-destructive and impulsive behavior in the patient with a borderline personality disorder: rethinking hospital treatment and management. *Archives of Psychiatric Nursing*, **6**, 178–82.

Gallop, R. (1997) Caring about the client: The role of gender, empathy and power in the therapeutic process. In: *The Mental Health Nurse: Views of Practice and Education* (ed. S. Tilley). Blackwell Science Ltd, Oxford.

Gallop, R. & Wynn. F. (1986) Difficult young adult chronic patients: Re-evaluating short-term clinical management. *Journal of Psychosocial Nursing and Mental Health Services*, **24**, 29–32.

Gallop, R., Lancee, W.J. & Garfinkel, P.E. (1989) How nurses respond to the label: Borderline personality disorder. *Hospital and Community Psychiatry*, **40**, 815–19.

Gallop, R., Kennedy, S., & Stern, D. (1994) The therapeutic alliance on an inpatient unit for eating disorders. *International Journal of Eating Disorders*, **16** (1).

Gallop, R., McKeever, P., Toner, B., Lancee, W. & Lueck, M. (1995) The impact of childhood sexual abuse on the psychological well-being and practice of nurses. *Archives of Psychiatric Nursing*, **IX** (3), 137–45.

Herman, J.L. (1992) *Trauma and Recovery*. Basic Books, USA.

Herman, J., Perry, C. & Van der Kolk, B. (1989) Childhood trauma in borderline personality disorder. *American Journal of Psychiatry*, **146**, 490–95.

Hurt, S.W. & Clarkin, J.F. (1990) Borderline personality disorder: prototypic typology and the development of treatment manuals. *Psychiatric Annuals*, **20**(1), 13–18.

Kroll, J. (1993) *PSTD/Borderlines in Therapy: Finding the Balance*. Norton, New York.

Linehan, M.M. (1987) Dialectical behavioral therapy: a cognitive behavioral approach to parasuicide. *Journal of Personality Disorders*, **1**, 328–33.

Linehan, M., Armstrong, H., Suarez, A., Allmon, D. & Heard, H. (1991) Cognitive behavioral treatment of chronically parasuicidal borderline patients. *Archives of General Psychiatry*, **48**, 1060–64.

Mahler, M. (1986) On the first three subphases of the separation-individuation process. In: *Essential Papers on Object Relations* (ed. Peter Buckley). New York University Press, New York.

Mahler, M. (1972) On the first three subphases of the separation-individuation process. *International Journal of Psycho-Analysis*, **53**, 333–8.

Masterson, J. (1976) Psychotherapy of the borderline adult: A developmental approach. Brunner/Mazel, New York.

Masterson, J. (1988) *The Search for the Real Self: Unmasking the Personality Disorders of Our Age*. The Free Press, New York.

Masterton, J. & Klein, R. (1989) *Psychotherapy of the Disorders of the Self: The Masterson Approach*. Brunner Mazel, New York.

May, D. & Kelly, M. (1982) Chancers, pests and poor wee souls: Problems of legitimation in psychiatric nursing. *Sociology of Health and Illness*, **4**, 279–301.

Merikangas, K., & Weissman, M. (1986) Epidemiolgoy of DMS – III Axis II personality disorders. *Annual Review of Psychiatry*, **V** (258–278) American Psychiatric Press Inc, Washington, DC.

Ogata, S.N., Silk, K.R., Goodrich, S., Lohr, N.E., Westen, D. & Hill, E.M. (1990). Childhood Sexual and Physical Abuse in Adult Patients with Borderline Personality Disorder. *American Journal of Psychiatry*, **147**, 1008–13.

Rogers, Carl (1957) The necessary and sufficient conditions of therapeutic personality change. *Journal of Counselling Psychology*, **21**, 95–103.

Rosenbluth, M. & Silver, D. (1992) The inpatient treatment of borderline personality disorder. In: *Handbook of Borderline Disorders* (eds D. Silver & M. Rosenbluth). International Universities Press, Madison, Conn.

Siever, L., Klar, H. & Coccaro, E. (1985) Biological response styles: Clinical implications. In: *Psychobiological Substrates of Personality* (eds L. Siever & H. Klar). American Psychiatric Press Inc, Washington, DC.

Stevenson, J. & Meares, R. (1992) An outcome study of psychotherapy for patients with borderline pesonality disorder. *American Journal of Psychiatry*, **149**, 358–62.

Stone, M. (1992) The borderline patient: Diagnostic concepts and differential diagnosis. In: *Handbook of Borderline Disorders* (eds D. Silver & M. Rosenbluth). International Universities Press, Madison, Conn.

Stone, M. (1993) *Abnormalities of Personality*. WW Norton & Co, New York.

Vaillant, G. (1992) The beginning of wisdom is never calling a patient a borderline; or: The clinical management of immature defenses in the treatment of individuals with personality disorders. *Journal of Psychotherapy Practice and Research*, **1**, 118–34.

Winnicott, D. (1965a) Ego distortions in terms of the true and false self. In: *The Maturation Processes and the Facilitating Environment*. Hogarth Press, London.

Winnicott, D. (1965b) The capacity to be alone. In: *The Maturation Processes and the Facilitating Environment*. Hogarth Press, London.

Winnicot,t D. (1965c) The theory of parent-child development. In: *The Maturation Processes and the Facilitating Environment*. Hogarth Press, London.

Winnicott, D. (1970) The theory of the parent-child relationship. *International Journal of Psycho-Analysis*, **50**, 711–17.

12 Suicide Prevention

Pierre Baume and *Michael Clinton*

Introduction

In the Western world suicide is ranked among the top ten causes of death. It is estimated that annually nearly one million people worldwide complete suicide (UNICEF, 1996). The rate of attempted suicide is thought to be up to 100 times more frequent than suicide. Thoughts of suicide have also become extremely prevalent in Western countries, with surveys reporting up to 60% of high school students having had suicidal thoughts and up to 7% having attempted suicide within the preceding 12 months.

The causes of suicide are complex and it is impossible to consider all the factors that have been implicated and how knowledge of them might be used to design suicide prevention programs. Therefore, suicide rates among young males aged 15 to 24 years in Australia have been chosen as the focus for this chapter. Suicide rates in this group have been singled out because Australia has a disproportionately high rate of suicide among young people and because the suicide rate for this group has risen four fold in the past 35 years. At a suicide rate of 16.4 per 100 000 young people aged 15 to 24 years, Australia has a higher suicide rate in this age group than Norway at 16.3, the United States at 13.2, Sweden at 12.2 and Japan at 7.0 (UNICEF, 1993).

Consideration of the factors that appear to contribute to the high rate of suicide among young people in Australia leads logically to consideration of prevention and crisis intervention. However, the model for suicide prevention presented and the discussion of crisis intervention that follows have been purposefully generalised to show their wider relevance. By focusing on the causation of completed suicide and attempted suicide in one age and gender specific group, it is possible to demonstrate the difficulty of accounting for why people take their own lives. There are factors that are clearly implicated, but it is yet to be shown why some people kill themselves while others experiencing similar challenges thrive and seem stronger for the experience. Perhaps the way forward is to study not only the factors that are implicated in suicide, but also the factors that explain why some countries have lower suicide rates. Greater understanding of these factors may assist with reducing the unacceptably high rate of suicide in countries like Australia, and wider knowledge of them among mental health nurses may assist with the development of more effective prevention and crisis intervention strategies.

The chapter refers to a wide range of literature to identify causal factors in suicide. Broad suicide prevention strategies that include roles for governments and health professionals are then considered. In the final section the management of people who are at risk of suicide is highlighted. Here the focus is on principles of crisis intervention and the development of timely and effective interventions. The interventions described are guidelines only, and should be modified according to the age, cultural background and specific needs of the person and their family or significant others.

Although people have died by their own hand throughout history, the term suicide emerged with the birth of science and the secular world of the mid-1600s (Shneidman, 1969). Before and since views on suicide have differed and some cultures have encouraged suicide. In Ancient Greece and Rome, convicted criminals were permitted to take their own lives. In India suicide is still tolerated and the voluntary suicide of an Indian widow (*suttee*) still occurs. However, suicide has been condemned by Islam, Judaism and Christianity, and suicide attempts in some countries are punishable by law. In Australia, it was not until the 1970s that the act of suicide was decriminalised. The act of attempted suicide remains a crime in the Northern Territory.

Prevalence

Suicide is now the leading cause of death from all external causes for all age groups in Australia, ahead of motor vehicle accidents and well ahead of homicides, which have remained relatively constant for the greater part of this century (ABS, 1996). Nearly 2500 deaths in Australia are recorded as suicide each year and this is probably an under-estimation of the true picture.

The most disturbing trend to have emerged in the past 30 years is the nearly four fold increase in the suicide rate for males aged 15 to 24 years (Baume, 1996). In the period 1960 to 1965 the suicide rates for young males increased from 6.8 to 27 per 100 000 and those for young females from 2 to 4 per 100 000 (Fig. 12.1). Twenty-five percent of all deaths among young males in the age group 15 to 24 years are now caused by suicide. The highest frequency of suicides in this age group occurs between 23 and 24 years of age (Fig. 12.2). The dramatic rise in the suicide rate for young males has not been matched by that for young females. Whereas the suicide rate for young women has fluctuated since it rose in the early 1960s, it has remained relatively constant at around 5 per 100 000 per year (Fig. 12.2).

The distribution of suicides across the States and Territories of Australia is not even, as Queensland and Tasmania have consistently higher rates. Much more research is required to explain this phenomenon, but rural isolation, patterns of gun ownership and the readily available means for carbon monoxide poisoning are factors to take into consideration.

Another cause of concern is the unacceptably high rates of suicide among Aboriginal Australians, especially as suicide was relatively uncommon

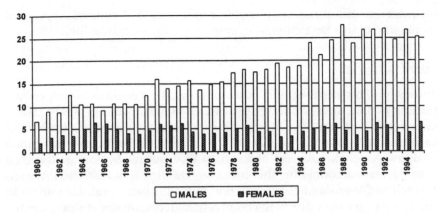

Fig. 12.1 Rates of suicide in Australia (1960–95): males and females 15–24 years. (*Source:* Australian Bureau of Statistics (1996) *Causes of Death in Australia.* Australian Government Publication Services, Canberra).

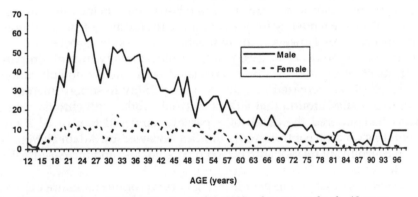

Fig. 12.2 Suicides registered in Australia. 1995 – by age at death. (*Source:* Australian Bureau of Statistics, unpublished data series, 1996).

among Aboriginal communities until recently. Urgent action is required because suicide rates for Aboriginal Australians are up to four times higher than those for the non-Aboriginal population (Baume, *et al.*, 1997). The suicide rate among young Aboriginal people aged 25 to 34 years is a particular cause for concern. Many of these deaths occur in custody; although the rate of deaths in custody for non-Aboriginal people was more than three times higher than that for Aboriginal people in the year to 31 December 1995 (Dalton, *et al.*, 1996). In that year there were 86 Aboriginal deaths in custody, representing a dramatic increase since 1992 when only two deaths occurred. The most frequent cause of death in custody was hanging, which accounted for 28 deaths. Such deaths are easily attributed to suicide, but it is far more difficult for a coroner to attribute intention in those deaths that are treated as accidental. Although suicide rates for older Aboriginal people remain low, this could change as the present cohort of young people ages. Moreover, the relatively low rate of deaths by suicide in the older age group reflects poor life expectancy. Put simply, Aboriginal people do not live long enough to complete suicide in later life.

Rural suicide

Studies have reported significant increases in the suicide of young people residing in rural areas, although the causes are not always generalisable to other regions (Baume & Clinton, 1997). Whereas the largest numbers of suicides occur in metropolitan areas, the sharpest rate of increase is in small rural towns with populations of less than 4000. Suicide by young men aged 15 to 24 years accounts for this increase (Dudley, *et al.*, 1992). However, research in Queensland has found few overall urban/rural differences in suicide rates, possibly due to the relatively high prevalence of suicide in the State. However, this finding is partly accounted for by regional variations in the suicide rates recorded for rural regions. There is some evidence that high rates are associated with the more deprived regions and low rates with more affluent rural areas (Baume, *et al.*, 1997).

A factor that may account for the steep rise in the suicide rates for rural areas may be the tendency for young people to stay away from traditional support networks. However, suicidal behaviour is often associated with a bereavement (Baume, *et al.*, 1997) and can reflect family turmoil. In particular, death of a parent has been associated with suicide, notably among young people at increased risk due to vulnerability to serious mental illness. Kosky (1983) found that 80% of suicidal youths with chronic mental illness had suffered the death of a parent, compared to 20% of a non-suicidal psychiatric control group. Studies reviewed by Adam (1990) also found a significant relationship between parental loss and increased risk of suicide.

The stressors that young people living in rural communities are exposed to include serious and often untreated mental health problems, stress related illnesses and overuse of prescribed drugs (Baume, *et al.*, 1997). High consumption of alcohol is another important risk factor (Bryant, 1992). Young people in rural areas also have easier access to firearms, which explains why there are more suicides by shooting in rural areas (Cantor, *et al.*, 1996).

Risk factors for suicide

Mental illness

Retrospective studies based on psychological autopsies (the reconstruction of events leading up to a suicide) and/or record linkage (review of the medical, psychological and social records of a person who has completed suicide) have reported the presence of a mental illness or a recent history of mental illness in a high proportion of people who have died by suicide, with estimates ranging from 31% to 92% (Baume, *et al.*, 1997).

Depression has been identified as the most frequent disorder in persons who complete suicide, affecting from 30% to 70% of those who die by suicide (Harris & Barraclough, 1997). More generally, mood disorders have been found to be associated with suicidal ideation, suicide attempts, and completed suicide (Brent, *et al.*, 1988). Depressive disorders are also over-represented among people who attempt suicide (Robbins & Alessi, 1985). However, since the majority of depressed people never attempt or complete suicide, it is clear that other factors must be involved in the causality of suicidal behaviour in people with depression. Such factors include previous suicidal behaviour, the risks for suicide discussed in this chapter, as well other forms of psychological distress.

Substance abuse disorders, personality disorders and schizophrenia are found more commonly among suicide completers than in the general population. That suicide is a major cause of premature death in persons with schizophrenia (Allebeck, 1989) is of concern because it is rarely attributable to psychotic symptoms (hallucinations and delusions) but is more likely to occur during periods of remission or improved functioning. Miles (1977), reviewing follow-up studies, concluded that as many as 10% of persons diagnosed with schizophrenia eventually die by suicide. However, there are large variations in the results of studies assessing suicide risk in people with schizophrenia, with estimates ranging from 15 to 75 times the risk found in the general population (Harris & Barraclough, 1997).

Conduct and personality disorders

Conduct and personality disorders are strongly implicated in explanations of suicide. In a sample of adult psychiatric outpatients, it was demonstrated that almost all suicide attempters had a comorbid DSM-IIIR Axis II diagnosis, regardless of their diagnosis on Axis I, suggesting a key role for personality disorders in suicidal behaviours (Sanderson, *et al.*,1992).

Though conduct disorder is not considered a personality disorder, it has been shown that a diagnosis of conduct disorder before the age of 15 years is the best predictor of an antisocial personality (Robins, 1978). Furthermore, psychological autopsy studies show that a diagnosis of conduct disorder is one of the main risk factors for completed suicide among males (Shaffer, 1988). Moreover, conduct disordered adolescent inpatients are significantly more suicidal than patients with major depression, even though they are significantly less depressed (Apter, *et al.*, 1988).

Substance abuse

Suicidal ideation and attempts have also been associated with both alcohol and substance abuse in adolescents (Lester, 1992), with high consumption often immediately preceding suicidal behaviour. Garfinkel, *et al.* (1982) found a tenfold higher rate of recent alcohol or drug use in adolescent suicide attempters than in controls. In some instances, intoxication is incidental to the suicide attempt, but in others it reflects the use of substances as part of the attempt itself (Schuckit & Schuckit, 1989). Therefore, substance abuse in young people appears both to increase the risk for multiple attempts at suicide and to add to the seriousness of each attempt, particularly for young people who are depressed (Robbins & Alessi, 1985).

Exposure to suicide

Several lines of evidence suggest that imitation can play a role in the pathogenesis of adolescent suicidal behaviour (Stack, *et al.*, 1994). Exposure to suicide is either direct person-to-person exposure (referring to the presence of suicidal behaviour within the family or other individuals close to the young person) or indirect exposure (referring to the influence of the media on the young person). Indirect exposure includes media coverage of fictional as well as real suicides. However, there is stronger evidence that suicidal behaviour in the family (Pfeffer, 1989a), or among peers (Lewinsohn, 1994) increases the risk of adolescent suicide.

Most evidence for an imitation hypothesis comes from epidemiological studies of suicide rates before and after exposure to media coverage of high profile suicides (Gould & Shaffer, 1986). Apparently there is a relationship between an increase in suicides and the publicity given in the media to suicide by celebrities, especially those in politics and entertainment; although the upsurge does not occur if suicides are not given major (front-page) attention (Phillips, *et al.*, 1992). Studies have also found an increase in suicides following televised accounts of fictional suicides, although there are other factors to take into account such as the way the suicide is portrayed and the information that accompanies the broadcast (Hafner & Schmidke, 1989). Therefore, media coverage of suicide, particularly repeated coverage of the suicide of celebrities, is a powerful inducement to imitation. However, the contagion effect is most likely to affect persons already at risk by influencing their choice of method rather than their decision to make an attempt (Skopek, 1997).

Evidence for a 'contagion' or 'imitation' effect stems from personal ties and emotional identification with a person who completes suicide, or exposure to media accounts of the suicide of a celebrity or fictional character. Sometimes the term, 'suicide clusters' is used to suggest a sequence of suicides in close geographical proximity. Suicide clusters have been reported to account for up to 10% of suicides in young people (Martin, 1996). There has been an increase in suicide clusters in recent years, and in Australia the phenomenon seems more common among Aboriginal young people (Baume, *et al.*, 1997).

Social and problem-solving skills

Suicide clusters and the other factors in suicide discussed so far raise the issue of social adaptability as another potential factor in explaining suicidal behaviour. The contribution of personal vulnerability, impaired social skills and poor peer relationships have been demonstrated to influence suicide behaviours (Pfeffer, *et al.*, 1993). For example, those who attempt suicide manifest more frequent and more serious interpersonal problems than either nonsuicidal psychiatric patients or non-hospitalised controls (Topol & Reznikoff, 1982). Furthermore, a strong relationship has been found between chronically impaired social adjustment, mood disorders and suicide (Puig-Antich, *et al.*, 1985a, 1985b). However, some studies using global measures of social adaptation have found no association between social impairment and suicidality (Brent, *et al.*, 1990).

Familial issues

The evidence that suicide tends to run in families must be taken into account by any model that seeks to explain suicide. Reviews by Roy (1992) and Lester (1992a) point out that it is difficult to differentiate between possible genetic factors involved in suicide, the presence of a family member as a role model for suicidal behaviour, and psychiatric disturbance in families. Furthermore, it is possible that, although suicide itself is not inherited, some families may have a greater probability of transmitting mental illnesses, thereby increasing the risk of suicide. In a review of family relations and suicide, Tousignant, *et al.* (1993) concluded that a poor relationship with parents is an important factor, but that coming from a divorced or separated family does not increase suicidal risk. However, neither environmental nor genetic influences alone may be sufficient to cause suicide. Twin studies and studies of children adopted at birth suggest a genetic link where the major inherited factor is an inability to control impulsive behaviour (Kety, 1990).

Suicide prevention

The previous section highlighted the complexity and interrelationships among the factors implicated in suicide. Therefore, any suicide prevention model needs to be based on current knowledge about suicide and its prevention, and practical enough to be of assistance to policy makers as well as to those involved in clinical practice. The complexity of the factors involved in suicidality and the further complexity of knowing how they might be influenced suggests that a model that provides a general framework for suicide prevention may be of more help than one that seeks to prescribe interventions yet to be validated by research.

As suicide is not a mental disorder and not a medical illness, at least until an attempt has been made, there is need for a suicide prevention model that builds on knowledge of the risk factors that have been discussed. Furthermore, for any suicide prevention model to be useful, it must be flexible enough to incorporate new research evidence, and it must itself be subjected to stringent evaluation. To meet these requirements it is necessary to identify the goals of suicide prevention, to state where the focus of prevention should be, to identify the target groups or individuals to be helped, and to describe the interventions appropriate to the integration of the model into systems that are already in place to prevent suicide.

Goal

The goal of the suicide prevention model shown in Fig. 12.3 is to reduce suicide rates for vulnerable groups and individuals by:

- Promoting the development of an infrastructure that will encourage social integration and contribute to a compassionate society
- Developing strategies to reduce the development of suicidal ideation and behaviour
- Providing appropriate management for those who have engaged in suicidal behaviour
- Assisting those who have been exposed to a suicide

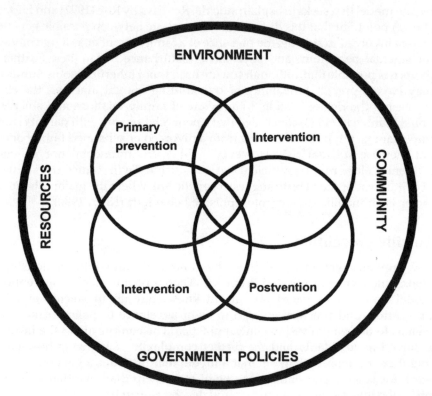

Fig. 12.3   An interactive model for the prevention of suicide (Baume, 1996).

Objectives

The objectives of the model are to ensure that suicide prevention initiatives are coordinated to achieve maximum benefit to the community by:

- Coordinating, monitoring and evaluating strategies to combat suicidality through an appropriate central point such as a Federal or State government department or a national reference centre such as the Australian Institute for Suicide Research and Prevention

- Linking services for suicidal persons or persons at risk for suicidal behaviour with other supports and services
- Disseminating information and/or providing training for relevant organisations/stockholders, and the general public
- Promoting, providing and improving access to relevant services
- Assembling scientific information and providing opportunities and resources for continuing research
- Encouraging full reporting of suicide events
- Improving the knowledge and skills of relevant care givers

Interventions

Four levels of intervention will be discussed:

- Primary prevention
- Early intervention
- Intervention
- Postvention

The approach described assumes that effective communication and shared commitment among professional services, community organisations and government departments will occur. The intersectoral nature of prevention and community participation is emphasised. Therefore stress is placed on the complementary roles of health professionals and carers as well as non-health service providers. It is also essential that all levels of government and the public and private health sector are involved.

Primary prevention

The strategies employed at this level are normally population based. Universal strategies are those designed for the whole population (for example, media campaigns to promote mental health). Selected interventions are targeted at sub-populations that share exposure to some commonly established risk factors (for example young males, Aboriginal Australians, people in custody, people who identify themselves as gay or lesbian, the mentally ill, the homeless, people living in rural areas).

Primary prevention strategies include information packages about suicidal behaviours that can be readily disseminated to services, local government agencies and the wider community. Other examples of primary prevention include the training of non-clinical professionals and members of the broader community in recognising risk signals for suicide and in discrediting myths relating to suicide. Primary prevention also encompasses measures such as reducing access to firearms, redesign of cars to reduce carbon monoxide poisoning, redesign of prison cells to diminish opportunities for death by hanging, changes to guidelines to limit access to prescription drugs, and other measures aimed at reducing access to the means of suicide. Particularly important with respect to the prevention of suicide among Aboriginal Australians is the role of governments in enacting legislation that promotes reconciliation and prevents discrimination on grounds of race, gender and ethnicity.

Early intervention

The goal of early intervention is the effective reduction of the intensity, severity and duration of risk behaviours for suicide. Therefore, early intervention strategies encompass improvement in the detection, assessment and management of people at risk. Early intervention strategies are targeted at individuals displaying general disorganisation in coping skills, stress reactions, depressive symptomatology, substance abuse, severe grief reactions and other kinds of personal vulnerability. They include more specific training for professionals, service providers and the wider community. Such training is directed at understanding and modifying behaviours which suggest that an individual may be vulnerable to suicidal behaviours and extends to ameliorating the personal vulnerabilities of those at risk by ensuring effective support programs and treatment. Individuals who display clusters of risk factors (excluding suicide attempters and people who deliberately self-harm, who require more focused intervention) are a particular focus of early intervention programs because their multiple needs make them vulnerable to poorly coordinated services.

Early intervention also addresses the need for improved cross-sectoral collaboration in minimising the risks of suicide. The services involved include telephone hotlines, other counselling services, support groups, community nurses, general practitioners and community health centres.

Intervention

Intervention or treatment involves provision of effective support to those at serious risk of suicide and those who have made attempts at suicide. Intervention strategies focus on the early detection, assessment and management of individuals with suicidal behaviours. They include the development of protocols for these purposes, training of personnel in their application, and the bedding in of effective treatment and management practices. These interventions are particularly important in accident and emergency departments, in 24 hour medical centres, and for health professionals dealing with attempts at suicide (general practitioners, community psychiatric nurses).

A further goal of intervention programs is the development of best practice models for clinicians dealing with people engaging in suicidal behaviours. Many people who attempt suicide never present to hospitals or other clinical staff, but care must be taken to ensure that those who do are not released without appropriate assessment and treatment. Improving access to mental health and other treatment services for people who attempt suicide presents a major challenge to the health care system. It also represents a window of opportunity for saving lives.

Postvention

Postvention is the support provided for those bereaved by a death resulting from suicide. Postvention activities recognise that the bereaved by suicide (the friends, family and peers of a person who has died as a result of suicide) may be particularly vulnerable to suicidal behaviours of their own as well as subject to severe grief reactions, at times leading to mental illness. Postvention strategies include setting up support groups for the bereaved, grief counselling, crisis response plans for schools and other institutions where a suicide has occurred, and training of professionals to sensitise them to the needs of those bereaved by suicide.

Management of the suicidal person

Immediate risk

When assessing the person who has made a suicide attempt, it is important to determine whether there is an immediate threat of another attempt at suicide or danger to another person that may require an immediate response. The most common immediate threats are drug overdose and self-mutilation. However, these are but two of the impending situations that may call for immediate intervention. All such situations require careful assessment and the making of a nursing assessment is critical. In cases of drug overdoses it is important to seek medical advice and often referral to an accident and emergency department is necessary. It is also important to collect as much information as possible about the drug(s) involved and the amount the person has taken. Wherever possible additional substantiating information should be sought. In other threatening situations consultation with the family and/ or police will be necessary.

Assessment

When there is no immediate risk/threat a more thorough assessment of the crisis should be considered. For any assessment it will be important to take into account:

Current state
It is not unusual for people presenting in a suicidal crisis to be under the influence of alcohol or some other substance. This is especially the case when stress has precipitated the use of alcohol or another drug. The effect of intoxication and poisoning is to impair judgement, sometimes sufficiently to result in destructive behaviour and an even more distressed mental state. In such circumstances an adequate assessment of the crisis may not be possible until intoxication has diminished. Hence, the primary goal is to ensure the safety of the person until a full assessment can be made.

Other factors that require careful assessment, and which may require stabilisation prior to adequate assessment, include acute psychotic states, delirium and confusion. Medical expertise is important in both the assessment and management of these states.

Situational factors

The purpose of assessing situational factors is to determine the extent to which the suicidal crisis is associated with a change in the external environment rather than an internal change in the capacity of the person to cope. While this is an artificial distinction, it is important to gauge the relative importance of these factors in order to make decisions about the likelihood of a further attempt at suicide or danger to another person. For example, a patient may be in a state of suicidal crisis because of the impending loss of a significant relationship. If the crisis is predominantly associated with a threat to the relationship, discussing the reasons for suicidal threats, the meaning of the relationship and options for the future may be helpful. However, if the problem of attachment has been precipitated by a general deterioration in coping associated with a relapsing psychiatric disorder, consideration of future options may be irrelevant or counter productive until the psychosis subsides.

Identification of resources and supports

Assessment of the person's resources for coping and support is an important next step. The most appropriate resources and supports will depend on the results of the assessment of environmental and personal factors. This is because the alleviation of any aspects of the suicidal crisis that are associated with external threats or difficulties will involve quite different resources from those required for the resolution of an internal crisis. For example, a patient who is in crisis due to the return of auditory hallucinations or other positive symptoms of schizophrenia may draw comfort from the prospect of an early appointment with a case manager or treating psychiatrist. On the other hand, a patient who is in crisis due to the break up of a relationship may be able to benefit more from the support of close friends. Where the presenting crisis involves both the return of psychotic symptoms and the breakdown of a relationship both interventions may be useful.

Assessment of protection needs

The crucial matter to be determined is whether as a result of a crisis the patient runs the risk of self-harm or of harming another person in the foreseeable future. Careful consideration of these possibilities is essential to the assessment of any person who has attempted or threatened suicide. It is not always possible to prevent harm or even to forecast whether or not harm is likely to occur. However, it is the responsibility of the clinician to assess any risk factors as thoroughly as possible. The assessment of suicide risk is discussed below. The assessment of intent is an important starting point.

Assessment of intent

Intent is an extremely difficult area to assess because it is often difficult to distinguish between an intention to commit suicide and a threat designed to convey a degree of distress rather than to signify the determination to self-harm. It is likely that clinicians will be more or less confident about their assessment of risk depending on their knowledge of the person. In general, it is advisable to be cautious and to take seriously any expression of an intention to self harm or to hurt another person, unless there are clear indications to the contrary.

Where there is no previous history of dangerous behaviour, a clear indication that there is no immediate intention to self-harm or to hurt another person should be sufficient to permit the assessment to proceed to the next phase. However, where there is a previous history of suicide attempts or an expression of the intention to harm someone, it is necessary to proceed with a more detailed assessment of protection needs by exploring the answers to key questions that should be put by the clinician. Such questions could include:

Assessment of resolve

How determined is the person to carry out their intentions? Issues of relevance to the assessment include the stability of the person's intent, the extent the person is concerned about the possible consequences of their behaviour for other people, the person's willingness to consider alternative ways of resolving their problems, and the person's willingness or otherwise to enter into an agreement not to harm themselves or others during an agreed period of time.

Assessment of planning and capacity

Does the person have a realistic plan to carry out their intention and do they have the means to execute their plan? Particular caution is needed if it appears the person has already made provision in the event of their death, or in the event of them facing criminal charges.

Assessment of presence or absence of protective factors

Does the person have significant others who are prepared to closely monitor their well-being and to provide close emotional support for as long as it might be needed? The absence of a support network clearly indicates the need for caution.

Assessment of previous behaviour in similar circumstances

Is there clear evidence of previous instances of life threatening behaviour? Previous history generally indicates a significantly higher level of risk.

The overriding question for each clinician is: Can I be reasonably assured of the safety of this person and their significant others? If the clinician cannot answer this question in the affirmative, it will be necessary to at least obtain a second opinion, and it may be necessary to proceed to acute inpatient admission, or, in cases where there is no evidence of psychiatric disorder, to involve family, friends or the police.

Evaluation

By the end of the crisis assessment a decision either to immediately transfer responsibility for care to another service or to make a less formal care arrangement involving family, friends or community based practitioners should be made. Depending on the outcome there will be differing but equally important responsibilities associated with the conclusion of the assessment.

In some cases the outcome will be transfer of care to a person or organisation with the ability to ensure the safety and/or treatment of the person. In these circumstances it is essential that there are:

- A clear and preferably written account of the results of the assessment and the reason for the decision to transfer management; *and*
- A transfer protocol which ensures that there will be no failure at key points. (In cases where involuntary admission is involved the key tasks are fulfilment of the requirements for regulation according to legislative requirements and the arrangement of appropriate transport.)

In the case of hospital admission, it is important for the nurse or other health care professional to discuss the admission process with the person and the person's family and/or friends. However, in most cases the person will be returned home to the care of family or friends or, perhaps, to care for themselves with appropriate follow up from a health professional. Before the patient can return home it is important to be confident that:

- The crisis is significantly ameliorated. This does not mean that the distress has resolved but that the patient and/or their family and carers feel confident that they can cope with the person's distress or difficulties.
- In the event of a return to a crisis state, the patient and/or their family and carers know what to do and where to turn for support.
- There is a plan for further assessment and an effective plan of action to resolve as far as possible the circumstances associated with the crisis. This plan could involve a broad range of actions according to the underlying issues ranging from counselling to psychiatric treatment.
- There is provision for follow up and a review of the person's progress in resolving the crisis. This might require the patient to telephone the clinician within a defined timeframe, such as within 48 hours, or an arrangement that the person visit their general practitioner. Where possible, a mobile after-hours team should visit the patient within 12 hours. The essential features of such follow ups are that arrangements are clear and structured to ensure that a review takes place. With less formal arrangements, it is essential that the nurse notes when a call from the person to the general practitioner is expected and whom to contact if the call is not received. If follow up is to be by the family doctor, it is essential that the doctor knows and agrees to provide support. Any request for the general practitioner to initiate contact with the person should be confirmed in writing.

The greatest challenge in crisis assessment is the evaluation of suicide risk. Suicidal thinking and behaviour are often associated with mental health crises and the consequences of completed suicide are irreversible and profoundly impact on the bereaved and the wider community. While suicide cannot always be prevented and may be difficult to anticipate, it is possible for people who attempt suicide to receive appropriate treatment if they are properly assessed.

Conclusion

Suicide is a complex behaviour and its prevention and management are equally complex. Fortunately, there are strategies that can reduce the risk of suicide, although they are not always effective, and more research is required to determine how they can be improved. Where an attempt at suicide is made, it is important that the person be adequately assessed and that they receive appropriate treatment. When a person successfully completes suicide, it is important to be alert to the possibility of other suicides and to ensure that their families, friends and loved ones have access to professional counselling and support.

It is also important to remember that the clinical perspective is not the only viewpoint from which suicide and its prevention can be considered. Although this will be the primary focus of the clinician and the mental health nurse, it is equally important to recognise that prevention strategies need to go beyond their focus on the individual and the family to direct attention at unemployment, abuse, discrimination and other institutionalised forms of inequality. Adequate support and appropriate assessment and treatment of the person are fundamental to assisting those who have attempted suicide and others who are at risk of suicide. However, it is equally important that legislation and social policy ensures an end to social inequalities that can be corrected through such means as better mental health services, positive discrimination in favour of rural areas and the ending of all forms of harassment, abuse and discrimination.

References

ABS (1996) *Cause of Death – Australia, 1995* (Catalogue No. 3303.0). Australian Government Publishing Service.

Adam, K.S. (1990) Environmental, psychosocial and psychoanalytic aspects of suicidal behaviour. In: *Suicide over the Life Cycle: Risk Factors, Assessment and Treatment of Suicidal Patients* (eds S.J. Blumenthal & D.J. Kupfer), pp. 39–96. American Psychiatric Press, Washington, DC.

Allebeck, P. (1989) Schizophrenia: A life shortening disease. *Schizophrenia Bulletin,* **15**(1), 81–9.

Apter, A., Bleich, A., Plutchik, R., Mendelsohn, S. & Tyano, S. (1988) Suicidal behaviour, depression and conduct disorder in hospitalised adolescents. *Journal of the American Academy of Child and Adolescent Psychiatry,* **27**(6), 696–9.

Baume, P. (1996) Suicide in Australia: Do we really have a problem? *Australian Educational and Developmental Psychologist,* **13**, 2, 3–39.

Baume, P.J.M., Cantor, C.H. & McTaggart, P. (1997) *Suicides in Queensland: A comprehensive study: 1990–1995.* Queensland Health Department.

Baume, P.J.M. & Clinton, M. (1997). Social and cultural patterns of suicide in young people in rural Australia. *Australian Journal of Rural Health,* 5(3). (In press)

Brent, D.A., Perper, J.A., Goldstein, C.E., Kolko, D.J., Allan, M.J., Allman, C.J. & Zelenak, J.P. (1988) Risk factors for adolescent suicide: A comparison of adolescent suicide victims with suicidal inpatients. *Archives of General Psychiatry,* 45, 581–8.

Brent, D., Zelenak, J.P., Bukstein, O. & Brown, R.V. (1990) Reliability and validity of the structured interview for personality disorders in adolescents. *Journal of the American Academy of Child and Adolescent Psychiatry,* 29(3), 349–54.

Bryant, L. (1992) Social aspects of the farm crisis. In: *Agriculture, Environment and Society: Contemporary Issues for Australia* (eds G. Lawrence, F. Vanclay and B. Furze). Macmillan, Melbourne.

Cantor, C.H., Turrell, G. & Baume, P.J.M. (1996) *Access to Means of Suicide by Young Australians.* A background report prepared for the Commonwealth Department of Health and Family Services, Youth Suicide Prevention Advisory Group, Canberra, Australia.

Dalton, V., Brown, M. & McDonald (1996) *Deaths in Custody Australia: No. 12. Australian Deaths in Custody and Custody-related Police Operations, 1995.* Australian Institute of Criminology, Canberra.

Dudley, M., Waters, B., Kelk, N. & Howard, J. (1992) Youth suicide in New South Wales: Urban rural trends. *Medical Journal of Australia,* 156, 83–8.

Garfinkel, B.D., Froese, A., & Hood, J. (1982) Suicide attempts in children and adolescents. *American Journal of Psychiatry,* 139, 1257–61.

Gould, M.S. & Shaffer, D. (1986) The impact of suicide in television movies: Evidence of imitation. *New England Journal of Medicine,* 315, 690–94.

Hafner, H. & Schmidke, A. (1989) Do televised fictional suicide models produce suicides? In: *Suicide Among Youth: Perspectives on Risk and Prevention* (ed. C.R. Pfeffer). American Psychiatric Press, Washington, DC.

Harris, E. & Barraclough, B. (1997) Suicide as an outcome for mental disorders. A meta analysis. *The British Journal of Psychiatry,* 170, 205–28.

Kety, S. (1990) Genetic factors in suicide: Family, twin and adoption studies. In: *Suicide over the life cycle: Risk factors, assessment and treatment of suicidal patients* (eds S.J. Blumenthal & D.J. Kupfer). American Psychiatric Press, Washington, DC.

Kosky, R. (1983) Childhood suicidal behavior. *Journal of Child Psychology and Psychiatry & Allied Disciplines,* 24(3), 457–68.

Lester, D. (1992) Alcoholism and drug abuse. In: *Assessment and Prediction of Suicide* (eds R.W. Maris, A.L. Berman, J.T. Maltsberger & R.I. Yufit). The Guildford Press, New York.

Lester, D. (1992a) *Why People Kill Themselves: A 1990s Summary of Research Findings on Suicidal Behavior.* Charles C. Thomas, Springfield, IL.

Lewinsohn, P.M. (1994) Psychological risk factors for future adolescent suicide attempts. *Journal of Consulting and Clinical Psychology,* 62, 297–305.

Martin, G. (1996) The Influence of Television in a Normal Adolescent Population. *Archives of Suicide Research,* 2, 2, 103–17.

Miles, C.P. (1977) Conditions predisposing to suicide: A review. *Journal of Nervous and Mental Disease,* 164(4), 231–47.

Pfeffer, C.R. (1989a) Life stress and family risk factors for youth fatal and nonfatal suicide behavior. In: *Report of the Secretary's Task Force on Youth Suicide: (Vol 2) Risk factors for youth suicide* (ed. L. Davidson & M. Linnoila). DHHS Pub. No. (ADM) 89–1622. US Government Printing Office, Washington, DC.

Pfeffer, C.R., Klerman, G.L., Hurt, S.W., Kakuma, T., Peskin, J.R. & Siefker, C.A. (1993) Suicidal children grow up: Rates and psychosocial risk factors for suicide attempts during follow-up. *Journal of the American Academy of Child and Adolescent Psychiatry*, **32** (1), 106–13.

Phillips, D.P., Lesyna, K. & Paight, D.J. (1992) Suicide and the media. In: *Assessment and prediction of suicide* (eds R.W. Maris, A.L. Berman, J.T. Maltsberger & R.I. Yufit). The Guildford Press, New York.

Puig-Antich, J., Lukens, E., Davies, M., Goetz, D., Brennan-Quattrock, J., & Todak, G. (1985a) Psychosocial functioning in prepubertal major depressive disorders: I Interpersonal relationships during the depressive episodes. *Archives of General Psychiatry*, **42**, 500–507.

Puig-Antich, J., Lukens, E., Davies, M., Goetz, D., Brennan-Quattrock, J. & Todak, G. (1985b) Psychosocial functioning in prepubertal major depressive disorders: II. Interpersonal relationships after sustained recovery from affective episode. *Archives of General Psychiatry*, **42**, 511–17.

Robbins, D.R. & Alessi, N.E. (1985) Depressive symptoms and suicidal behavior in adolescents. *American Journal of Psychiatry*, **142**, 588–92.

Robins, L.N. (1978). Study of childhood predictors of adult antisocial behavior. *Psychological Medicine*, **8**, 611–22.

Roy, A. (1992) Genetics, biology and suicide in the family. In: *Assessment and Prediction of Suicide* (eds R.W. Maris, A.L. Berman, J.T. Maltsberger & R.I. Yufit). The Guilford Press, New York.

Sanderson, W.C., Friedman, T., Wetzler, S., Kaplan, M.L. & Asnis, G.M., (1992 November) *Personality disorders in patients with major depression, panic disorder and generalised anxiety disorder*. Paper presented at the Annual Meeting of the Association for the Advancement of Behavioral Therapy, Boston, MA.

Schuckit, M.A. & Schuckit, J.J. (1989) Substance use and abuse: A risk factor in youth suicide. In: *Report of the Secretary's Task Force on Youth Suicide* (Vol. 2). Risk factors for youth suicide (eds L. Davidson & M. Linnoila). DHHS Pub No. (ADM) 89-1622. US Government Printing Office, Washington, DC.

Shaffer, D. (1988) The epidemiology of teen suicide: An examination of risk factors. *Journal of Clinical Psychiatry*, **49**(9, Suppl.), 36–41.

Shneidman, E. (1969) *On the Nature of Suicide*. Jossey-Bass, San Francisco.

Skopek, M. (1997) Carbon monoxide poisoning: Management implementations. *Australian and New Zealand Journal of Psychiatry*. (In press.)

Stack, S., Gundlach, J. & Reeves, J. (1994) The heavy metal subculture and suicide. *Suicide and Life-Threatening Behavior*, **24**(1), 15–23.

Topol, P. & Reznikoff, M. (1982) Perceived peer and family relationships, hopelessness, and locus of control as factors in adolescent suicide attempts. *Suicide and Life-Threatening Behaviour*, **12**, 141–50.

Tousignant, M., Bastien, M.F. & Hamel, S. (1993) Suicidal attempts and ideations among adolescents and young adults: The role of father's and mother's care of parental separation. *Social Psychiatry and Psychiatric Epidemiology*, **28**(5), 256–61.

UNICEF (1996) *The Progress of Nations, 1996*. United Nations International Children's Emergency Fund, New York.

UNICEF (1993) *The Progress of Nations*. United Nations International Children's Emergency Fund, New York.

13 Forensic Psychiatric Nursing

Tom Mason and *Dave Mercer*

Introduction

Forensic nursing has now emerged as a specialist professional territory throughout the psychiatrised world. An ongoing expansion in its field of operations, in parallel with the trend to medicalise criminality, increasingly embroils nursing staff in the dual systems of mental health and criminal justice. A growing body of literature testifies to the search for a *professional identity*, yet ironically this has typically been at the expense of *professional practice*. In the contemporary health-care marketplace, characterised by performance indicators, outcome measures and evidence-based interventions, the forensic enterprise has survived on anecdote and assumption. To ask why this should be so, or ask how it might be remedied, are the concerns of this chapter. We will suggest that forensic nursing is best understood, in postmodern terminology, as a *discursive practice*; that the apparent contradictions of clinical care and political control are a textually interwoven domain.

The first part of this chapter (*Theoretical Foundations*) charts the historical development of, and inextricable linkage between, *knowledge* and *power* in constructing a version of forensic *truth*. This is the dominant discourse of science, of psychiatry, psychology and criminology; an *objective reality* which powerfully defines the reality of the *objects* of its attention. Despite the diversity of settings in which forensic nurses now work, from maximum security institutions to community based initiatives, the role remains an adjunct of medicalised deviance. Fundamental contradictions, crystallised in nineteenth century medico-legal developments, belie the sophistry of present day practice. The 'dangerous individual' is now enshrined as a central tenet of forensic behavioural science and its allied professional disciplines. The critical analysis presented here suggests that therapeutic claims on the 'soul' of the offender–patient entangle the health care *agent* in a larger web of societal policing and public hygiene.

Derived from the above theoretical foundations, the second part of the chapter (*Practice Issues*) focuses on the subjective experience of caring for the mentally disordered offender and, more recently, the survivors of violence and abuse. It explores the tensions which, inevitably, underscore the nurse–patient relationship in custodial forensic environments; indeterminate sentencing, compulsory detention, and enforced treatment. This set of power relations, it is argued, have outlasted institutional reform and radical restructuring of service delivery. Genuine advances in clinical practice will depend upon critical research and political awareness which questions the assumed neutrality of therapeutic language. In the interactional sphere of nurse and patient another set of discourses can be heard, if one chooses to listen. From the roof-top protest to the therapeutic dialogue, recipients of forensic services enact resistance as a form of em*pow-er*ment. The forensic nursing profession, in critically addressing its role and function, must reverse the adage that silence is golden.

THEORETICAL FOUNDATIONS

Medicalisation

The relationship between the law and psychiatry is nowhere more sharply focused than in the branch of mental health known as 'forensic'. Although riven with tensions this association is embedded in the discursive practice of both professions, legal and psychiatric, by the conjoining of the two states of criminality and mental disorder. Whether it be the terminological structuring of 'criminal behaviour and mental health' or 'mental abnormality and offending behaviour' matters little. It is the fact that the legal and psychiatric are linked together which produces an affiliation in both lay and scientific, and popular and professional, language. Furthermore, this coupling of clearly delineated social states, criminality and madness, suggests, *a priori*, a causal relationship between the two. Although never clearly established in empirical terms the association enjoys a popularised credence, witnessed in film, fiction and the media. Notwithstanding, this correlational perspective belies a historical, and contemporary, claim on the criminal which has raged for centuries.

From a classical position offending behaviour belonged to the domain of the law, whether the perpetrators were mad, bad, or both; punishment for the transgression reflected a rational calculus of social harm and deterrence, irrespective of mental state considerations (Young, 1981). Compassion, a periodic gift in some cases, was a sparse commodity amid the profusion of penance and retribution, and unrelated to the *treatment* of offenders in the sense of penological modernism (Garland, 1990). The European reformist movement of Pinel and Tuke had little impact on mentally disordered offenders, and legislation ostensibly borne out of public and professional concerns merely reflected competitive conflicts between the legal and psychiatric spheres. Not until the mid-nineteenth century was the criminal, as object and subject, embraced by psychiatry; a professional colonisation paralleled by a new technology of disciplinary control, which focused upon the criminal rather than the crime. The contemporary dilemma of punishing the body, or treating the mind, echoes the rehabilitative moral therapy of the carceral society (Mercer & Mason, 1998).

In a seminal paper, Foucault (1978) argued that the concept of the 'dangerous individual' emerged in nineteenth century legal psychiatry as a result of psychiatric testimony being heard, and more importantly, taken notice of, in certain criminal cases across Europe between the years of 1800 and 1835. It was not that the alienists of an inchoate psychiatry had not previously given evidence in courts, as on the contrary their judgements regarding insanity were regularly reported; it was the fact that in these unusual cases they were taken seriously. The six cases representing Foucault's analysis are deemed to share common features that converge to allow psychiatry to envelop them. They constructed a picture of insanity very different to what had hitherto constituted an understanding of madness; they were all very serious crimes usually accompanied by cruel or bizarre events, they were offences committed against nature, against the 'heart', against familial relationships and across generations, and finally they were committed without reason.

Thus, psychiatry laid claim to a knowledge of these crimes that no-one else could fathom. The reasons that underpinned these heinous acts were beyond the judiciary, the jurors and the public, but psychiatry professed to comprehend their rationale. Insanity, when raised as an issue in relation to penal law usually involved imbecility or furor, the afflicted person being considered as obviously mentally impaired or 'raving mad'. These cases, argued Foucault, lacked the visibility of either, and psychiatry of the time created a condition to account for their lack of passion or reason. This new category was called *homicidal monomania*, being 'a derangement which would have no symptoms other than the crime itself, and which could disappear once the crime had been committed' (Foucault, 1978, p. 5). Later discounted as fictional, *homicidal monomania* convinced the magistrates of the time of the expertise of psychiatrists and the scientificity of their work. In so doing, criminal psychiatry, as a mode of *public hygiene* penetrated not only the judicial arena of the courtroom but the larger societal body; a professional territory that symbolised a field of knowledge, a modality of power and a technology of discipline (Foucault, 1978).

Thus, for almost 200 years, the crime and the criminal have been melded into one conjoint figure – the mentally disordered offender. Furthermore, the manner of this accomplishment alluded to a focus upon a supposed relationship between mental disorder and criminal behaviour. The expansion of forensic psychiatry, predicated upon this affiliation, wrested 'danger' from the domain of public and social space with the promise of the therapeutic 'gaze'; that through the application of the science of psychiatry it could be measured, managed and manipulated by the medical enterprise. Forever navigating and mapping out the uncharted regions of human behaviour, forensic psychiatry is a paradoxical venture; the success of its involvement rarely equalling the success of its evolvement (Bursztajn, *et al.*, 1994). For some, these disappointments reside in unrealistic expectations and the need for a reinterpretation of scientific knowledge:

'Increasingly, as the field keeps pace with post-modern scientific understanding, competence assessment is becoming highly focused and differentiated, identifying impairments of specific capacities and functions that result from mental illness and traumatic experience'.

(Bursztajn, *et al.*, 1994, p. 612)

Others, with some wit, might conjecture that the current and future directions of forensic practice are as fictional as its past.

This medicalisation, or psychiatrisation, of the criminal is routinely comprehended through a processural mechanic rather than an understanding of structural content. The medicalisation process relates to the manner in which the target group, the criminally insane, are brought under the authority of psychiatry. For this to be achieved it must induce a conviction of expertise. To take an example from general medicine, something is observed as being abnormal, or different in some way, and then categorised as similar to other disease types. The aetiology of this abnormality is then explored and established, concluding in a diagnosis of some description. Following this, there is likely to be an application of therapy, an intervention, some administration of treatment. Finally, a prediction would be made concerning the likely outcome of the disorder. This process can be illustrated in the following way:

Identification = classification = diagnosis = treatment = prognosis

Seen in terms of the mentally disordered offender, we can discern the process by which medicalisation is accomplished in relation to deviant behaviour. An abnormality is identified, which can be cloaked in the irrationality of the crime, its lust, its fervour, its horror; or obscured in the criminal, in his madness, his callousness, his silence. This 'oddness' is classified according to an ever expanding nosology of disorder, giving the illusion that sophisticated categorisation equates with *knowing* a disease. Once indexed, forensic interventions can be applied and predictions made as to the relapse and recidivism of such offenders. We can see from the structure of this process that although forensic psychiatry is able to satisfy the first three stages of this process, identification, classification and diagnosis, it struggles to fulfil the expectations of the latter two, treatment and prognosis. Or, perhaps given the amount of false positives and false negatives, forensic psychiatry does not know what it is doing as much when it gets things right as it does when it gets things wrong. Therefore, we conclude that it is more about process than content.

Defining forensic nursing

It was the medical model of the nineteenth century asylum which framed the emergence of mental health nursing. Instruction and education for nurses, in this era, was circumscribed by an intellectual climate of positivism, directed at a scientific understanding, prediction and control of pathology: 'Trained nurses enhanced medical credibility, but did not progress the care of the mentally ill because their training did not imply or encourage a questioning of the positivistic basis of psychiatric treatment'

(Chung & Nolan, 1994, p. 226). In relation to the forensic field it has been suggested that somatic theories about mental illness, incorporated within a broader doctrine of degeneracy, had political as well as clinical significance. As sick offenders were spared the gallows, and removed from prisons, psychiatry enacted a regime of social control which was masked by the pretext of objectivity and scientific status:

> 'The doctor became accustomed in the first instance to relating crime to mental illness and, subsequently, to an anatomical lesion, thereby increasing the standing and social influence of the medical profession in general and of psychiatrists in particular'.

> (Huertas & Martinez-Perez, 1993, p. 461)

Similarly, in the USA, the origins of legislative provision for disordered offenders was embroiled in conflicting definitions of mental disease, and a distinction between the 'insane criminal' and the 'criminally insane' (Quen, 1994). These early antagonisms, expressed in neurological and psychological discourse, find a contemporary variant in the controversy surrounding psychopathic disorder as a treatable condition (Blackburn, 1993).

The *archaeology of ideas* is more than an historical excursion into the roots of professional practice. In a Foucauldian sense, the 'past' becomes a medium for understanding the 'present'; both how things *are*, and how they might *otherwise* be (McHoul & Grace, 1995). The detrimental effects of the medical 'gaze' for those labelled mentally ill, and for mental health nursing, have been noted as '... the power to focus on to a subject a body of knowledge so that the subject is no more than the sum of that knowledge' (Ashmore & Ramsamy, 1993, p. 46). Madness is reduced to the signs and symptoms of the *clinic*, a denial and devaluation of the temporal and spatial contexts of individual experience. The language of the clinic does not simply *describe*; through the application of dominant knowledges, it *constructs* the recipients of its gaze. For forensic nurses, the Foucauldian thesis offers a rich discursive terrain:

> 'It also enters into his investigations of those forms of knowledge which are much less official, such as the knowledges which medical and psychiatric patients, criminals and sexual perverts, for example, have of themselves'.

> (McHoul & Grace, 1995, p. 4)

Critical analyses of the asylum and the prison (Foucault, 1973, 1977; Ignatieff, 1978) disentangle the knowledge-power equation that framed forensic practice, and witnessed the evolution of a transcarceral system (Menzies, 1987).

An international perspective on the concept of forensic nursing reveals a multiplicity of role functions and responsibilities within a diverse range of practice settings. While the emergence of this ill-defined discipline resides in the commonality of medicalised criminality, current developments indicate, both, global expansion and increasing specialisation; focused upon the response to societal violence in a climate of litigation (Scales, *et al.,*

1993). Nursing staff in accident and emergency departments, casualty, and crisis centres are increasingly faced with the challenge of caring for the victims of violent and abusive behaviour. A parallel trend has seen the growing use of mental health legislation to process and manage offenders, with nurses playing a key role in assessment, pre-trial evaluation, diversion from criminal justice, and therapeutic intervention. Nursing staff may be institutionally located, or dispersed within a network of community based units and agencies; contractually demarcated by the patronage of mental health or criminal justice/corrections systems (Peternelj-Taylor & Johnson, 1995). Yet, regardless of this diversity, the demands of clinical practice are unified around a shared set of legal, ethical, political, administrative and professional concerns (Scales, *et al.*, 1993).

If forensic nursing has long been associated with the, carceral, care and treatment of the 'criminally insane', the application of bio-technical advances in forensic science has radically redefined professional territories; with a distinction between 'living' and 'dead' forensic patients (Lynch, 1993). Thus, in the USA the recognition of forensic nursing as a discrete discipline has been attributed to a formal address (Lynch, 1986) at the American Academy of Forensic Science (AAFS) concerned with the nursing function in death investigation (Standing Bear, 1995). The bio-medical underpinning of nurse education, it is suggested, ideally equips health care staff to undertake investigative duties that were formerly the province of law-enforcement officers; from the collection of forensic evidence at the scene of crime, to the medico-legal management of both survivors and perpetrators. This professional convergence of a humanistic nursing philosophy and forensic science (Lynch, 1993) is idealised as a sensitive and empathic response to societal problems; maintaining the integrity of two independent roles, counselling and criminalistics. Not without irony, it appears that a new role dilemma is emerging to rival the *therapeutic custody* debate. Thus, it has been noted that the co-optation of a professional ethic into the conservative, macho, and prosecution orientated sub-culture of police work 'threatens to rob forensic nursing of its very soul' (Standing Bear, 1995).

The scope of forensic nursing practice

The difficulty for forensic mental health workers is the tripartite structure that needs to be addressed in any risk assessment of mentally disordered offenders; an arrangement involving the offender, the professional, and the victim. In other words, it engrosses complex considerations of the nature of, both, the crime and the mental disorder, the character of the forensic work being undertaken, and the necessity of protecting the public. In general psychiatry, where a patient is not considered a danger to others, the main concern is a compromise between the patient and the professional. One can act in the best interests of the patient while operating ethical professional practice given that the patient wishes to engage psychiatry and volunteers his or her acquiescence. However, when a third party is entrenched in the equation the focus of decision-making is more complex and bristles with ethical difficulties. When a person is a danger to another, no matter how rational or irrational this may be, there is a drive to protect the third party by detaining the patient against their will. Thus, the hospitalisation is as much for the benefit of the public as it is for the patient. Again, a subtle nuance reveals itself here, in that, the law does not generally make allowance for prisoners to be detained indefinitely for reasons of their being considered dangerous. Yet, mental health legislation, generally, does. Within this perplexing cauldron the forensic mental health nurse operates, and we now ask what is the nature of this work?

There appear to be subtle differences, at an international level, as to the main focus of forensic work which is dependent upon the emphasis on the tripartite pattern illustrated above. Part of forensic work entails addressing the psychopathology of the patient, either alone or within the family setting, and this has two main motivations. First, there are those who consider that the person's mental state is the focus of attention and not the criminal activity, while secondly, there are others who argue that by dealing with the mental disorder the criminality is resolved. This latter point, of course, assumes a relationship between crime and mental disorder. There are other forensic mental health workers who believe that the main area of mediation should entail offence specific work. By this it is usually meant that the nature of the crime should be the focus of therapeutic intervention. The antecedents to the violation should be known and understood by both the patient and the therapist, the motivations of the crime should be explored, and the consequences of the act should be comprehended. Offence work also involves a focus on the integrity of others, the values of society, and personal empathy towards the suffering of victims. Another dimension to the work of forensic mental health professionals involves work with the victims themselves, in which survivors are supported and helped to overcome the traumas of their ordeal.

A global assault on the asylum system, as the precursor to enlightened mental health provision generally, has re-shaped the structural framework, both locus and focus, of forensic practice. In the UK, for example, social policy (DoH/HO, 1992) has linked the disposal of mentally disordered offenders to a community care model within a larger lexicon of empowerment, citizenship and human rights. If the implementation of Charter standards (DoH, 1992) and consumerist philosophies into high security settings has been problematised (McKeown & Mercer, 1995), the equation is no less challenging within the contemporary climate of de-institutionalisation. Indeed, the relationship between social care and social control, fused in the construction of forensic practice, becomes evermore invisible and invidious (Schrag, 1980). As the technology of surveillance, rather than the technology of containment, comes to define the nursing role there is a need for practitioners to understand the nature and operation of power within the societal body politic (Foucault, 1988). Forensic nurses are now deployed in police stations, prisons, law courts and diversion schemes, where the community represents a site of professional convergence and therapeutic surveillance (Mason & Mercer, 1996).

It is these political tensions which complicate the concept of client advocacy in relation to the forensic nurse–patient relationship (Burrow, 1991). Yet, the *ideal* of an advocacy role illustrates the wide ranging, and dualised, dimensions of (post) modern forensic nursing practice; from the re-humanisation of the asylum, rehabilitation and reintegration of offender–patients into the community on one hand; to the prosecution of perpetrators and the legal/therapeutic support of their victims on the other. In this sense, Coram (1993) delineates 'physiologically orientated forensic' and 'psychiatric forensic' nursing; for each the nurse–patient relationship is premised on criminal action, the distinction residing in the status of the client as, respectively, victim or perpetrator. As violence and criminal behaviour are drawn into the mental health system, forensic nurses find themselves situated on a continuum; from the scene of the crime to the sentencing outcome, and beyond. Examples would include the collection and recording of genetic evidence such as blood, tissue, or semen (Hoyt & Spangler, 1996); forensic photo-documentation of trauma wounds and injuries like bruising or bite marks (Pasqualone, 1996); sexual assault examination, postvention suicide work and grief/bereavement counselling (Lynch, 1993).

Psychiatric forensic nursing in the USA is, largely, concerned with pre-trial evaluation and assessment of clinical and legal sanity; to establish diminished capacity, or offer therapy to regain competency for the courtroom. By contrast, correctional forensic nursing is seen as providing for the physical health care needs of convicted, incarcerated, criminal populations (Coram, 1993). Outside of the criminal law, forensic responsibilities are defined even more widely in terms of the legal nurse consultant. Here the application of clinical expertise is applied to civil cases, with registered nurses acting as independent consultants for attorneys in areas of overlap between the law and medicine; such typically embrace medical malpractice, product liability, personal injury, workers compensation and probate (Wetther, 1993).

PRACTICE ISSUES

Ethics

The mad versus bad debate is an old and extremely well rehearsed one. In medical and legal terms it centres on the extent to which a person is considered *compos mentis* (of sound mind) and thus responsible for their actions (McCall-Smith, 1987). For a person to be guilty, in law, there must be evidence that they are *actus reus* (guilty by act) and *mens rea* (guilty in mind). The assessment of this is based on rational thought which can be defined as thought endowed with reason in which conclusions are drawn from premises. However, immediately we see problems with this.

The divided debate

Dangerous individuals, as aberrant members of the societal body, have been dealt with differently over time and between cultures. Whether explication is sought in professional expertise, or lay notions of evil, it is the search for explanation that makes the criminally insane vulnerable to the insertion of medical power. This causal quest lies at the heart of what is considered *reason* in our society, and directly determines what is understood as *justice*. Although justice is a particularly difficult concept to define it is commonly thought of in two ways: 'justice as "fairness" and justice as "appropriate punishment for wrongdoing"' (Seedhouse, 1986, p. 109); each of value in relation to the mentally disordered offender. If a person is seen as non-reasoning they are not held responsible for their actions. Conversely, if a person is considered to have reasoned thought they are deemed to be responsible for their behaviour; in the former, they are perceived as mad, and in the latter as bad. In both explanations the next stage is a question of justice. This forms the dividing point in the polarised debate.

Societal mechanisms exist to confine the bad to imprisonment and the mad to treatment. However, when both are conjoined, through the criminal offence, the mentally disordered offender is dually sentenced. Too often, the treatment ethic is used as a piece of professional chicanery in order to confuse and confound the fact that the treatment *is* the punishment and that the confinement *is* the imprisonment. Just as the mad and the bad are rolled into one in the form of the mentally disordered offender, the treatment becomes the punishment in the form of incarceration. At a practical level we can see this operationalised in the shifting trends between a treatment focus and a secure philosophy (Neilson, 1992).

Consent, competence and confidentiality

Within a system of compulsory detention and enforced psychiatric treatment, the general ethical principles of consent, competence and confidentiality are clearly compromised. To speak of consent within forced detention is to severely limit it to minor inconsequential matters, given the structural overriding of autonomy derived from a legislative framework and a physical confinement. This imbalance of power (Sines, 1993) inevitably safeguards the greatest number but at the forfeit of the few; a utilitarian and paternalistic system. In contrast to this, other moralists have offered counter ethical propositions to account for such confinement. These would include an emphasis on individualism in which the patient is foremost; a beneficent and non-maleficent approach aimed to 'relieve a patient's suffering'; and an idealistic philosophy in which the patient's dangerousness receives scientific attention through the application of medicine. This belief in the curative force of psychiatry lies at the heart of the rationalisation of compulsory detention for forced treatment.

Forced treatment is also of central concern in the issue of competence. It is not so much a problem of what constitutes reasoned and rational thought, but more to do with the mechanisms of overriding the principle of autonomy for compulsory psychiatric intervention. Society has invested powers in psychiatric workers to decide when a person is considered unreasonable and irrational, and to convert this assessment into an evaluation of dangerousness. This, then justifies compulsory confinement and the use of psychiatry in creating compliance (Holm, 1993). The assessment of competence relies upon the subjective interpretation from one value system onto another's. This is merely a question of power in which the micro politics of the body (and mind) become the economy of psychiatry (Foucault, 1988). Assessing competence means to be judgemental, paternalistic and idealistic.

Confidentiality, again, is a concept which is grossly mutated within a system of compulsory detention. It usually refers to professional workers respecting and keeping the 'secrets' of the patient and is: 'one of the most venerable moral obligations of medical ethics' (Gillon, 1985, p. 106). While such represents a core professional responsibility, there will be times in forensic practice when those boundaries are not so clearly defined. For example, if a compulsorily detained psychiatric patient informed a member of staff of violent sexual fantasies, with the risk of these being acted out, nursing staff would need to balance confidentiality with the safety of others. A failure to act on this information would invert the moral and constitute unethical behaviour.

However, confidentiality in the compulsory detention of dangerous individuals is mutated further. Part of the role of the forensic psychiatric mental health worker is to gather information on the patient's mental state in relation to the assessment of dangerousness. This involves investigation of fantasy structures, attitudes to potential victims, levels of remorse, abilities to understand consequences to behaviours emitted, etc. This exploration involves a search for 'clues' to offending behaviours, which once identified are reported, recorded, and presented as evidence to justify continued incarceration; an 'ambivalent logic' in which utopian intentions are fused with totalitarian consequences on the basis of a psychiatric identification (Owen, 1991). Therefore, any information which the patient offers, from casual conversation to therapeutic exchange, is a re-affirmation of past detention and a justification for future detention. This is a breach of the principle of confidentiality no matter how justified. Little wonder that confidentiality has been called a 'decrepit concept' (Siegler, 1982).

Advocacy, negotiation and empowerment

Within the concept of compulsorily detaining patients for forced treatment the notions of advocacy, negotiation and empowerment appear absurd; unless these are adopted from the perspective of an intermediary who is attempting to act on behalf of the patient *against* the system of captivity. Advocacy, in its truest sense, can only be undertaken by those who are external to the system of control (Brandon, 1991). Mental health workers within the organisation of compulsory detention can only advocate for the patient from a biased position as an agent of that control. This is not to devalue the feelings of sympathy and empathy that many mental health workers express pertaining to the lot of the compulsorily detained, but merely to highlight that the task of the true advocate from within the system is an impossible one. One can do one's best but it cannot be true advocacy as there is a clear conflict of interests.

Negotiated care is a popular term. Unfortunately, again, it is extremely limited within compulsory detention. It can only take place with reference to the micro politics of everyday living in which the captive client can gain minor benefits as a trade-off for compliance (Berman & Segal, 1982). Major negotiation regarding treatment and discharge operates above and beyond the patient level. Behavioural bartering occurs at the patient interface only around trivial decisions, giving a pretence that the patient has the power, and right by charter, to be involved in negotiated care delivery. This is similar to the ideal of empowerment in which patients are given the illusion that they have the puissance to affect major decisions regarding their captive career but in reality can only adjust the minor aspects of their lives within detention (McDougall, 1997).

Advocacy, negotiation and empowerment give the impression that the patient has some degree of autonomy, can act on free will, and self-determine personal events. Forensic services, based upon the views of 'users', have begun to consider ways of reversing a tradition of insularity and task orientated custodial containment; in-service training, the involvement of patients in staff selection and education, partnership and collaboration (Russell & Kettles, 1996). However, such initiatives will remain a naive fantasy unless the centrality of power differentials is recognised: 'The manner in which service users perceive and refer to their bodies is controlled by the concepts, theories and symbols that have been supplied by health care professionals' (Morrall, 1996). As the communication of professional discourses, and the technology of security, become ever more sophisticated the voices of the marginalised are lost in cyberspace.

Therapeutic custody

For institutionally based forensic nurses throughout the psychiatrised world, *therapeutic custody* is a debate rehearsed to the point of stagnation. It is, typically, presented as the hallmark characteristic of a profession charged with managing the delicate equation between health needs and security demands; with nursing staff cast in the 'unenviable hybrid' role of carer and custodian (Burrow, 1993a). This binary opposition, rooted in history, remains an important issue for clinical practitioners, yet the axiomatic exclusivity of the dominant discourses precludes alternative accounts. Thus, in attempting to unravel the social reality of forensic nursing, it can be suggested that the *text* of a theory-practice gap is eclipsed by the *texturing* of a discursive-practice.

At one level we clearly see the dichotomous roles involved in those whose task is caring for the mentally ill in secure psychiatric establishments and in those whose job is to maintain that security. In some forensic settings these two roles are performed independently by two sets of staff, i.e. nurses and security aides (Bernier, 1986). In this system there are clear boundaries between the two groups with nursing staff avoiding the entanglement of control and discipline and the security staff eluding the complication of care and compassion. However, this system is not without its problems as tensions and conflicts can occur between carers and custodians who both feel that their function takes precedence. The distance between the two groups can be considerable (Maier, 1986). In another approach the two roles are the responsibility of one group of staff, i.e. nurses. This puts great onus on the ability of nursing staff to function in each set of behavioural repertoires and an implicit expectation that patients can respond to therapeutic encounters with staff who manage security and the control of aggression. The fact that a custodian can be compassionate, and a nurse a disciplinarian, is not disputed as quite clearly these functions exist in most people. However, what is not clear, and has received little debate, is the extent to which it is the custody itself which is therapeutic, or alternatively it is the therapy which is custodial.

Workers in the forensic field are supposed to vacillate between therapy and custody (Burrow, 1993b) while, in reality, the activity is more akin to a form of societal policing under the guise of nursing (Mason & Chandley, 1990). In Britain these dual roles are incorporated into one person in the form of the forensic psychiatric nurse. What is important in these presumed dichotomous functions is that no such boundaries exist, they are, in fact, one and the same thing. This is how society can construct the management of dangerousness; through the medicalisation of punishment, legitimated by a mental health act, by compulsory detention for treatment, and through the ransom of professional explanation, they become medical hostages (Mason & Jennings, 1997).

Rehabilitation

As mentioned earlier, it is the latter two stages of the medical model that forensic psychiatry appears to have most difficulty in fulfilling; the application of therapeutic interventions and the assessment of prognosis. These aspects fall neatly into the notion of the rehabilitation of the mentally disordered offender. However, there are two further dimensions to this debate that need to be considered; the extent to which therapeutic interventions are, in fact, applied, and how effective they are when implemented.

Assessing the issue of *what* therapeutic interventions are utilised is analogous to negotiating the edge of an abyss that dissects the professional territory of forensic health care. The sentiments of this chapter reflect personal involvement with three fundamental ingredients of progressive practice; a review of the literature, research findings, and clinical experience. Published material on therapeutic work with mentally disordered offenders is sparse indeed; the majority is provided by colleagues in psychology and psychiatry, with a much smaller contribution from psychiatric nurses. That which is reported in the literature mainly concerns short-term research studies, and ranges from drug trials to more esoteric therapeutic engagements. However, this is not the important point. The portentous concern is that there is much less evidence that this, albeit growing body of discourse, translates into the clinical arena. Without doubt, innovative individuals and groups have attempted to apply into practice some meaningful interventions, but sadly this mainly involves the goodwill of staff, professional motivation, and a concern for the patients in their care. In real terms, overall strategies are, typically, disjointed, lack a cohesive policy, and fail to encompass an appropriate outcome evaluation. A heavy reliance upon medication, and the abstruse milieu therapy, is no longer convincing; yet, neither is the retort of outraged conservatives reciting a 'menu' of 'goodies' from the contents page of the latest psychiatric textbook. Therapies there may well be, their application in the forensic field is spartan.

A few optimistic sources, generally referred to as the 'what works' debate, suggest that some therapies may offer a degree of success. Developing techniques in interviewing, counselling, support, information sharing, trust formation, and group-leadership skills, indicates how a systematic approach might contribute significantly to the health careers of mentally disordered offenders (Priestly & McGuire, 1983). Ross, Fabiano and Ewles (1988), for example, over many years have developed a Reasoning and Rehabilitation Program which claims a markedly significant reduction in recidivism for this group of offenders. More focused work on specific personality traits has reported some success, for example, McDougall, *et al.* (1987) using cognitive-behavioural techniques, or Carson (1979) applying cognitive-interpersonal methods. These latter approaches have more recently been embraced within the nascent enterprise of forensic psychotherapy (Cordess & Cox, 1996).

A distinction also needs to be drawn between *treatment*, as a specific corrective technology, and the broader philosophical ideal of *rehabilitation*. If a semantic confusion surrounds the use of these terms at a conceptual level, it is manifestly experienced at a clinical level; and most acutely, perhaps, by nursing staff. Advanced practice in secure settings, alongside mainstream psychiatry, has embraced a plethora of 'psycho-therapeutic' modalities. From offence-specific group work to individual counselling sessions, *talk* rather than *tablets* signifies the catalyst of both personal change and institutional reform. *Intervention* has replaced *treatment* as the defining dynamic of a client–therapist relationship; mentally disordered offenders accepting responsibility for their behaviours, and practitioners facilitating growth rather than administering cures. A critique of the language that proclaims these trends as progressive needs to decode the discourses which construct the text: 'Discourses provide frameworks for debating the value of one way of talking about reality over other ways' (Parker, 1992, p. 5).

The insertion of 'talking therapies', as discursive strands, into forensic environments can be problematised at a series of levels in relation to practice. At a structural level concerns about the emergence of a therapeutic state have been well documented in the last three decades (Conrad & Schneider, 1980). The incorporation of behaviours such as child abuse and sexual violence into a model of pathological deviance are frequently cited examples of de-politicised criminality as the territory of experts (Dobash & Dobash, 1992); of social issues translated into individual problems in a web of mystification and myth (Hillman & Ventura, 1992). At an organisational level, it has been noted how the ethical underpinnings of a therapeutic relationship are compromised by the spatial and temporal dynamic of the *captive client* (Berman & Segal, 1982; Pilgrim, 1988). In this sense forensic practice, of which nursing is one component, cannot be divorced from institutional culture, power relations and ideology. If the historical development of dominant discourses have constrained and controlled those to whom they refer, *resistance* (Foucault, 1980), as an inversion of the therapeutic gaze, offers a more genuine mode of empowerment.

Two examples of discourse analysis from a forensic practice setting can be used to, briefly, illustrate how the narrative exchanges of patients and staff contribute to understanding and change; in this way a philosophical position, and methodological approach, can shape care delivery.

(1) Interventive work with sexual offenders
Relapse prevention programs, as an interventive technique with sexual offenders (Laws, 1989), are now a well established initiative in the penal system, secure hospitals, and community forensic services. The move, influenced by feminist scholarship, away from conceptualising rape as individual sickness allows a confrontation of societal and institutional sexism (Brownmiller, 1975; Wyre, 1993). Nursing staff who act as group facilitators, sharing the 'sexual stories' (Plummer, 1995) and 'hate speech' of rapists (Kellett, 1995), have an opportunity to deconstruct discourses which reinforce offender identities and gendered inequality. This must entail a critical exploration of the occupational culture within which any offence-focused work takes place. Challenges can be directed at, for instance, strategies of collusion, the diminished role and status of female staff, or the consumption of pornographic materials and negative representations of women (Mercer & McKeown, 1997).

(2) Women as objects of knowledge and power
In stark contrast to the male perpetrators discussed above, women who find their way into the forensic services are often the victims and survivors of sexual abuse and violence (Potier, 1993). Disrupted lives, low self-esteem, and a common experience of being disbelieved and disempowered, is typically exacerbated by the conditions of their detention (Adshead & Morris, 1995). Following savage criticism of the treatment of female patients in the British Special Hospital System (HMSO, 1992), the

construction of more appropriate services was placed high on the political and professional agendas (SHSA,1995). At the same time, though, there needs to be a critical appraisal of the discourses which underpin institutional care; to shift resources without shifting knowledges is a redundant exercise (McKeown & Mercer, 1998). A textual archaeology of dominant knowledges reveals the psychiatrisation of female offenders as a complex interaction between discursive structures and patriarchal power (Allen, 1987). Nowhere is the experience of a language which *silences* more acutely felt than in the context of individual and group work at ward level. Again, it is the narrative voices of women, so often unheard or dismissed, that hint at points of resistance to the power relations which construct and constrain their lives.

Ethnographic studies of ward cultures in forensic hospitals offer a rich insight into the power relations within which practitioners operate, with enormous implications for treatment and rehabilitation (Richman, 1989). The discourse dynamics of staff and patients evidence tension, dissent and conflict; where the notion of 'therapy' as 'an undifferentiated moral essence' is one part of the professional rhetoric of medical and nursing staff (Richman, 1998).

Risk assessment

There are few areas of health care in which the issue of a 'third party' is of such paramount importance as it is in the forensic mental health arena. The tripartite relationship between professional, patient and victim is further complicated by wider public debate relating to the victims' right to justice, and the publics' right to protection. For forensic psychiatry to be considered an effective mode of mental health care it must demonstrate its worth by eliminating, or at least reducing, the likelihood of recidivism. If the criminal justice system is not considered appropriate, and incarceration alone is deemed unacceptable, then the notion of a dynamic progression through a mental health career, via a process of treatment intervention, brings into stark relief the issue of risk.

Risk is a term that has its etymological roots in sixteenth century civil law relating to insurance (Foucault, 1978). However, in this era the concept of risk dealt mainly with individual dangers on a one-to-one basis without the addition of third party involvement. With increased industrialisation there came third party risks incurred by, for example, employers and transport companies who exposed others to work-related accidents. This was linked to a form or error, but a minor error such as inattention, negligence, or lack of precautions; established through a chain of cause and effect rather than attempts to establish fault. This ushered in the notion of no-fault liability. Parallel to the physical and medical risks of early urban life, 'dangerousness' assumed an epidemic status to which 19th century legal psychiatry responded (Foucault, 1978).

Contemporary forensic psychiatry is concerned with, both, risk assessment and risk management, which is underscored by the clinical prediction of dangerousness (Prins, 1996). Although the individual assessments undertaken for the prediction of such risks are too numerous to mention here, we can briefly outline what has become known as the first and second generations of dangerousness assessments (Monahan, 1984). The 'first generation' refers, in the main, to the number of outcome studies of released mentally disordered offenders from varying institutions. Known, collectively, as the follow-up studies they show that the majority of those released did not go on to re-offend. In particular, there are the 'Baxstrom' studies which were based on a group of 969 released offenders by order of a United States Supreme Court who deemed one such patient, Johnny Baxstrom, as being illegally detained. This legal ruling triggered a series of released offender patients and further outcome research (Steadman & Keveles, 1972). Although these studies have a number of flaws they began to sow doubt as to the mental health professionals' ability to accurately predict dangerousness. The 'second generation' of research aimed to establish a more predictive accuracy of assessments through attention to issues of validity and reliability. However, the research demonstrated that the notion of dangerousness was an increasingly complex one and not readily accessible to research efforts. In conclusion, it seems that 'predictive accuracy remains to be demonstrated even in the short term...' (Blackburn, 1993, p. 332).

Inquiries

Mistakes, malpractice and mistreatment occur in all forms of health care environments. However, they have a certain added poignancy when those patients receiving care are doing so against their wishes and reside in the setting against their will. Vulnerable groups, such as the elderly, children and the mentally impaired, by dint of their inability to speak out, or be heard, call for careful monitoring of systematic, institutional or individual abuse. Similarly, mentally disordered offenders in a variety of forensic mental health locations are vulnerable to misuse. In some settings the system inhibits their speaking out against mistreatment, with complaints dismissed as symptomatic of their disordered thinking (HMSO, 1992). There is often a disparaging feeling amongst some forensic care workers that the offenders deserve what they get in retribution for their crimes; patients may well be coerced into silence out of a fear of continuing incarceration should they become known as 'trouble-makers'. Furthermore, it is often difficult to separate out in the forensic mental health worker the socialisation of the public person from the value system of a professional identity.

Operating at the interface between professional codes and social influences is the media, reflecting the values of the social group that it represents. For the media to do this it must observe society very carefully and, to paraphrase a philosophical author on the issue, it achieves this in the following way: 'you don't only read the newspapers, the newspapers read you, and you don't only watch the television the television watches you'

(Baudrillard, 1987). It is for this reason that the media can produce contrasting headlines referring to the same patient population, the mentally disordered offender, linking into a perceived differing value system merely reflecting what society wishes to hear. Two recent examples, from British tabloids, would include 'Slack Security Let Crazed Rapist Flee Rampton' (*The Sun*, 1994) and 'Storm Over Bid To Free Sex Killer' (*Daily Mail*, 1985). At other times the same newspapers are happy to publish headlines which champion the 'poor unfortunates' brutalised by nurses. Such vacillation exhibits a changing perception regarding the nature of madness and badness, a confusing area which often leads to the situations that inquiries are built upon.

Inquiry reports feature large in many institutions that hold people against their will, for whatever reason, and include prisons, psychiatric hospitals, forensic units, children's homes, and a spectrum of secure settings. The main focus of such inquiry reports pertain to:

(1) escapes, with or without the escapee engaging in harm to others
(2) deaths of detainees while in institutional care, either suicidal, homicidal or by maltreatment
(3) allegations of mistreatment or poor conditions
(4) riots, with or without injury and destruction, and
(5) patients officially released who go on to cause harm to others.

Here, we will restrict ourselves specifically to the forensic environments in which the number of official inquiry reports are growing steadily.

It should not be surprising that people who are compulsorily detained, or forced to undergo treatment that they otherwise would not wish to receive, should attempt to escape. Nor should it come as a revelation that the same group of offenders engage in strategies of non-compliance such as roof-top incidents, dirty protests, and resorting to silence. Moreover, some degree of empathy on our part should appreciate the depths of despair that incarcerated patients feel; either through insight into their offending behaviour, or a contemplation of their apparent bleak futures which sometimes precipitates suicide. However, what is difficult to come to terms with is the human suffering caused by the forensic institution itself, where processes, a lack of resources, or the workforce contribute to the deaths of patients in custody.

In a series of British inquiries into forensic establishments common threads emerge. The Boynton Report (Rampton) (HMSO, 1979) highlighted organisational abuse through systems of patient treatment that became culturally legitimated, and accepted practice, in the management of violence and aggression. Extended too far, the application of control through intimidation, brutality and fear, embroiled many staff in allegations of mistreatment. The Inquiry into Complaints about Ashworth Hospital (HMSO, 1992) investigated many charges of abuse including sexual misconduct, brutality and the death of a patient in seclusion. This report ushered in sweeping reforms at the high security forensic hospital; managerial reorganisations, and the employment of a number of external staff were used to create a groundswell of culture change. Unfortunately, these measures appear to have been less than effective as, at the time of writing, Ashworth Hospital is undergoing yet another inquiry (by Judge Fallon) following allegations of the establishment of a paedophile ring, by inpatients, who were served by visitors bringing in children (Rose, 1997). Broadmoor Hospital was rocked by a series of investigations following deaths of three patients in seclusion over a number of years. All three patients were Afrocarribean which led to serious charges of racism. Each of the reports subsequently identified systems of poor practice relating to patient care and the lack of a caring attitude from the organisation.

In Australia a series of inquiries into allegations of unsafe, unethical and unlawful practices in Ward 10B of the Townsville General Hospital Psychiatric Unit spanned the years between 1986 to 1991. They were first initiated by a politician who maintained systematic political pressure over this extended period to investigate the practice of psychiatry at that unit. An unauthorised release of clinical and confidential documentation to the media ensured that professional bodies were under public scrutiny to act against individuals involved. Through a political and media campaign suicides and child abuse, deaths and injuries, soared in the local town. The name of Ward 10B evoked terror in patients destined to be admitted. The main psychiatrist concerned in the allegations was to write a book entitled *Ward 10B: The Deadly Witch-Hunt*, in which he argued that the politician concerned fuelled the allegations through the media coverage (Lindsay, 1992).

These public inquiries show clearly the powerful relationship between political concern, media coverage, public awareness and professional consequences. The emergent theme, in all these reports, is the subjugation of the patient to organisational objectives aimed at the management and control aberrant behaviour in its most extreme forms. Sadly, in the absence of effective treatment approaches, research or education, those who are charged with the responsibility for maintaining order appear at a loss to effect this function without recourse to abuse.

Multidisciplinary team working

Multidisciplinary team working lies at the heart of forensic mental health care, possibly more so than in any other branch of professional practice. On the face of it multidisciplinary collaboration has many advantages; it affords a number of professions to debate issues relating to patient care, it pools together areas of knowledge and expertise, it expands the breadth of interpretations relating to the patients' mental state or behaviour, and it shares decision-making, responsibility, and risk. In an otherwise rigidly structured hierarchy of professional class divisions the multidisciplinary team concept epitomises an equitable fraternity of multi-professions operating in a democratic framework. As individuals they each have strengths and weaknesses, but as a team those strengths are compounded and the weaknesses minimised. The main difficulty that usually arises involves the operationalising of the multidisciplinary team concept. Professional boundaries and occupational differences are often contested territories which, in this budding branch of health care, are fiercely defended.

However, there may well be other factors at play in the multidisciplinary forensic team which have more practical ramifications (Burrow, 1994). The inchoate nature of the forensic psychiatric profession is such that those two main areas of practice, which suggest a sphere of expertise, are found wanting; that is, the efficacious application of interventions and the accuracy of prognosis. Entwined within these are issues relating to the assessment of dangerousness, risk management, non-compliance, resistance to treatment, and third party risk. The multidisciplinary team offers some protection against public outcry, professional enquiry and litigation in the event of disputation. Although the sharing of responsibility provides some degree of security against litigation it should be remembered that in British Law the Responsible Medical Officer is ultimately accountable for patient care, including nursing care. The area of forensic mental health care is an area of professional practice with few rewards as the majority of patients are detained against their wishes. The family and friends of patients are often antagonistic to the organisational staff; victims, and their relatives, may understandably feel that the perpetrator has 'got off lightly' and be hostile to the idea of a treatment disposal rather than a punitive one. Coupled to the issues of compulsory detention and forced treatment this makes for a sensitive area in relation to human rights and abuse, providing a rich ground for the litigious. Multidisciplinary team working offers some defence to this.

Community

The expansion of services for forensic patients has now taken us full circle with the development of community provision; the community being that very place in which the mentally disordered offenders execute their crimes, become socially stigmatised, and from which they are excluded via hospitalisation or incarceration (Mason & Mercer, 1998). Now, with the fragmentation of the asylum, and the drive to community care, the mentally disordered offender is returned, once again, to the society whose values, and laws, they have transgressed. However, the community service developments share a common theme; that of an increased technology of psychiatric surveillance through varying degrees of supervision. There are a growing number of court diversion and court liaison schemes whereby those offenders considered to be suffering from some form of psychiatric disorder or learning difficulty can be diverted from the criminal justice system to the mental health system (Hillis, 1993; Kitchener, 1996). There is the location of psychiatric nurses in police stations and prisons which is now regarded as a growth industry, at least in Britain (Backer-Holst, 1994). There is also an expansion of professional development in terms of forensic probation officers, social workers and community psychiatric nurses who work in a wide range of settings from out-patient clinics and daycare centres to residential hostels and private forensic services (Vaughan & Badger, 1995).

Within this expansion of community services there are two broad areas which we would wish to outline. The first refers to Case Management, which has become an internationally popular term in a relatively short period of time (Bergen, 1992). Case Management is concerned with maintaining mentally ill persons in the community at the initial point of contact and can be broken down into various approaches. First, the service brokerage model in which the mental health professional attempts to organise the most appropriate services for the offender; second, the social entrepreneurship approach which involves a close collaboration with the offender and his needs; and third, the extended co-ordinator model which involves expanding the role of the professional (Beardshaw & Towell, 1990). Case Management is usually depicted in stages which, typically, include:

- Case identification
- Assessment
- Need analysis
- Service design
- Implementation
- Monitoring
- Evaluation
- Re-assessment

Forensic Case Management carries specific problems relating to the types of offending behaviours, increased liability in the event of relapse/recidivism, and extended responsibilities that fall outside the usual clinical-therapist relationship.

The second area is concerned with assertive and passive outreach which involves the marrying of patients' needs to community service provision. While in the former (assertive outreach) it involves ensuring the maximum provision in a more determined manner by actively following-up and tracking-down patients who fail to attend for appointments, in the latter (passive outreach) the professional is more likely to wait for the patient to turn-up or to anticipate developments in a deteriorating situation without actively intervening. Forensic outreach, because of the potentially dire consequences of relapse and recidivism tends to be assertive in nature.

Conclusion

Forensic mental health care is a relatively new branch of psychiatric practice which is still in the throes of attempting to stand as an independent sphere of expertise. Its early conceptualisation was founded on the creation of a fictional diagnostic category, homicidal monomania, which was used to convince others of a supposed proficiency by the psychiatric fraternity. Two hundred years later we see contemporary forensic psychiatry engaged in a similar chicanery in which the main thrust of psychiatric activity is concerned with the elaborate production of a mythical enterprise. This endeavour, typically, relies on convincing others of a forensic expertise by evading the thorny issues of forensic practice. In this chapter we have sought to address this deficit by illuminating the theoretical foundation and exploring the practical issues. By doing so we hope to have drawn the theory and practice together, to some degree, and to have given ourselves an anchorage point for future development. As we turn to the next century forensic mental health practice may well evolve into a scientific discipline. However, before this can occur we will need to undergo a painful process of casting off; we will need to explode the myths, shed the fantasies, and discard the forensic fiction.

References

Adshead, G. & Morris, F. (1995) Another Time, Another Place. *Health Service Journal.* 9 February 24–6.

Aiken, F. & Tarbuck, P. (1995) Practical, Ethical and Legal Aspects of Caring for the Assaultive Client. (In Press.)

Allen, H. (1987) *Justice Unbalanced: Gender, Psychiatry and Judicial Decisions.* Open University Press, Milton Keynes.

Ashmore, R. & Ramsamy, S. (1993) The Concept of the 'Gaze' in Mental Health Nursing. *Senior Nurse,* **13** (1), 46–9.

Backer-Holst, T. (1994) A New Window of Opportunity: The Implications of the Reed Report for Psychiatric Care. *Psychiatric Care.* March/April, 15–18.

Baudrillard, J. (1987) *The Evil Demon of Images.* Power Institute of Fine Arts, Sydney.

Beardshaw, V. & Towell, D. (1990) Assessment and Case Management: Implications for the Implementation of 'Caring for People'. *King's Fund Institute Briefing Paper 10.* King's Fund, London.

Berman, E. & Segal, R. (1982) The Captive Client. *Psychotherapy, Research and Practice.* **19,** 31–6.

Bernier, S.L. (1986) Corrections and Mental Health. *Journal of Psychosocial Nursing,* **24** (6), 20–25.

Blackburn, R. (1993) *The Psychology of Criminal Conduct: Theory, Research and Practice.* John Wiley and Sons, Chichester.

Brandon, D. (1991) Listen to the Real Experts. *Nursing Times,* **87,** (49), 33.

Brennan, A. (1989) Clinician's Conundrum ... Informed Consent Among Mentally Ill Patients. *Nursing Times,* **85** (20), 48–9.

Brownmiller, S. (1975) *Against Our Will: Men, Women and Rape.* Simon and Schuster, New York.

Burrow, S. (1991) The Special Hospital Nurse and the Dilemma of Therapeutic Custody. *Journal of Advances in Health and Nursing Care,* **1** (3), 21–38.

Burrow, S. (1993a) The Treatment and Security Needs of Special Hospital Patients: A Nursing Perspective. *Journal of Advanced Nursing,* **18** (8), 1267–78.

Burrow, S. (1993b) The Role Conflict of the Forensic Nurse. *Senior Nurse,* **13**(5), 20–25.

Burrow, S. (1994) A Source of Conflict at the Heart of the Team: The Role of the Forensic Multidisciplinary Care Team. *Psychiatric Care,* **1**(5), 192–6.

Bursztajn, H., Scherr, A. & Brodsky, A. (1994) The Rebirth of Forensic Psychiatry in Light of Recent Historical Trends in Criminal Responsibility. *Psychiatric Clinics of North America,* **17** (3), 611–35.

Carson, R.C. (1979) Personality and Exchange in Developing Relationships. In: *Social Exchange in Developing Relationships* (eds R. Burgess & T. Huston). Academic Press, New York.

Chung, M. & Nolan, P. (1994) The Influence of Positivistic Thought on Nineteenth Century Asylum Nursing. *Journal of Advanced Nursing*, **19**(2), 226–32.

Conrad, P. & Schneider, J. (1980) *Deviance and Medicalisation: From Badness to Sickness*. C.V. Mosby, London.

Coram, J. (1993) Forensic Nurse Specialists: Working With Perpetrators and Hostage Negotiation Teams. *Journal of Psychosocial Nursing*, **31** (11), 26–30.

Cordess, C. & Cox, M. (1996) *Forensic Psychotherapy: Crime, Psychodynamics and the Offender Patient*, Vols 1 and 2. Jessica Kingsley, London.

Department of Health (1992) *The Patient's Charter*. HMSO, London.

Department of Health/Home Office (1992) *Review of Health and Social Services for Mentally Disordered Offenders and Others Requiring Similar Services*. HMSO, London.

Dobash, R. & Dobash, R. (1992) *Women, Violence and Social Change*. Routledge, London.

Foucault, M. (1973) *The Birth of the Clinic: An Archaeology of Medical Perception*. Tavistock, London.

Foucault, M. (1977) *Discipline and Punish: The Birth of the Prison*. Penguin, London.

Foucault, M. (1978) About the Concept of the 'Dangerous Individual' in 19th Century Legal Psychiatry. *International Journal of Law and Psychiatry*, **1** (1), 1–18.

Foucault, M. (1980) *The History of Sexuality: An Introduction*. Vintage, New York.

Foucault, M. (1988) *Power/Knowledge: Selected Interviews and Other Writings, 1972–1977*. Harvester Press, London.

Garland, D. (1990) *Punishment and Modern Society: A Study in Social Theory*. Clarendon Press, Oxford.

Gillon, R. (1985) *Philosophical Medical Ethics*. John Wiley & Sons, Chichester.

Hillis, G. (1993) Diverting Tactics. *Nursing Times*, **89**(1), 24–7.

Hillman, J. & Ventura, M. (1992) *We've had a Hundred Years of Psychotherapy – and the World's Getting Worse*. Harper, San Francisco.

HMSO (1979) The Boynton Report (Rampton). HMSO, London.

HMSO (1992) *Report of the Committee of Inquiry into Complaints about Ashworth Hospital*, Vols 1 and 2. HMSO, London.

Holm, S. (1993) What is Wrong with Compliance? *Journal of Medical Ethics*, **19**, 108–10.

Hoyt, C. & Spangler, K. (1996) Forensic Nursing Implications and the Forensic Autopsy. *Journal of Psychosocial Nursing*, **34** (10), 24–31.

Huertas, R. & Martinez-Perez, J. (1993) Disease and Crime in Spanish Positivist Psychiatry. *History of Psychiatry*, **4** (16), 459–81.

Ignatieff, M. (1978) *A Just Measure of Pain: The Penitentiary in the Industrial Revolution, 1750–1850*. Columbia University Press, New York.

Kellett, P. (1995) Acts of Power, Control and Resistance: Narrative Accounts of Convicted Rapists. In: *Hate Speech* (eds R. Whilcock & D. Slayden). Sage, London.

Kitchener, N. (1996) Forensic Community Mental Health Nurses and Court Diversion Schemes. *Psychiatric Care*, **3**(2), 65–9.

Laws, R. (1989) *Relapse Prevention with Sexual Offenders*. Guilford Press, New York.

Lindsay, J. (1992) *Ward 10B: The Deadly Witch-Hunt*. Wileman Publications, Queensland.

Lynch, V. (1993) Forensic Nursing: Diversity in Education and Practice. *Journal of Psychosocial Nursing*, **31** (11), 7–14.

Maier, G. (1986) Relationship Security: The Dynamics of Keepers and Kept. *Journal of Forensic Sciences*, **31** (2), 603–608.

Mason, T. & Chandley, M. (1990) Nursing Models in a Special Hospital: A Critical Analysis of Efficacy. *Journal of Advanced Nursing*, **15**, 667–73.

Mason, T. & Mercer, D. (1988) *Critical Perspectives in Forensic Care: Inside Out.* Macmillan, London.

Mason, T. & Mercer, D. (1996) Forensic Psychiatric Nursing: Visions of Social Control. *Australian and New Zealand Journal of Mental Health Nursing*, **5** (4), 153–62.

Mason, T. & Jennings, L. (1997) The Mental Health Act and Professional Hostage Taking. *Journal of Medicine, Science and the Law*, **37** (1), 1–10.

McCall-Smith, A. (1987) Commentary: Exoneration of the Mentally Ill. *Journal of Medical Ethics*, **13**, 201–208.

McDougall, T. (1997) Patient Empowerment: Fact or Fiction? *Mental Health Nursing*, **17** (1): 4–5.

McHoul, A. & Grace, W. (1995) *A Foucault Primer: Discourse, Power and the Subject.* UCL Press, London.

McKeown, M. & Mercer, D. (1995) Is a Written Charter Really the Answer? Human Rights in Secure Mental Health Settings. *Psychiatric Care*, **1** (6). 219–23.

McKeown, M. & Mercer, D. (1998) Fallen From Grace: Women, Power and Knowledge. In: *Critical Perspectives in Forensic Care: Inside Out* (eds T. Mason & D. Mercer). Macmillan, London.

Menzies, R. (1987) Cycles of Control: The Transcarceral Careers of Forensic Patients. *International Journal of Law and Psychiatry*, **19** (3), 233–49.

Mercer, D. & McKeown, M. (1997) Pornography: Some Implications for Nursing. *Health Care Analysis*, **5** (1), 56–61.

Mercer, D. & Mason, T. (1998) From Devilry to Diagnosis: The Painful Birth of Forensic Psychiatry. In: *Critical Perspectives in Forensic Care: Inside-Out* (eds T. Mason & D. Mercer). Macmillan, London.

Monahan, J. (1984) The Prediction of Violent Behaviour: Toward a Second Generation of Theory and Policy. *American Journal of Psychiatry*, **141**(1), 10–15.

Morrall, P. (1996) Clinical Sociology and the Empowerment of Clients. *Mental Health Nursing*, **16**(3), 24–7.

Neilson, P. (1992) A Secure Philosophy. *Nursing Times*, **88**, 31–3.

Owen, D. (1991) Foucault, Psychiatry and the Spectre of Dangerousness. *Journal of Forensic Psychiatry*, **2**(3), 238–41.

Parker, I. (1992) *Discourse Dynamics: Critical Analysis for Social and Individual Psychology.* Routledge, London.

Pasqualone, G. (1996) Forensic RNs as Photographers: Documentation in the ED. *Journal of Psychosocial Nursing*, **34** (10), 47–51.

Peternelj-Taylor, C. & Johnson, R. (1995) Serving Time: Psychiatric Mental Health Nursing in Corrections. *Journal of Psychosocial Nursing*, **33**(3), 12–19.

Pilgrim, D. (1988) Psychotherapy in British Special Hospitals: A Case of Failure to Thrive. *Free Associations*, **7**, 11–26.

Plummer, K. (1995) *Telling Sexual Stories: Power, Change and Social Worlds.* Routledge, London.

Potier, M. (1993) Giving Evidence: Women's Lives in Ashworth Maximum Security Psychiatric Hospital. *Feminism and Psychology*, **3** (3), 335–47.

Priestly, P. & McGuire, J. (1983) *Learning to Help: Basic Skills Exercises.* Tavistock, London.

Prins, H. (1996) Risk Assessment and Management in Criminal Justice and Psychiatry. *Journal of Forensic Psychiatry*, **7**(1), 42–62.

Quen, J. (1994) Law and Psychiatry in America Over the Past 150 Years. *Hospital and Community Psychiatry*, **45** (10), 1005–10.

Richman, J. (1989) *Psychiatric Ward Cultures Revisited: Implications for Treatment Regimes*. Paper presented to the British Sociological Society Annual Conference.

Richman, J. (1998) The Ceremonial and Moral Order of a Ward for Psychopaths. In: *Critical Perspectives in Forensic Care: Inside Out* (eds T. Mason & D. Mercer). Macmillan, London.

Rose, D. (1997) Child Sex Probe at Ashworth. *Daily Post*, February, 8, 1.

Ross, R.R., Fabiano, E.A. & Ewles, C.D. (1988) Reasoning and Rehabilitation. *International Journal of Offender Therapy and Comparative Criminology*, **32** (1), 29–35.

Russell, J. & Kettles, A. (1996) User Views of a Forensic Service. *Psychiatric Care*, **3** (3), 98–104.

Scales, C., Mitchell, J. & Smith, R. (1993) Survey Report on Forensic Nursing. *Journal of Psychosocial Nursing*, **31** (11), 39–44.

Schrag, P. (1980) *Mind Control*. Marion Boyars, London.

Seedhouse, D. (1986) *Health: The Foundations for Achievement*. John Wiley & Sons, Chichester.

SHSA (1995) *Service Strategies for Secure Care*. SHSA, London.

Siegler, M. (1982) Confidentiality in Medicine: A Decrepit Concept. *New England Journal of Medicine*, **307**, 1518–21.

Sines, D. (1993) Balance of Power. *Nursing Times*, **89**, 52–5.

Standing Bear, Z. (1995) Forensic Nursing and Death Investigation: Will the Vision be Co-Opted? *Journal of Psychosocial Nursing*, **33** (9), 59–64.

Steadman, H.J. & Keveles, G. (1972) The Community Adjustment and Criminal Activity of the Baxstrom Patients: 1966-1970. *American Journal of Psychiatry*, **129**, 304–10.

Vaughan, P.J. & Badger, D. (1995) *Working with the Mentally Disordered Offender in the Community*. Chapman and Hall, London.

Wetther, K. (1993) Forensic Responsibilities of the Legal Nurse Consultant. *Journal of Psychosocial Nursing*, **31** (11), 21–5.

Wyre, R. (1993) Pornography and Sexual Violence: Working with Sex Offenders. In: *Pornography: Women, Violence and Civil Liberties* (ed. C. Itzin). Oxford University Press, Oxford.

Young, J. (1981) Thinking Seriously about Crime: Some Models of Criminology. In: *Crime and Society: Readings in History and Theory* (eds M. Fitzgerald, G. McLennan & P. Pawson). Routledge and Kegan Paul, London.

14 Recovery, Mental Illness and Mental Health Nursing

Michael Clinton and *Sioban Nelson*

Introduction

What is recovery from mental illness? Is it a return to premorbid functioning or just feeling well? Should it be understood as 'in remission' or as 'absence of disorder'? Has the patient really recovered or was the diagnosis incorrect in the first place? In this chapter we consider these questions. We turn our focus to the notion of recovery, examine its historical variants and highlight the porosity of mental health nursing practice to the shifting discursive structurings of mental illness. The argument is staged that understandings of recovery delimit the therapeutic encounter and frame mental health nursing practice. This mental health nursing practice is argued to represent a complex and multiple, as opposed to unitary, social form. We argue against notions of an evolutionary development of mental health nursing practice and propose a layered and contingent structuring of practice.

Let us take schizophrenia as our example. Over the past ten years, it seems, recovery from schizophrenia has been the subject of consideration by the American Psychiatric Association (APA). The DSM-IIIR noted that: 'Full remissions do occur, but their frequency is currently a subject of controversy' (APA, 1987, p. 191). Moreover, the APA concedes a shift from 'in remission' to 'recovery' with great caution:

> 'Differentiating Schizophrenia in Remission from No Mental Disorder requires consideration of overall level of functioning, length of time since the last episode of disturbance, total duration of the disturbance, and whether prophylactic treatment is being given'.
>
> (1987, p. 195)

Eight years later the APA was of somewhat firmer, and more sceptical, opinion:

> 'Complete remission (i.e.: a return to premorbid functioning) is probably not common in this disorder'.
>
> (1995, p. 282)

Nonetheless, the case for recovery, it seems was convincing enough to introduce a *new* course specifier: 'single episode in full remission'. According to APA (1995) then, there does exist a subset of patients with schizophrenia who fall ill once, for long enough to satisfy diagnostic criteria, and then appear to recover.

Thus a tiny window of opportunity presents itself within the prognostic realm of possibility for persons with a diagnosis of schizophrenia – some patients get better. This modest concession is worthy of reflection. What has occurred within the authoritative discourse that governs the medical model of mental illness to affect such a development? How do such changes relate to treatment, and, by consequence, nursing care?

To answer this question it is necessary to look at the notion of recovery, and the unstable place it has held in conceptualisations of mental illness. As we will see, in the nineteenth century during the time of 'moral treatment', recovery resulted in the transformation of the lunatic into the useful Christian citizen. In the various strains of talking therapies (from Freud to R.D. Laing) recovery involved a deep psychic resolution, a moment of truth that freed the subject from pain and disorder. Later, the notion of recovery began to disappear altogether as the biological model came to dominate diagnosis and treatment. The mentally ill person became the victim, the intersecting point of genetic, biochemical and (perhaps) social stressors, treatment focused upon neutralising manifestations of the disease process. The 1990s find the person with a diagnosis of mental illness less happy to be the victim of circumstances and more inclined to find recovery in the personal growth and empowerment movement. In what follows we will describe in detail both the history of these discursive framings of mental illness and their impact on nursing therapeutics.

Therapy and power

These questions open a discussion about therapeutic certainty, therapeutic authority and power. In examining these questions we will consider the insights of Michel Foucault (1991, p. 102) on government and power. Foucault described government as the:

'... ensemble formed by the institutions, procedures, analyses and reflections, the calculations and tactics that allow the exercise of this very specific albeit complex form of power, which has at its target the population.'

In his work on governmentality Foucault provided a framework and a vocabulary with which to examine power as the 'action on the action of others' (Miller & Rose, 1994, p. 35). Foucault suggested:

'... that successful government of others depends, in the first instance, on the capacity of those doing the government to govern themselves. As for the governed, to the extent that it avoids the extremes of domination, their government must aim to affect their conduct – that is, it must operate through their capacity to regulate their own behaviour. In this respect too, successful government of others is often thought to depend upon the ability of those others to govern themselves, and must therefore aim to secure the conditions under which they are enabled to do so.

(Hindess, 1996, p.105)

It is this idea of power as something that can occur remotely, as opposed to directly and obviously, that connects our discussion of therapeutics and power. In this chapter the concept of recovery and its place within the treatment models – moral treatment, illness model, antipsychiatry model, empowerment/autonomy model – will be historicised. Nursing's relationship to these models – the history of practice in relation to dominant discourses will be subjected to analysis. Of consistent interest to this discussion will be the interrelationship between power and knowledge and the relationship between nursing practice and this power/knowledge axis.

People suffering from mental illness have long been subject to analysis by psychiatrists, psychologists, historians, sociologists, political economists and philosophers. (Indeed, Foucault in *Madness and Civilization* (1967) made a major contribution to the antipsychiatry movement, particularly in Europe. Foucault was concerned with the role of the madman and the constitution of the other, historicising lunacy and the asylum movement in those terms.) For mental illness, perhaps more than any other disorder, can be and is interpreted through a grid of normative, economic and social imperatives. The logic that binds lunacy to demonic possession or moral depravity or social disadvantage can only be understood by reference to the dominant interpretive models and discursive frameworks of the time. In the light of these observations, this chapter seeks to attempt to understand the (re)emergence of one element in mental health discourse: the element of recovery.

Historicising the notion of recovery may help explain its tentative elevation to the bounds of the possible in the prognosis for schizophrenia. The idea of recovery, we will argue, is not as self-evident as it may appear. Recovery has come to mean quite different things at different times. For a time, it seems, it even disappeared altogether. The return of recovery for those diagnosed with schizophrenia illustrates our argument that recovery can only exist within a discursive framework that allows for the release of the subject from therapeutic authority. But the issues in our discussion are far broader than our example of schizophrenia and gain little from adherence to diagnostic criteria which are themselves products of a particular history and discursive structuring. In fact, an exploration of the idea of recovery provides us with a powerful device to use as an indicae of the relationship between knowledge and power, of the role of agency and of the emergence of the recovered, self-regulating subject.

The self-regulating subject can be understood through an analysis of the power and knowledge nexus through which it is constituted – the discursive space through which practices and knowledges define the subject and constitute the subject as self-defining. Discourse in this context is taken to mean the means by which it is possible to say something about a subject or person. It is this that enables one to speak of 'medicine' or even 'society' as single intelligible entities. Discourse defines the realm of possibility and it is a contingent and complex force, both constituting and dependent upon historical, social and political framings. It is the connection between discourse and practice that was of particular interest to Foucault. According to him:

> '...the target of analysis wasn't institutions, theories or ideology, but practices – with the aim of grasping the conditions which make these acceptable at a given moment; the hypothesis being that these types of practice are not just governed by institutions, prescribed by ideologies, guided by pragmatic circumstances – whatever the role these elements actually play – but possess up to a point their own specific regularities, logic, strategy, self-evidence and "reason". It is a question of analysing a "regime of practices" – practice being understood as places where what is said and what is being done, rules imposed and reasons given, the planned and the taken for granted meet and interconnect.'
>
> (Foucault, 1991, p. 75)

In relation to recovery the notion of discourse allows for discussion of the constituting factors within the various forces that have shaped mental health, and with them the idea of recovery. The power of discourse as a disciplinary force, is one which forms part of the complex of government.

> 'In addition to acting directly on individual behaviour, it [government] thus aims to affect behaviour indirectly by acting on the manner in which individuals regulate their own behaviour. In this respect, too, government involves an element of calculation – and a knowledge of its extended object – that is not necessarily present in every exercise of power.'
>
> (Hindess, 1996, p. 106)

The regulation of behaviour, no less than the regulation of the behaviour of others, is here seen to be dependent upon the knowledge of the subject. This idea of the subject as the object of calculation brings in the idea that rather than the subject representing an individual will with freely chosen choices of self-regulation, there is a disciplinary power at play, the object of which is the subject. It was Foucault's intention to explore in this work on government and discipline the constitution of the humanist subject:

> '...that is, the conception of the human individual as endowed with a soul, consciousness, guilt, remorse, and other features of an interiority that can be worked on by other agents. This humanist subject came to be seen as the locus of usable energy and, therefore, as the focus of instrumental control: the focus, in other words, of discipline...'
>
> (Hindess, 1996, p. 115)

It is through the notion of recovery that the government, rather than control or management, of the subject can find exemplary expression. For rather than the moral therapeutics of the nineteenth century or the brutal reworkings of the premodern period, mental illness by the late twentieth century has become reconstituted as a problem of government and the nurse's prime role that of assisting the patient to self-regulation.

Discourses on recovery

In this section discourses on recovery are considered against the background of psychiatry as the dominant discipline influencing mental health nursing practice. The examples are presented in chronological order. This is not intended to imply that notions of recovery have evolved from one another, nor that the latter notions have surpassed earlier ones. Neither is it to suggest that shifts in emphasis have worked only in the direction of progress. Every change in mental health practice has brought unforeseen problems that are still to be resolved. The statistic that five out of every ten people with schizophrenia in the United States are living in a boarding house or nursing home, or are in hospital, homeless or in jail (Warner, 1994, p.191) makes the point.

In the first of the following sub-sections, it will be shown that 'recovery' was inexplicable in the absence of a standardised approach to psychiatric diagnosis and treatment. In the next sub-section it will be shown how concerns about the integrity of the self and human freedom became issues as the discipline of psychiatry came under challenge from both sides of the Atlantic. It will be argued that these concerns led on to the more contemporary notion of recovery as a process for reconstituting the self.

With the rise of modern psychiatry there was a return to conceptualising mental illness as a personal affliction amenable to treatment, as opposed to a demoniacal affliction (Whitwell, 1936, p.133). The return of this ancient notion of madness as an 'affliction' amenable to treatment was accompanied by early attempts to define a science of psychiatry based on medicine and gave rise to the need to explain why some patients recovered while others did not. If medicine was a science, it should have been possible to predict who would recover and to generalise predictions to categories of patients. However, success in treatment was piece meal and belied explanation.

In 1888, Dr Strahan, Assistant Medical Officer at the Northampton County Asylum in England, published an article on four 'cases' of recovery. It is clear from his account that recovery in his terms equated to a decline in symptomatology and the ability to return to roles outside the asylum. But his account is not only of interest because of what it implies about what recovery was taken to be at the time, but also because it emphasises that recovery was a rare event:

> 'They [the records of patients who recover] are rarely of any practical value. They are, nevertheless, always cheering ... They occasionally light up in [the] mind [of the asylum medical officer] a ray of hope, and stimulate him to still further efforts in the treatment of any of his chronic cases who may show even the slightest tendency toward recovery. But, unhappily, in the great majority of cases his [sic] best efforts are of little avail, and his patient remains with him until Death ...'

> (Strahan, 1888, p. 1)

Of even more interest is the possible explanation for 'cases' of recovery implied by Strahan. On noticing that three of the four 'cases' he was about to describe were associated with the patients being transferred from another asylum, he ingeniously posed questions that enabled him to point to a possible explanation without inviting the scorn of his colleagues:

> 'Had, then, the change in residence had any share in bringing about the happy result? . . . the unexpected peep into the long-forgotten world of reality, and the hurry and hubub of a railway journey – had all these coming suddenly and unexpectedly proved such a moral shock as to wake up the dreaming brain to healthier action?'

(Strahan, 1888, p. 1)

However, that all four cases were women alerted Dr Strahan to another explanation:

> 'We know that the climacteric [the menopause] with its many nervous troubles is a most fruitful source of mental disorder, and it is just possible that in the great change undergone in this period, which in the female, often amounts to a tearing down and rebuilding of the nervous system, the disordered brain, which has been incapable of healthy thought for years, may, like other organs, as the stomach, etc., quit abnormal and once more take on normal action.'

(Strahan, 1888, p. 3)

Strahan was encouraged in these thoughts by the knowledge that such luminaries as Bucknill and Tuke had said that the 'change of life' can exercise 'a beneficial influence on those already insane' (Strahan, 1888, p. 3). This is not to attribute to Strahan an attitude to 'lunacy' totally imbued with a physiological explanation of recovery. Rather it is to draw attention to both his difficulty in explaining recovery and his bias in favour of an ultimately physical, and therefore, 'scientific' explanation. However, his comments on the role of 'moral shock' in mediating between the train journey and its effect on the nervous system leaves open a role for social and psychological factors in triggering systemic change. Thus, the problem for Strahan was to explain the inexplicable in the absence of a convincing scientific framework.

Strahan's difficulty arose out of the lack of scientific evidence to support the claim that medical treatments had any beneficial effects (Chung & Nolan, 1994, p. 226) and the related problem of explaining recovery in the absence of such evidence. After all, he was writing 10 years before Krae-pelin became influential in the taxonomy of mental illness and 23 years before Bleuler asserted a more systematic, but still incomplete, description of schizophrenia. The German psychiatrist, Kraepelin was the first to describe the separate identity of *dementia praecox*, thus anticipating the later diagnosis of schizophrenia and bringing to an end the era of psychiatry which was dominated by the notion that madness consisted of one com-prehensive disorder manifesting in different forms. This view was replaced with the notion of discrete and distinct illnesses (Clare, 1976), a process well elucidated by Foucault in his study of the rise of modern medicine, *The Birth of the Clinic* (1973).

The Swiss psychiatrist, Bleuler later suggested that the term, *dementia praecox*, be replaced by that of schizophrenia to recognize the 'rending' or 'splitting' of the psychic functions that he took to be the outstanding feature of the disorder. Bleuler was also instrumental in exploring the life experiences as well as the symptomatology of people with one or other of the group of illnesses he was later to refer to as the schizophrenias (Clare, 1976). But at the time of Strahan's article (1888) positivist science had contributed little to the evolving practice of psychiatry and our understanding of mental disorder (Chung & Nolan 1994, p. 229). It was this absence of an effective science for the diagnosis and treatment of mental illness that was to have important consequences for the practice of mental health nursing, as will be demonstrated later in this chapter.

Recovery as treatment outcome

With the development of psychiatric taxonomies and the resultant consistent diagnostic systems certainty came to replace mystery. By the twentieth century the rare and quixotic view of recovery had been replaced by the notion of recovery as an outcome of effective treatment. Yet if the diagnosis and treatment of schizophrenia is taken as an example, twentieth-century literature on the effectiveness of psychiatry shows an interesting paradox: the greater precision in diagnosis and treatment led to less than impressive clinical outcomes. Substantial clinical improvement occurred in less than half the patients diagnosed and treated (at follow up averaging almost six years) (Hegarty, *et al.*, 1994, p. 1409). In the half century 1920–70, a favourable outcome in the treatment of people diagnosed with schizophrenia increased from an average of less than 25% to an average of a little over 50% (Hegarty, *et al.*, 1994, p. 1412). Such gains have been attributed by authors such as Hegarty, *et al.*, to the introduction of neuroleptic medication and an increased emphasis on family and community interventions (1994, p. 1412).

However, the recent trend in successful treatment outcomes is down to levels familiar prior to the 1950s due to stricter diagnostic criteria and changes in the provision of psychiatric services, including deinstitutionalisation. Furthermore, the view that neuroleptic medication has been successful in the treatment of schizophrenia has been challenged. Recovery rates for patients admitted since the advent of neuroleptics in Europe and North America are no better in the 1990s than for those admitted after World War II or during the first two decades of the century (Warner, 1994, p. 81). Furthermore, the rate of mental hospital bed occupancy as a proportion of the general United States population was already declining before the introduction of antipsychotic drugs (Warner, 1994, p. 100). Moreover, there is evidence that some people with schizophrenia would do better if they were not medicated and that the long term use of antipsychotic medication makes the underlying biochemical deficits of schizophrenia worse (Warner, 1994, p. 243). Thus, the second half of the twentieth century produced stricter diagnostic criteria, better controlled treatment methods and more specific clinical outcomes. And while the move to standardise these elements of mental health practice strengthened the scientific status of psychiatry, the outcomes were less spectacular than would have been hoped for by Strahan and his contemporaries.

Recovery as ontological security

Psychiatry has not only been undermined by the less than spectacular results that have been achieved in the treatment of serious mental illnesses such as schizophrenia, it has also been criticised from within. Laing (1960; 1964) was prominent among psychiatrists of his generation in the United Kingdom in calling into question the nature of mental illness and the practice of psychiatry. He did so by offering a radically different reading of what it means to be mentally ill and what it means to practise as a psychiatrist. One of the strongest features of the writing by Laing, was his ability to get inside the experience of people with a psychosis. According to him, what was lacking was a primary 'sense of ontological security', by which he meant that people experiencing psychosis lacked the personal resources to protect themselves from being treated as mere objects in the environments of others. Part of the insight of Laing was to understand what passes for psychotic illness as an existential crisis. He was also a critic of what he thought of as the impersonal social forces, including psychiatry, that fostered this irredeemable sense of alienation. The links Laing had with the counter culture, and his personal use of drugs, notably LSD, were enough for him to be dismissed as a crank by his fellow psychiatrists and others with more conservative views.

Recovery as freedom from deception and exploitation

Szasz (1960; 1973) was no less controversial than Laing in that he accused his fellow psychiatrists in the United States of manufacturing madness for their own ends. He made an important distinction between madness, a label conferred arbitrarily by psychiatrists in the pursuit of their own interests, and 'problems in daily living', the sorts of challenges that everyone experiences, but which are overwhelming for the more vulnerable. For Szasz any notion of recovery involves freedom from psychiatrists with their repressive forms of treatment and inclination to bestow labels that determine the fortunes of the stigmatised and oppressed. Unlike Laing, Szasz had no commitment to an explicit ontology to ground his critique of psychiatric practice. His arguments were couched more in terms of a critique of the values of modern psychiatry, and by implication the mores of the United States, in which one group of people, psychiatrists, can live by the deception and exploitation of another group of people, patients.

Central to such deception and exploitation is what Szasz regarded as two fundamental errors in thinking about mental illness as a fact. The first error is to confuse what happens in the physical structures and physiological processes of the brain with the mental experiences of the person. For example, to confuse deficits in neurological processes with beliefs that the person takes to be true, such as the belief that his or her insides are rotting (Szasz, 1973, p. 12). The second error consists in interpreting communications about people and the world, including statements about mental states, as symptoms of neurological functioning. According to Szasz (1973, p. 18) both errors lead psychiatrists to attribute the label 'mental illness' to people in the absence of any sense of the social and ethical context in which they make their attributions, and in ignorance of the part played by their own preferences and prejudices. What Szasz sought to emphasise was not that the problems psychiatrists label as 'mental illness' do not exist, but that they are categorised as diseases at our peril because in such classifications we mistake a metaphor for a fact (Szasz, 1973, p. 23).

Recovery as the reconstitution of the self

A more realistic assessment of what psychiatry can and cannot achieve, successive waves of deinstitutionalization and the rise of the consumer movement have led to a redefinition of the relationship between the mental health professional and the mental health 'consumer'. The notion of the mental health 'consumer' is important here because it signals a much needed change in status for those who use mental health services. Fundamental to this change is the notion of people with mental illness as partners in their own treatment and care (Palmer-Erbs, 1996; Palmer-Erbs & Manos, 1998). The challenge for them has become one of reconstituting an enduring sense of self which empowers them to take control of their lives (Davidson & Strauss, 1992, p. 131). Once achieved, the reconstituted self becomes both a refuge from the illness and a foundation for further recovery. A sense of self-efficacy and of a strong internal locus of control are particularly important in this regard (Davidson & Strauss, 1992, p. 132). Other characteristics of the reconstituted self include more tolerance of personal strengths and more determination to overcome the detrimental effects of mental illness (Davidson & Strauss, 1992, p. 134).

These intrapersonal aspects of recovery are complemented by literature that promotes self-care and skills development among people who have a mental illness. The methods of self-care advocated are generally regarded as coping efforts that complement rather than replace psychiatric treatment, however they are regarded also as a means of compensating for the limitations and adverse affects of medication:

> 'One of the most compelling arguments for [this] skills training rehabilitation model of chronic psychiatric disorders comes from the failure of antipsychotic drugs to remediate the negative symptoms of mental disorder (Schooler, 1986); the serious side effects of neuroleptics which often evoke noncompliance (Van Putten, 1974; Kane 1985); and the fact that medications by themselves cannot teach patients the coping skills they require for survival.'

> (Liberman, *et al.*, 1986, p. 631)

An emerging trend in this perspective is the encouragement that consumers have received to regulate their illness by paying closer attention to the onset of returning symptoms or an increase in their intensity (Hamera, *et al.*, 1991, p. 630). Family intervention programs have taken a similar educative role and have been found to be successful in fostering change in coping strategies both on the part of consumers and members of their families (Lee, *et al.*, 1993, p. 177). A key element in the success of such programs is an approach to treatment and rehabilitation that empowers consumers (Tobias, 1990, p. 357). Such perspectives on 'recovery' transform notions of disability and pessimism into resources for capability and hope (Kerser, 1994, p. 337). The outcomes in this way of understanding 'recovery' are not 'cure' and freedom from symptoms. Rather, the outcomes are those of a process of lifelong learning that enables the person to develop ego strength and positive identity structures to replace those of a victim of mental illness.

Notions of recovery

These ideas about 'recovery' and many others can be regarded as making claims about how and where change is accomplished in mental illness. A Foucauldean reading of them suggests that the notion of recovery has to be regarded as contested by forms of social practice. At the time Strahan (1888) was writing at the end of the nineteenth century, the progress of science was not seen to have proceeded far enough to account for the apparent recovery of four patients with chronic insanity. Writing more than a century later Hegarty et al. (1994) were able to show how the standardisation of methods of diagnosis and treatment outcomes have paradoxically raised the important issue of the relative ineffectiveness of psychiatry. The critiques by Laing (1960; 1964) and Szasz (1960; 1973) bring into question the assumptions made by Hegarty, *et al.* (1994) in that the two former thinkers posit forms of recovery that are outside orthodox psychiatry. For Laing, recovery is ontological security. For Szasz it is freedom from deception and exploitation. For Laing and Szasz, then, although each of these authors takes a throughly distinctive approach, recovery can be understood as a recovery of the self.

An important thrust of our analysis is to here draw attention to the practices of 'governmentality' that in this context can be understood to constitute the interiority of people with a mental illness as they work to reconstitute themselves (Davidson & Strauss, 1992). In its weak form the 'governmentality' argument of Foucault implies that in each age of mental health care there will be forms of practice that operate through social practices, such as the regime of the asylum, that encourage people with a mental illness to regulate their behaviour (see the earlier quotation from Hindess, 1996, p. 105.) However, the governmentality argument enables a stronger inference to be made. To the extent that self regulation has become the dominant form of social control involving people with a mental illness, it can be suggested that current practices of self-care and symptom control on the part of people with a mental illness are more effective methods of social control than those of the asylum and illness eras they have begun to replace. For by engaging in self-care, people with a mental illness not only seek to recover themselves, but also to regulate themselves and their behaviours in more deeply penetrating ways than was possible when psychiatric practice was at its most coercive. In this way it is possible to argue that the external controls of the asylum system have been replaced by more subtle practices in which the consumers of mental health services have become agents in their own control (Clinton, 1993). The implications of this analysis for mental health nursing practice will be taken up in the next section.

Discourses and mental health nursing practice

It is impossible to present a detailed analysis of the relationship between discourses on recovery and mental health nursing practice in a chapter of this length. A complete analysis would require detailed consideration of the social practices in which each element of the discourse described is embedded, as well as an exploration of the relationship between these practices and wider social formations. However, it is possible to indicate the forms of mental health nursing practice that are associated with the ways of speaking about recovery that have been described without implying a strict chronological ordering of their emergence and influence on mental health nursing practice. What follows is a loose summary of major themes in mental health nursing practice in the late nineteenth and twentieth centuries.

Practice as 'points of character'

The transition from the 'madhouse' to the asylum that was in progress when Strahan was writing in 1888 brought with it an intended change in practice that was signalled in the guidance given to the predecessors of mental health nurses, the asylum attendants. The very, term, 'asylum', itself, was chosen to replace the old term of 'madhouse' to signify, a *place of protection*.

The term 'patient' was also intended to signal a change in attitude, in that it was meant to indicate that the person formally known as a 'madman' or as a 'lunatic' was, in fact, ill and in need of treatment. That the attitudes associated with the former terminology were recognized as being difficult to change was reflected in the pains that were taken in the *Handbook for Attendants of the Insane* (Medico-Psychological Association, 1911) to stress that it is easy to forget that a person who is strong in bodily health is ill, when that person is 'causing plenty of trouble, apparently for no other reason than from a wish to cause trouble' (p. 315). Thus the first principle of the 'general nursing care of the insane' was to recollect to one's self that the purpose of the 'asylum' was to afford protection to the 'patient'. The second principle was to understand that the 'proper treatment' was important not only in the moral sense of protection from harm, but also in the sense of recognising that the chances of recovery were good if the patient was treated properly. Proper treatment in this context referred not to medical intervention, but to the avoidance of neglect and 'injudicious management'. However, in keeping with the views of Strahan, recovery was seen in many 'cases' to be but a 'small prospect' (Medico-Psychological Association, 1911, p. 315).

A major focus of practice in the 'asylum' was 'true medicine' of a moral nature, the advice and control essential to effective discipline. Indeed, the discipline and routine of the asylum were likened to the hygiene of an 'ordinary hospital'. The analogy was carried so far as to claim that excitement and disorder are to a 'patient' in an asylum what microbes are to a patient with wounds or sores (Medico-Psychological Association, 1911, p. 315). In the absence of effective clinical interventions, the attendants were encouraged to develop not technical skills in the sense that thera-peutic interventions would be understood today, but *moral qualifications* that would assist in maintaining good order and discipline. Primary among the moral qualifications required were the personal habits of morality, decency, sobriety and honesty. These 'points of character' were regarded as essential for advancement in the asylum system as they engendered the trust and respect of superiors. On these strong foundations were to be built the habits of endurance and cheerfulness that could cope with the 'dull routine' of asylum life and 'make the best of things' for attendants, fellow attendants and patients alike. Firmness of mind was important also because it was easier for the patients to 'respect and obey' the attendants who knew their own minds. No less important was self-control because an 'appeal to physical force' was 'not to be thought of for one moment', as the respected attendant needed to display the ability to 'withdraw from any wrangle from which an advantage could not be claimed' (Medico-Psychological Association, 1911, p. 319). At the same time practice was thought of primarily in terms of the 'protection of the patient' by 'proper treatment' which could lead to recovery and in the perfection of moral qualifications that would be best suited to maintaining discipline and control. Both principles of practice can be explained in part by the absence of effective medical or psychiatric interventions for what today would be regarded as mental disorder. Without effective treatments, 'protection from harm' could in some unknowable circumstances contribute to recovery in ways that could not be easily explained. In the absence of any systematic understanding of the process of recovery, appropriate practice for the attendant was to develop those moral qualifications of character that best contributed to the good order and discipline of the asylum.

Practice as 'effective treatment'

The transition from the asylum to the mental health services of today has replaced the role of the asylum attendant with that of the mental health nurse. These changes have been accompanied by the emergence of a dis-course on practice that emphasises the importance of effective psychiatric treatment. The emergence of physical treatments (Insulin Therapy and

Unmodified Electroconvulsive Therapy) involved the mental health nurse in providing assistance to the psychiatrist. The role of the nurse in Electroconvulsive Therapy still involves preparation of the patient, assistance with administering the treatment and management of the patient in the recovery period (Weir & Oei, 1996). Later, the introduction of antipsychotic, antidepressant and antianxiety agents required nurses to dispense medication, to monitor therapeutic effects and to be vigilant for side effects. The role of the mental health nurse in supporting psychopharmacological treatments is still a dominant one (Weir & Oei, 1996) and has gained new impetus from the reintroduction of Clozapine (McAllister & Chatterton, 1996) as a treatment for schizophrenia.

Mental health nursing practice has also been strongly influenced by the psychotherapeutic treatments that came into widespread use in the 1950s and 1960s. These therapies led to the development of specialised forms of therapy to meet the needs of individual and groups of patients. Modified forms of group therapy emerged as marital therapy (Miller & Rose, 1994) and family therapy (Miller & Rose, 1994). At the same time other forms of psychosocial intervention became popular, especially behaviour therapy (Barker, 1982; Bandura, 1969; Eysenck, 1960) and cognitive therapy (Ellis, 1984; Beck, 1976; Ellis, 1973). At first the role of the mental health nurse was to support psychiatrists and psychologists in the conduct of these 'talking therapies', but as nurses became proficient they began to take on the role of primary therapist (Marks, 1985; Marks, *et al.*, 1977). This move was complemented by a burgeoning literature on the principles and practice of psychosocial nursing. The contribution of Hildegaard Peplau (1952) is an important example of a theoretical framework for therapeutic mental health nursing practice that remains influential. Such psychosocial approaches to intervention have become so dominant that there has been a recent call for the reintegration of the biological perspective into mental health nursing practice (McBride & Austin, 1996).

Therefore the dominant analogy of the disordered biopsychosocial system that can be restored to harmony by skilled intervention has emerged to join the moral hygiene analogy as a discourse on practice. At the same time the development of therapeutic skills in the practitioner has come to share the same importance as that formerly given to moral qualifications. That the increasing importance of the technical skills of the mental health nurse has not displaced the importance of *character* completely is demonstrated by contemporary recognition of the personal attributes necessary for a mental health nurse to be effective in the role of therapist as well as in the role of assistant to the psychiatrist. Therefore, the principle of effective treatment has come to challenge rather than to replace the principle of 'proper treatment' in contemporary discourses as is attested to by nurse scholars who state that:

> 'The role of the psychiatric nurse has three important elements: that relating to custodial care, that which is supportive to the medical model of care, and that

which requires psychiatric nurses to personally influence the mental health status of patients.'

(Reynolds & Cormack, 1990, p. 6)

Practice as 'a shared humanity'

The development of mental health nursing practice was strongly influenced by the dominant discourse on effective treatment that became the *raison d'être* of psychiatry as it emerged as a medical specialty. At first the role of the nurse was to provide custodial care and to assist psychiatrists in the treatment of patients. Later the role of the nurse changed to place greater emphasis on the importance of the nurse-patient relationship. The new role emerged partly to overcome the limitations imposed on nursing practice by the constraints of custodial care and partly to overcome frustration at involvement in physical treatments over which nurses had little control. The dual influence of the antipsychiatry movement stimulated by Laing and Szasz and the work of nursing scholars such as Orem (1980), Altschul (1972), and Peplau (1952), who sought to find new ways of conceptualising the role of the nurse, brought about a change in nursing values. Gradually the discourse on mental health nursing practice changed to accommodate humanistic and ontological concerns for the patient. Patients were no longer to be seen as the passive recipients of custodial care and treatments, but as people who shared a common humanity with the nurse. The challenge for mental health nurses was to transform their work into practices complementary to rather than subordinate to biologically orientated psychiatry (Reynolds & Cormack, 1992, p. 9)

In this discourse the first principle of mental health nursing practice is competence in human relationships. The word competence is used here in preference to effectiveness to recognise the nurse–patient relationship as an important end in itself. The primary function of mental health nurses within this discourse is to capitalise on the opportunities that arise to confer therapeutic benefit by becoming aware of, reflecting on, and considering the possible consequences of the quality of their interactions (Peplau, 1992; 1988; 1987). Primacy in this discourse is given to nurse–patient dialogue because the:

> 'Talking that occurs during these nurse–patient interactions serves such purposes as therapeutic work, teaching, planning or review of patient programmes or schedules, planning for discharge...'

(Peplau, 1992, p. 90)

Such dialogue occurs in the often informal and casual encounter between nurse and patient and sits largely outside the formal interactions found in the more formal interventions associated with the discourse on effective treatment.

Conferring therapeutic benefit in this wider sense broadens the scope of what can be regarded as recovery and is a reciprocal process in which the process of improvement extends to the nurse. Speaking in this way about recovery and mental health nursing practice, de-emphasises the analogy of the harmonious biopsychosocial system characteristic of the discourse on effective treatment by asserting that of a shared humanity. Central to the refocused ontology is the notion of selfhood, the autonomous identity that requires support and nurturing if each human being is to fulfil their potential and experience the security of being understood, loved and valued in mutually positive relationships with others (Laing, 1960). With this shift in emphasis, to be a sensitive, caring person became the hallmark of competence in nursing practice. This move marked a return to the importance of *character* associated with the asylum era. However, the *character* to be developed by the nurse now was intended to be free of the trappings of repression.

Practice as 'empowerment'

Mental health nursing practice was subtly influenced by the discourse on freedom associated with Szasz. His thoughts on the repression of people with a mental illness caught the *zeitgeist* of the 1960s as the discontent of the post war generation questioned every orthodoxy and promoted what seemed at the time to be radical ideas (Hobsbawm, 1994, p. 298). Against this background, mental health nurses re-examined their attitudes. The outcome was unease with the still largely authoritarian regime of the psychiatric hospital despite its partial amelioration by the rise of the therapeutic community movement (Rogers, *et al.*, 1993). At the same time community mental health nursing practice developed apace in the wake of deinstitutionalisation. As a result the scope of practice of community based mental health nurses was broadened to place greater emphasis on over-coming the effects of the lack of community resources. Slowly the concept of recovery became redefined to reflect the emerging focus on the ability of the person with a mental illness to live a reasonably independent life in the community. The dominant analogy in this discourse became the empowerment of the person with mental illness (Anthony, 1993). Empowerment was to be achieved by equalising the nurse–patient relationship, by integrating people with mental illness back into the com-munity, and by ensuring access to income support and accommodation. Later the discourse on empowerment was strengthened as the setting up of self-help groups broadened into a wider community movement (Jewell & Posner, 1996). The adoption of the terms 'consumer', or the more political 'survivor' (McLean, 1994), in preference to the term 'patient' reflected this sea change. Within this discourse the concept of recovery was redefined to include the ability of people with a mental illness to speak up on their own behalf and to enjoy the same freedoms as other members of the community (Jewell & Posner, 1996).

Conclusion

In this chapter we have emphasised the multiple discursive framings of mental illness and subsequent mental health nursing. The role shift for the carer of the person with mental illness from asylum attendant to mental health nurse did not put an end to custodial care. Neither did the emergence of the therapeutic role of the nurse extinguish altogether the role of the custodian. Still less has the current concern for the empowerment of the person with a mental illness disempowered the mental health professional. At each moment in mental health nursing practice, the attitudes of the past have lingered to weave the mutiplicity of contemporary practice.

The discursive formation of mental health practice continues to remain open as new mental health workers enter the field (see Chapter 6) and as people with a mental illness take on roles in support of other former patients (see Chapter 1) (Salem, 1990; Gyulay, *et al.*, 1994; McLean, 1994). Therefore, the discourses on mental health nursing practice described in this section are best regarded as a discursive formation consisting in ways of speaking that have rules about how nurses, patients and nursing practice are to be talked about. It follows that discourses on mental health nursing practice should be regarded as different complex ways of determining what can and cannot be said about what mental health nurses do and seek to achieve. Each new emphasis has emerged to reflect changes in social values and in the attitudes of mental health nurses as discursive formations on mental health nursing practice incorporate new ideas and rework nuances reflecting changed thinking about mental illness. Thus the role of recovery and its effect on mental health nursing practice must be understood as constituted by past, present and future discursive framings of madness, treatment and power.

References

Altschul, A. (1972) *Patient–nurse Interaction: A Study of Interaction Patterns in Acute Psychiatric Wards*. Churchill Livingstone, Edinburgh.

American Psychiatric Association (1987) *Diagnostic and Statistical Manual of Mental Disorders*, 3rd edn Revised. APA, Washington, DC.

American Psychiatric Association (1995) *Diagnostic and Statistical Manual of Mental Disorders*, 4th edn. APA, Washington, DC.

Anthony, W.A. (1993) Recovery from mental illness: the guiding vision of the mental health service system in the 1990s. *Psychological Rehabilitation Journal*, **16**(4), 11–23.

Bandura, A. (1969) *Principles of Behaviour Modification*. Holt, Rinehart and Winston, New York.

Barker, P.J. (1982) *Behaviour Therapy Nursing*. Croom Helm, London.

Beck, A.T. (1976) *Cognitive Therapy and the Emotional Disorders*. International Universities Press, New York.

Chung, M.C. & Nolan, P. (1994) The influence of positivistic thought on nineteenth century asylum nursing. *Journal of Advanced Nursing*, vol. 19, pp. 226–32.

Clare, A. (1976) *Psychiatry in Dissent: Controversial Issues in Thought and Practice*, Tavistock Publications, London.

Clinton, M. (1993) On reflection: Towards a critique of reflective practice as a strategy for the development of nursing practice. *Australian and New Zealand Journal of Mental Health Nursing*, vol. 2, no. 4, pp. 162–9.

Davidson, L. & Strauss, J.S. (1992) Sense of self in recovery from severe mental illness. *British Journal of Medical Psychology*, **65**, pp. 131–45.

Ellis, A. (1973) *Humanistic Psychotherapy: The Rational-Emotive Approach*. Julian Press, New York.

Ellis, A, (1984) *Rational-Emotive Therapy and Cognitive Behaviour Therapy*. Springer, New York.

Eysenck, H.J. (1960) *Behaviour Therapy and the Neuroses*. Pergamon, Oxford.

Foucault, M. (1967) *Madness and Civilization*. Vintage, New York.

Foucault, M. (1973) *The Birth of the Clinic*. Tavistock, London.

Foucault, M. (1991) Governmentality. In: *The Foucault Effect* (eds G. Burchill, C. Gordon & P. Miller). University of Chicago Press, Chicago.

Gyulay, R., Mound, B. & Fanagan, E. (1994) Mental health consumers as public educators: a qualitative study. *Canadian Journal of Nursing Research*, 26(2), 29–42.

Hamera, E.K., Peterson, K.A., Handley, S.M., Plumlee, A.A. & Frank-Ragan, E. (1991) Patient self-regulation and functioning in schizophrenia. *Hospital and Community Psychiatry*, **42**(6), 630–31.

Hegarty, J.D., Baldessarini, R.J., Tohen, M.T., Waternaux, C. & Oepen, G. (1994) One hundred years of schizophrenia: A meta-analysis of the outcome literature. *American Journal of Psychiatry*, **151**(10), 1409–16.

Hindess, B. (1996) *Discourses of Power*. Routledge, London.

Hobsbawm, E. (1994) *Age of Extremes: The Short Twentieth Century 1914–1991*, Michael Joseph, London.

Jewell, K. & Posner, N. (1996) A consumer focus. In: *Mental Health and Nursing Practice* (eds M. Clinton & S. Nelson). Prentice Hall, Sydney.

Kerser, S.M. (1994) The consumer perspective on family involvement. In: *Helping Families Cope with Mental Illness* (eds H.P. Lefley & M. Wasow). Harward Academic Publishers, USA.

Laing, R.D. (1960) *The Divided Self: An Existential Study of Sanity and Madness*. Tavistock, London.

Laing, R.D. (1964) *Sanity Madness and the Family*. Tavistock, London.

Lee, P.W.H., Lieh-Mak, F., Yu, K.K. & Spinks, J.A. (1993) Coping strategies of schizophrenic patients and their relationship to outcome. *British Journal of Psychiatry*, **163**, 177–82.

Liberman, R.P., Mueser, K.T., Wallace, C.J., Jacobs, H.E., Eckman, T. & Massel, H.K. (1986) Training skills in the psychiatrically disabled: Learning, coping and competence. *Schizophrenia Bulletin*, **12**(4), 631–47.

Marks, I. (1985) *Psychiatric Nurse Therapists in Primary Care: The Expansion of Advanced Clinical Roles in Nursing*. Royal College of Nursing, London.

Marks, I., Hallam, R.S., Connelly, J. & Philpott, R. (1977), *Nursing in Behavioural Psychotherapy*. Royal College of Nursing, London.

McAllister, M., & Chatterton R. (1996) Clozapine: Exploring clients' experiences of treatment. *Australian and New Zealand Journal of Mental Health Nursing*, **5**(3), 136–42.

McBride, A.B. & Austin, J.K. (1996) *Psychiatric-mental Health Nursing: Integrating the Behavioural and Biological Sciences*. W.B. Saunders Company, Philadelphia.

McLean, A. (1995) Empowerment and the psychiatric consumer/ex-patient movement in the United States: contradictions, crisis and change. *Social Science and Medicine*, **40**(8), 1053–71.

Medico-Psychological Association (1911) *The Handbook for Attendants of the Insane,* 6th edn. Bailliére, Tindall & Cox, London.

Miller, P. & Rose, N. (1994) On therapeutic authority: psychoanalytical expertise under advanced liberalism. *History of the Human Sciences,* **7**(3), 29–64.

Orem, D. (1980) *Nursing concepts of practice,* 2nd edn. McGraw-Hill, New York.

Palmer-Erbs, V.K. (1996) A call to action for all psychiatric-mental health nurses: It's time to create collaborative partnerships with consumers of mental health services and their families. *The Clinician,* **1**(1), 13–14.

Palmer-Erbs, V.K. & Manos, E. (1998) Are we there yet? When will we be there? Designing collaborative plans for future psychiatric rehabilitation nursing practice. *Journal of Psychosocial Nursing and Mental Health Services,* **36**(4).

Peplau, H.E. (1952) *Interpersonal Relations in Nursing.* G.P. Putmans Sons, New York.

Peplau, H.E. (1987) Interpersonal constructs for nursing practice. *Nurse Education Today,* vol. 7, pp. 201–8.

Peplau, H.E. (1988), *Interpersonal Relations in Nursing.* Macmillan, London.

Peplau, H.E. (1992) Interpersonal relations model: Theoretical constructs, principles and general applications. In: *Psychiatric and Mental Health Nursing: Theory and Practice* (eds W. Reynolds & D. Cormack). Chapman & Hall, London.

Rogers, A., Pilgrim, D. & Lacy, R. (1993) *Experiencing Psychiatry. User Views of Services.* Macmillan Press, MIND, Basingstoke.

Salem, D.A. (1990) Community-based services and resources: The significance of choice and diversity. *American Journal of Community Psychology,* **18**(6), 909–15.

Schooler, N.R. (1986) The efficacy of antipsychotic drugs and family therapies in the maintenance treatment of schizophrenia. *Journal of Clinical Psychopharmacology,* **6**, 11S–19S.

Strahan, S.A.K. (1888) Recovery from chronic insanity: Four cases. *The Journal of Mental Science,* July.

Szasz, T. (1960) The Myth of Mental Illness. *The American Psychiatrist,* vol. 15, pp. 113–18.

Szasz, T. (1973) *Ideology and Insanity.* Penguin Books Ltd, Harmondsworth.

Tobias, M. (1990) Validator: A key role in empowering the chronically mentally ill. *Social Work,* **35**(4), 357–9.

Warner, R. (1994) *Recovery from Schizophrenia: Psychiatry and Political Economy.* Routledge, London.

Weir, D. & Oei, T. (1996) Treatment and nursing interventions. In: *Mental Health & Nursing Practice* (eds M. Clinton & S. Nelson). Prentice Hall, Sydney.

Whitwell, J.R. (1936) *Historical Notes on Psychiatry.* H.K. Lewis & Co, Ltd., London.

Index